Medical Bacteriology

Practical Approach Series

For full details of Practical Approach titles currently available, please go to www.oup.com/pas.

The following titles may be of particular interest:

Molecular Epidemiology (No 251)
Edited by Mary Carrington and Rus Hoelzel

"Each chapter has been written with new researchers in mind, with an easily navigable layout and succinct definitions of specialist terms. The examples provided are presented well and the authors successfully avoid redundant statements, making the information accessible and easy to digest ... Molecular Epidemiology was a delight to read and would be invaluable for an undergraduate module." *Journal of Biological Education*
October 2001 0-19-963811-X (Hbk); 0-19-963810-1 (Pbk)

Basic Cell Culture (No 254)
Edited by John Davis

"I think that this is a very useful book, and I recommend it not only to beginners, but also to more experienced cell culture workers, who will find many new hints and pieces of information, presented in a readily accessible way." *Experimental Physiology*
January 2002 0-19-963854-3 (Hbk); 0-19-963854-3 (Pbk)

Epitope Mapping (No 248)
Edited by Olwyn Westwood and Frank Hay

Epitope mapping is a unique compendium of current methodology on epitope mapping that is both comprehensive and authoritative. As such, it is an invaluable laboratory manual and reference guide for all researchers involved in epitope mapping.
March 2001 0-19-963653-2 (Hbk); Paperback 0-19-963652-4 (Pbk)

Monoclonal antibodies
Edited by Phil S. Stepherd and Christopher Dean

"An authoritative team of investigators brings together a series of concise and proven methods used in laboratories around the world which can be used by both basic scientists and researchers interested in the clinical application of monoclonal antibodies. An experienced molecular biologist without much expertise with immunochemical methods and immunologists, pathologists and others will find this book very helpful. For undergraduate and graduate students this inexpensive book is a good source of information on methods, which are shown in the form of concise protocols and well referenced" *Cell Biology International*
May 2000 Series No: 227 0-19-963722-9 (Hbk); 0-19-963723-7 (Pbk)

No. 265

Medical Bacteriology

Second Edition

A Practical Approach

Edited by

Peter Hawkey

Health Protection Agency,
West Midlands Public Health Laboratory,
Birmingham and Solihull NHS Trust,
Birmingham B9 5SS, UK
and
Division of Immunity and Infection,
University of Birmingham,
Birmingham B15 2TT, UK

Deirdre Lewis

Health Protection Agency South West,
Department of Microbiology,
Gloucestershire Royal Hospital,
Gloucester GL1 3NN, UK

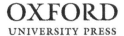

OXFORD
UNIVERSITY PRESS

*This book has been printed digitally and produced in a standard specification
in order to ensure its continuing availability*

OXFORD
UNIVERSITY PRESS

Great Clarendon Street, Oxford OX2 6DP

Oxford University Press is a department of the University of Oxford.
It furthers the University's objective of excellence in research, scholarship,
and education by publishing worldwide in

Oxford New York

Auckland Cape Town Dar es Salaam Hong Kong Karachi
Kuala Lumpur Madrid Melbourne Mexico City Nairobi
New Delhi Shanghai Taipei Toronto
With offices in
Argentina Austria Brazil Chile Czech Republic France Greece
Guatemala Hungary Italy Japan South Korea Poland Portugal
Singapore Switzerland Thailand Turkey Ukraine Vietnam

Oxford is a registered trade mark of Oxford University Press
in the UK and in certain other countries

Published in the United States
by Oxford University Press Inc., New York

Oxford is a registered trade mark of Oxford University Press
in the UK and in certain other countries

Published in the United States
by Oxford University Press Inc., New York

© Oxford University Press 1989
© Oxford University Press 2004

ISBN 0-19-963778-4

Dedication

This book is dedicated to Les White and Annie Bushell

Having worked with **Les White** in Bristol in the early 1980s, I can honestly say that he was one of the nicest colleagues with whom I have ever worked. He was kind, amusing, extremely intelligent, and always pleased to share his considerable knowledge. Les was able to develop rapidly and quality assure any new antimicrobial assay and it was no surprise that he became the national expert in this field. Hence our delight when he agreed to co-author, with David Reeves, the chapter on assays. As would be expected of an author of his calibre, his contribution was clear, authoritative and required almost no editing. It was a great shock to us all when Les died on 16th April 2002, after a short illness. He is, and always will be, hugely missed by all who knew him

(Deirdre Lewis)

When I asked **Annie Bushell** to write a chapter on soft tissue and wound infections for the first edition of this book, it was because of her breadth of knowledge combined with a quick eye for what was both practical and most importantly significant. The result was one of the best and most comprehensive chapters in the book. Above all, Annie was a perfectionist and it shows in the quality of her work, even now nearly fifteen years after it was written. In revising the chapter, I have had the assistance of another very able young microbiologist, who has many of Annie's qualities and I am sure Annie would have approved of the chapter and Nicky! I first met Ann in Bristol as a newly appointed registrar and she guided me patiently and tactfully through the intricacies of learning clinical microbiology. Both Ann and her husband David became close personal friends from that time forth. It was a series of tragic events that led to both their deaths within four months of each other in 2002.

(Peter Hawkey)

Preface

It is perhaps not surprising that in the fourteen years that have elapsed since the completion of the first edition of this book, there have been a substantial number of developments in the diagnosis and management of bacterial infections. It has therefore been necessary to make significant amendments to many of the chapters. We hope however that the book retains its essentially practical nature, which we have been told made the first edition so useful to those studying for membership of the Royal College of Pathologists, BSc degrees in Medical Microbiology, and other similar examinations.

As in the first edition the methods described in each chapter reflect the personal choice of the author(s) and therefore all available methods may not have been included.

The emphasis in some chapters has altered markedly since the first edition. For example antimicrobial assays are now performed using predominantly "black box" technology and so the principles of the biochemical basis of a test are given rather than a description of how to use a machine, which is best acquired from the manufacturer's instructions. On the other hand new methods are included in the antimicrobial susceptibility-testing chapter, which are directed at achieving greater methodological standardisation in the UK.

We are grateful to all the authors for working so hard to produce chapters with current and relevant information and Mrs Jane Moore for co-ordinating and assisting our editorial work. It is to be hoped that the second edition will be found to be as useful to the clinical microbiologist in their daily laboratory work as the original edition.

Contents

Bacteriology of the genital tract *93*

Catherine A. Ison, Alun J. Davies, and Peter M. Hawkey

Bacteriology of superficial and deep tissue infection *121*

Nicola Baker, Ann Bushell, and Peter M. Hawkey

CONTENTS

Principles of biochemical tests for the identification of bacteria   387

Epidemiological questionnaire   397

Protocol list

High performance liquid chromatography (HPLC)

Bacterial typing systems

Abbreviations

ACB	antibody-coated bacteria
AFB	acid-fast bacilli
BV	bacterial vaginosis
CAMLiC	continuous automated mycobacterial liquid culture
CFT	complement fixation test
cfu	colony-forming units
CIE	counterimmune electrophoresis
CLED	cysteine lactose electrolyte-deficient
CNS	coagulase negative staphylococci
CPE	cytopathic effect
CSF	cerebrospinal fluid
CVC	central venous catheter
EDI	electronic data interchange
EIA	enzyme immunoassay
EPR	electronic patient record
EQA	external quality assessment
FPIA	fluorescence polarization immunoassay
FTA	fluorescent treponemal antigen
GI	gastrointestinal
GLC	gas–liquid chromatography
HPLC	high performance liquid chromatography
HVS	high vaginal swab
IT	information technology
LRT	lower respiratory tract
MIC	minimum inhibitory concentration
MRSA	methicillin-resistant *Staphylococcus aureus*
MSU	midstream urine
NVS	nutritional variant streptococcus
PCR	polymerase chain reaction
PDE	peritoneal dialysis effluent
PID	pelvic inflammatory disease
RDS	rapid diagnostic sera
SOP	standard operating procedures
THA	treponeme haemagglutination
TNase	thermostable deoxyribonuclease
UCP	urine collection pads
VDRL	venereal disease reference laboratory
ZN	Ziehl–Neelsen

Contributors

J.M. Andrews
Department of Microbiology,
City Hospital NHS Trust,
Birmingham, B18 7QH, U.K.

N. Baker
West Midlands Public Health
Laboratory, Health Protection Agency,
Birmingham Heartlands Hospital,
Birmingham B9 5SS, U.K.

D. Brown
Health Protection Agency
East of England, Cambridge
Laboratory, Microbiology,
Addenbrooke's Hospital, Hills Road,
Cambridge, CB2 2QW, U.K.

A.C. Bushell (deceased)
Department of Microbiology
Withybush Hospital, HaverfordWest,
Oxford.

P.K. Curly
Department of Microbiology,
Leeds General Infirmary,
Gt George Street, Leeds,
LS1 3EX, U.K.

A.J. Davies
Sandwell District General Hospital,
Lyndon, West Bromwich,
West Midlands, B71 4HJ, U.K.

E.M. Davies
Microbiology, Cardiff
National Public Health Service,
Wales, Cardiff and Vale,
NHS Trust, Health Park,
Cardiff CF14 4AX, U.K.

R. Freeman
Health Protection Agency, North East,
General Hospital, WestGate Road,
Newcastle upon Tyne, NE4 6BE, U.K.

Clive Graham
Department of Microbiology,
Royal Victoria Hospital,
Newcastle Upon Tyne,
NE1 4LP, U.K.

P.M. Hawkey
Health Protection Agency,
West Midlands Public Health
Laboratory, Birmingham Heartlands
Hospital, Birmingham B9 5SS, U.K.

W.A. Hyde
Independent Consultant, 2 Calder
Avenue, Hindley Green, Wigan,
WN2 4TR, U.K.

C.A. Ison
Department of Infectious Diseases &
Microbiology, Imperial College
London, St Mary's Campus,
London W2 1PG, U.K.

K.G. Kerr
Consultant Microbiologist,
Department of Microbiology,
Feloston wing, Harrogate District
Hospital, Lancaster Park Ro
Harrogate, HG2 75X, U.K.

D.A. Lewis
Health Protection Agency South West,
Department of Microbiology,
Gloucestershire Royal Hospital,
Gloucester GL1 3NN, UK

A. Lovering
Department of Medical Microbiology,
Southmead Hospital, Bristol,
B10 5NB, U.K.

J.A. Lowes
Health Protection Agency SouthEast,
Southampton Laboratory,
Southampton General Hospital,
Southampton SO16 64D

A.P. MacGowan
Department of Medical Microbiology,
Southmead Hospital, Bristol,
B10 5NB, U.K.

O.M. Murphy
Pathology Department,
Bon Secour Hospital,
College Road, Cork,
Ireland.

Steve O'Hara
Health Protection Agency SouthEast,
Southampton Laboratory,
Southampton General Hospital,
Southampton SO16 64D

S.R. Palmer
Department of Epidemiology,
Statistics and Public Health,
University of Wales, College of Medicine,
Health Park, Cardiff LF14 4XN

S.J. Pedler
Department of Microbiology,
Royal Victoria Infirmary,
Queen Victoria Road, Newcastle upon
Tyne, NE1 4LP, U.K.

D.S. Reeves
Department of Microbiology, Southmead
Hospital, Bristol, BS10 5NB, U.K.

E.G. Smith
Health Protection Agency,
West Midlands Public Health
Laboratory, Birmingham Heartlands
Hospital, Birmingham B9 5SS, U.K.

L.O. White (deceased)
Department of Microbiology,
Southmead Hospital, Bristol,
BS10 5NB, U.K.

T. Winstanley
Department of Microbiology,
Royal Hampshire Hospital,
Glossop Road, Sheffield, S10 2JF, U.K.

Chapter 1
Bacteriology of urine

Eleri M. Davies
Microbiology, Cardiff National Public Health Service Wales, Cardiff and Vale NHS Trust, Health Park, Cardiff CF14 4AX, UK.

Deirdre A. Lewis
CDSC South West, Public Health Laboratory, Gloucestershire Royal Hospital, Great Western Road, Gloucester GL1 3NN, UK.

1 Introduction

The urinary tract above the level of the distal urethra is normally sterile but infection at any site within the tract is possible, from the kidney to the urethra, the commonest site of infection being the urinary bladder. In general micro-organisms gain access to the urinary tract from neighbouring sites, most commonly the perianal region, resulting in ascending infection, although spread by the haematogenous route is usually responsible for infections by *Salmonella* spp., and *Mycobacterium tuberculosis*.

The aim of laboratory diagnostic procedures in urinary tract infection should be the detection of the abnormal presence of bacteria at any site within the tract together with evidence of inflammation. In this chapter the practical aspects of the laboratory diagnosis of urinary tract infection, from the time of specimen collection to that of issuing the final report, is presented.

2 Specimen collection and transport

2.1 Collection

Specimen collection normally occurs in the clinical setting, either in the community or in hospital. Urine is a relatively easy specimen to obtain, but contamination of the sample by commensal flora adjacent to the urethra is common, and unfortunately these organisms are also the ones that cause true infection. Thus scrupulous care in the collection of the sample is required. Clear instructions must be given to patients and staff on how to take a specimen and the importance of sterile containers stressed.

2.1.1 Types of specimen

The following types of urine specimens may be collected and submitted to the laboratory for analysis:

(a) *Midstream urine (MSU)*—see Protocol 1 for method of collection. This is the commonest urine specimen received, appropriate for most patients. At one time it was thought necessary to collect urine from females by catheterization but when it was recognized that catheterization itself introduced a risk of infection this practice was stopped. Contamination of the MSU however is a particular problem in female patients hence the external genitalia should be cleaned with soap and water before the specimen is collected. Antiseptics should not be used for cleaning as any residue may adversely affect the culture result. The first passage of urine should remove commensals from around the urethra leaving the midstream urine relatively free of contaminants. The reliability of a positive result from a properly taken MSU in a female has been found to be 80% after one specimen, 90% from two consecutive specimens, and 100% if three specimens give the same result. In males a single specimen is sufficient, as contamination is much less likely.

(b) *Catheter specimen of urine (CSU)*. A CSU should be obtained by aspirating urine aseptically using a syringe and needle from the lumen of the catheter near to the patient, via the port present for this purpose. Specimens taken from the catheter bag should be discouraged.

(c) *Suprapubic aspirates (SPA)*. This specimen is obtained by aseptically aspirating urine directly from the bladder in the midline above the pubic ramus. The bladder must be palpable. This technique is particularly useful in babies and young children. Contamination of this specimen is not an issue, therefore any growth from a SPA should be considered significant.

(d) *Clean catch urine (CCU)*. Collection of this specimen, particularly from babies, requires patience as a sterile container is held ready to catch any urine when passed.

(e) *Bag urine (BU)*. A sterile collection bag is applied to the cleansed perineum to catch urine, which must then be drained into a sterile container. Again this is commonly used in infants. Culture results are difficult to interpret as contamination is common with this method of specimen collection.

(f) *Urine collection pads (UCP)* (see Protocol 2 for method of collection). This method of collecting a urine specimen is increasingly finding favour in paediatric units as an alternative to CCUs and BU. Small studies have confirmed comparability (1). They are less nurse-intensive than CCUs, but the urine should be aspirated from the pad as soon as possible after voiding to maximize detection of pyuria as the UCP traps white cells over time (2). For urgent urine microscopy specifically to assess pyuria a CCU may be preferable.

(g) *Other specimen types.*
   i. Specimens from ileal conduits should be collected by careful catheterization of the stoma. They should only be taken if there is an indication for treatment such as pyrexia or constitutional upset.

ii. Ureteric urine may be sampled via a cystoscope.

iii. Urine from the kidney from a nephrostomy.

Protocol 1

Method for collection of MSU

Equipment and reagents

- Soap and water
- Sterile container

Method

1 Preferably collect the first specimen of the day.

   (a) *For females.* Clean the external genitalia with soap and water and then holding the labia apart pass urine, discarding the first part of the stream.

   (b) *For males.* Cleaning the external genitalia is unnecessary but retract the foreskin in uncircumcised males and disregard the first part of the stream.

2 Place a sterile container in the line of flow and collect a midstream sample of at least 20 ml.

3 After completing micturition, transfer urine aseptically to a specimen container. When boric acid is used fill the container to the mark indicated.

4 Send the specimen plus the request form to the laboratory as soon as possible.

Protocol 2

Method for collection of urine from UCP

Equipment

- UCP
- Sterile container
- Sterile syringe

Method

1 Clean the baby's perineum with warm water.

2 Place the UCP in the nappy towards the front.

3 Check the pad every 10–15 min to see if urine has been passed. An enuresis alarm could be used to alert staff.

4 When wet, wearing gloves, remove the pad, put the tip of a sterile syringe into the pad, and draw up a sample of urine.

5 Transfer urine into sterile container for transport to laboratory.

2.1.2 Timing of specimen collection

For MSUs the first sample of the day is the best as bacteria will have had an opportunity to grow overnight in the bladder. To diagnose renal tuberculosis three early morning urine specimens should be submitted to the laboratory.

Schistosoma haematobium may be seen in urine taken to coincide with maximum egg secretion between 1000 and 1400 hours or from a 24 hour collection of the terminal portion of voided urine.

2.2 Transport

Once collected the urine should be cultured with minimal delay, ideally within one hour of collection. Refrigeration at 4 °C will arrest any bacterial growth, therefore where delay in transport is likely specimens should be refrigerated or alternative ways of preventing bacterial multiplication during transport should be considered. These are:

(a) *Specimen containers with boric acid.* A midstream sample of urine is collected in a sterile receptacle (Protocol 1) and then transferred to the boric acid container, which is filled to a given mark so that the final concentration is 1.8% (w/v) (3, 4). It is important that this concentration is achieved as boric acid has some antibacterial activity when more concentrated. In fact even at a concentration of 1.8% (w/v) it may decrease the number of organisms, particularly of some *Pseudomonas* spp. The necessity to collect 15 ml of urine to achieve the correct concentration of boric acid means that this method poses problems when collecting urine from babies and small children.

(b) *Dip inoculum technique*—(see Protocol 3). The plastic slide may carry a variety of culture media, but one of the most commonly used is a combination of MacConkey agar on one side and cysteine lactose electrolyte-deficient (CLED) agar on the other (5). Culture by this method eliminates the problem of overgrowth and may also allow better survival of some organisms between collection and examination in the laboratory. The disadvantages of this method are:
   - i. Cost.
   - ii. Quantification and identification of organisms are more difficult than when urine is spread on larger agar plates.
   - iii. No urine is received, therefore cell counts cannot be performed.

Protocol 3

Dip inoculum technique[a]

Equipment and reagents

- See Protocol 1
- Double-sided slide carrying culture media

Protocol 3 continued

Method

1 Collect MSU as previously described (Protocol 1).

2 Dip the double-sided slide carrying culture media into the urine.

3 Allow to drain and then place in a closed sterile container for transport to the laboratory.

[a] Micturation directly onto the double-sided slide should be discouraged because of the uneven distribution of bacterial growth which may cause interpretation difficulties.

3 Microscopy and other rapid screening methods

A sample of urine is the commonest specimen received by most microbiology laboratories. To process fully all urine samples takes much time and effort and up to 80% of the specimens will yield no growth. As workloads and cost pressures increase some laboratories have developed selection criteria based on microscopy, use of reagent strips, and turbidity of samples to eliminate some samples from the full process. Other laboratories continue to process all specimens received. Developments in automated methods for detection of bacteriuria allow results to be produced more quickly and may further change the way urine is processed in the future. Selection of urine for processing also occurs at a stage before a specimen is even sent to a laboratory. Partly in response to increasing costs and partly because of the need for overnight culture medical practitioners, and indeed some hospital practitioners, recommend the use of reagent strips to determine whether or not to send a urine sample for culture (6, 7).

3.1 Reagent strips/dipsticks

The commonest reagent strips used for diagnosing urinary tract infections are the leukocyte esterase and nitrate reductase (Greiss) tests.

3.1.1 Leukocyte esterase test

This is the detection of leukocyte esterase released from leukocytes in urine using strips containing indoxyl carboxylic acid ester (8). The method is sensitive (88–94%) at detecting white blood cell counts of >10 per mm^3, it will also remain positive even when the white cells are lysed due to transport delay for example. However, vitamin C, cephalosporins, gentamicin, nitrofurantoin, high levels of protein or glucose, and high specific gravity may interfere with the reaction.

3.1.2 Nitrate reductase (Greiss test)

Gram-negative organisms that commonly cause urinary tract infections convert dietary nitrate to nitrite. This dipstick test detects nitrite in urine. The positive predictive value of the test is high, but it has a low sensitivity (detecting only between 40% and 80% of positives) (9). This may be due to the absence of nitrate reductase in some organisms notably, enterococci, Group B streptococci, and *Pseudomonas* spp.; there may be insufficient nitrate in the patient's diet; or the frequency of passing urine may not allow sufficient time for the nitrates to be converted to nitrite (takes 4 h). The inability of the test to pick up Group B streptococci makes it particularly inappropriate as a screening test for asymptomatic bacteriuria of pregnancy (10). Alone it is not a reliable indicator of urinary tract infection.

Combining the two tests gives high sensitivity, specificity, positive and negative predictive values for colony counts of 10^5 cfu (11, 12).

Although reagent strips offer a cheap alternative to full processing in the laboratory they have some drawbacks:

(a) When used at the point of care they are often used by personnel not trained in medical laboratory sciences. This can be addressed by improving staff training and following guidance issued by the Joint Working Group on Quality Assurance in Near Patient Testing (13).

(b) Differentiation between contamination and true infection cannot be made.

(c) An assessment of cell type, species of bacteria, presence of casts or crystals cannot be made.

(d) They cannot be considered reliable for early infections or infections due to low numbers of organisms (11).

3.1.3 Automated reading of reagent strips

Visual assessment of colour changes on reagent strips is subjective and can result in a variation of interpretation. To combat this automated reading systems are available such as the Aution™ family of analysers (Meranini Diagnostics, Berkshire, UK) and the Ames Clinitek 100 reflectance spectrophotometer (Bayer Diagnostics, UK).

3.2 Microscopy

Microscopy of urine may be performed on centrifuged or uncentrifuged urine. The presence of leukocytes, erythrocytes, casts, squamous epithelial cells, crystals, bacteria, other organisms, and cellular components are looked for. Microscopy of uncentrifuged, unstained urine by the microtitre tray and inverted microscope method or a disposable counting chamber are the commonest methods used currently in UK laboratories.

3.2.1 Uncentrifuged urine methods

(a) *The microtitre tray and inverted microscope method* (Protocol 4). This method is attributable to Rant and Shepherd (Public Health Laboratory, Norwich). It is quick and very reproducible. It can be used to detect casts. Modifications have been made to the method to incorporate culture by filling some microtitre wells with CLED agar. The urine being transferred from the microscopy well to the culture well by a multipoint inoculater.

(b) *The haematocytometer chamber (Fuchs–Rosenthal or Neubauer)* see Chapter 2. This is an accurate method for quantifying the cellular content of urine, but is more accurate than is really required for routine purposes. Its main disadvantages for repeated use are that it is laborious and time-consuming and the chambers have to be cleaned and disinfected between use. Breakage of counting chambers is also relatively expensive. Disposable versions avoid the need for cleaning/disinfection and breakage is not a problem. However mass use in a large laboratory can be costly.

(c) *The three-coverslip counting chamber method* (14). In effect a cheap alternative to the haematocytometer chamber, but rarely used for mass processing of urine. Casts cannot be detected by this method.

Protocol 4

The microtitre tray and inverted microscope method for urine microscopy

Equipment

- Fixed volume pipette (60 μl)
- Disposable plastic tips
- Flat-bottomed plastic microtitre tray
- Inverted microscope with ×20 objective lens

Method

1 Attach disposable tip to the pipette and draw up 60 μl of urine from a well-mixed sample. Dispense into the appropriate well of the microtitre tray making sure that the sample covers the whole bottom surface.

2 Allow a minimum of 5 min for the cells to settle, then examine under ×20 objective of the inverted microscope. Scan several fields to check for even distribution of cells and urine.

3 Estimate the average count per field of each cell type.

4 Convert count per field to count per mm^3 by multiplying by a conversion factor detailed by calibrating the microscope.

$$N \text{ (conversion factor)} = \frac{\text{cells/mm}^3}{\text{average cells/field}}$$

5 Note the presence of bacteria, casts—identify what type and crystals.

3.2.2 Staining of uncentrifuged urine

Although not in common use as a routine procedure in the UK, staining of urine is a rapid and inexpensive method for estimating bacteriuria at $\geq 10^5$ colonies/ml. One or more organisms per oil immersion field has a sensitivity of 85–95% and a positive predictive value of up to 98% when correlated with a colony count of $> 10^5$/ml (15).

A drop (50 μl) or 10 μl loop full of urine is allowed to dry on a slide, then Gram stained and examined with a ×100 objective oil immersion lens. This method provides information on types as well as numbers of bacteria.

3.2.3 Staining of centrifuged urine

Again not routinely performed in UK laboratories centrifugation techniques can be difficult to standardize, time-consuming, and messy. However stained centrifuged urine can be used to detect casts and provide information on the type of bacteria present. Also in comparison with other rapid screening methods for the detection of bacteriuria it is both sensitive (90–96%) and specific (90%), with a positive predictive value of 60–70%, negative predictive value 96–99% (13, 16, 17).

3.2.4 Other staining methods for urine

Gram stain is the commonest stain used (method Appendix I). Acridine orange has been used (18), but offers no real advantage over Gram staining. The Ziehl-Neelsen stain for acid-fast bacilli can be applied to urine (Appendix I) but it is probably best not to use it because of the relatively common positive findings due to the presence of *Mycobacterium smegmatis*. Urine should be cultured for *Mycobacterium* spp. without performing microscopy.

3.3 Automated screening methods for urine

3.3.1 Automated microscopy

The Yellow IRIS™ (International Remote Imaging Systems Inc.) was the first automated analyser to be used to streamline urine microscopy (19). Compared with conventional microscopy it detected more abnormalities and was well standardized, however throughput was slow and variable and the system was expensive. There are now other automated systems available, for example: UF-100™ (Sysmex UK Ltd., Berkshire) which uses flow cytometry and DC impedance technology and promises precision data three-fold better than conventional microscopy, a handling capacity of 100 specimens per hour, with recognition and quantitation of all elements completely automatic without any human interaction. (20); Questor™ (Difco Laboratories Ltd., Surrey) uses an automated single channel impedence particle counter method to count and categorize particles in urine (21). When compared with conventional methods it performed with a sensitivity of 93%, specificity 74%, PPV 43%, NPV 98%. Questor takes approximately one minute to process each sample. All these systems offer accurate, rapid results allowing negative results to be produced quickly, and reducing the numbers of urine specimens requiring full culture. The capital costs appear to be the main disadvantage.

3.3.2 Automated methods for detection of bacteriuria

Various automated and semi-automated methods have been evaluated but have had little success in the UK. They include:

(a) Colorimetric filtration: urine is passed through a negatively charged filter which electrostatically attracts bacteria retaining them on the filter. Safranin O dye is used to stain the trapped cells. This method forms the basis of the disposable system, Filtra Check-UTI (Meridian Diagnostics, Cincinnati, Ohio) (22) which gives a positive or negative result based on a pink colour change in a microtitre well.

(b) Bioluminescence: this method is based on the enzymatic bioluminescent reaction of bacterial adenosine 5'-triphosphosphate (ATP) mixed with luciferin and luciferinase, which is measured by a luminometer. UTI screen (CORAL Biomedical, San Diego, California) (23) incorporated this method.

4 Interpretation of findings on microscopy

4.1 Leukocytes

However the microscopy is performed the laboratory should report the results as number of cells per mm^3 or define the number of cells per high power field (hpf) that correlates with the 'normal' excretion of leukocytes by calibration of the microscope (see Protocol 4). Little (24) showed that a concentration of 10 leukocytes/mm^3 correspond to a white cell excretion rate of 150 000–200 000 per hour, which is considered to be the upper limit of normal. Using the inverted microscope method ($\times$20 objective) 5 leukocytes per hpf generally correlates with 10 leukocytes/mm^3. $\geq$20 leukocytes per hpf can therefore be considered to be abnormal. Raised leukocyte counts in urine may be due to infection, but can also be found in all forms of inflammation. The leukocyte count may be elevated in relation to a catheter, tumour, or calculi (stones), or may represent contamination from the vagina in females. Persistent pyuria in the presence of sterile urine is often because the patient has already started a course of antibiotic since pyuria can persist for several days after the bacteria have been eliminated. Otherwise sterile pyuria should alert the clinician to the possibility of infection due to fastidious organisms, sexually transmitted infections (particularly *Chlamydia trachomatis*), calculi, or bladder neoplasms. Renal tuberculosis is far less common, but should be considered if the clinical picture seems appropriate. Leukocytes are vulnerable to the hypotonicity of urine, therefore if microscopy is delayed the cell count may be artificially low. Leukocytes also disintegrate in alkaline urine, thus in infections caused by *Proteus* spp. There may be no apparent pyuria.

Differences in urine flow will also result in differing cell counts. Essentially microscopy of urine must be interpreted with great caution as the presence of pyuria is not always indicative of infection and the absence of pyuria does not rule out infection.

4.2 Red cells

Haematuria is not a normal finding, although red cells in urine samples from females may have come from the vagina. When associated with inflammation of the urinary tract, leukocytes are almost invariably present. Haematuria as an isolated finding is more commonly associated with stones or tumour, or occasionally with tuberculosis or fungal infections of the urinary tract. Red cells also lyse in hypotonic or hypertonic urine, therefore dipstick tests for haemoglobin may be positive when the microscopy is negative. On occasions requests will be received for urine microscopy looking for dysmorphic red cells as an indicator of site of origin (glomerulonephritis). This analysis is best done by phase-contrast microscopy (25).

4.3 Epithelial cells

Usually described as absent, scanty (+/−), +, and ++/+++, their presence should be noted and is suggestive of contamination of the urine specimen by contact with skin.

4.4 Bacteria

When seen they are usually predictive of a positive culture, but they cannot be used to differentiate contamination from true infection. If no growth results from a specimen in which bacteria have been seen, this is an indication for a Gram stain of a centrifuged deposit of the urine (see Section 3.2.3).

4.5 Casts and crystals

The detection of casts and some crystals can be helpful in the diagnosis of conditions other than urinary tract infection.

4.5.1 Casts

These are cylindrical protein moulds formed by precipitation of protein within the renal tubules, they are often indicative of renal pathology. An atlas of urinary sediment, such as Lippman (26), will provide good photomicrographs of casts. Types of cast and their associated pathology are given in Table 1.

4.5.2 Crystals

Many different crystals can be found in urine (Table 2). In most cases the finding is not significant, however occasionally and particularly when in large numbers they may be significant such as in cases of ethylene glycol poisoning (calcium oxalate crystalluria) or acute uric acid nephropathy (large numbers of uric acid crystals). Certain drugs such as aciclovir and sulfadiazine produce interesting crystalluria. Crystals are also seen in association with renal calculi, but are not diagnostic of the condition.

Table 1 Types of cast and their significance[a]

Cast type	Main associated conditions
Hyaline	May be seen in normal individuals (after strenuous exercise)
	Any parenchymal renal disease
Granular	Any parenchymal renal disease
	Diabetic nephropathy
Erythorocyte (red cell)	Necrotizing glomerulonephritis
Myoglobin	Renal failure 2° to rhabdomyolosis
Waxy	Renal failure
Leukocyte (white cell)	Acute pyelonephritis
	Acute proliferative glomerulonephritis
Epithelial	Acute tubular necrosis
	Acute interstitial nephritis
	All types of glomerulonephritis
Fatty	Nephrotic syndrome

[a] Modified from ref. 27.

Table 2 Types of crystals commonly seen in urine

Acid urine	Alkaline urine
Calcium oxalate bihydrate	Calcium phosphate
Calcium oxalate monohydrate	Calcium phosphate (plates)
Uric acid	Triple phosphates
Amorphous urates	Amorphous phosphates

5 Culture

5.1 Choice of media

The media chosen for urine culture must support the growth of common urinary pathogens, prevent the swarming of *Proteus* spp., and contain an indicator for lactose fermentation to aid identification. A combination of blood agar and MacConkey agar has been used, but has been superseded in most laboratories by CLED (cysteine lactose electrolyte-deficient) agar (28), which fulfils all the requirements for a single urine culture medium. Blood agar does not inhibit the swarming of *Proteus* and MacConkey agar inhibits the growth of many Grampositive species. Urine samples such as suprapubic aspirates, ureteric urine obtained via a cystoscope, urine from patients with bladder tumours, or any urine obtained by aseptic surgical methods should have extra agar plates put up in addition to the routine CLED plate.

(a) Suprapubic aspirates, ureteric urine, surgically obtained. Add blood agar, chocolate agar, Sabarouds agar +/−, anaerobic plate.

(b) Urine from patient with bladder tumour. Add an anaerobic plate.

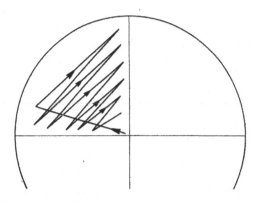

Figure 1 Method of streaking urine to obtain single colonies, using one agar plate for four samples.

5.2 Culture methods

5.2.1 Calibrated loop technique

A standard bacteriological loop, commonly a 2 μl size, is used to deliver a fixed volume of urine onto an agar plate (29). The urine is then streaked to obtain single colonies onto full plates, half-plates, or quarter-plates (Figure 1). For certain specimens, such as suprapubic aspirates, ureteric urine, or other surgically obtained urine specimens low organism counts are considered to be significant, therefore larger volumes of urine, e.g. 100 μl should be cultured so as not to miss low numbers of organisms.

5.2.2 Paper foot method (30)

This is a screening method suitable for quick processing of large numbers of urines. The method's limit of detection is down to 5×10^3 cfu/ml (see Protocol 5).

5.2.3 Multipoint inoculator method (31)

This method uses a multipoint inoculator to transfer urine from a microtitre tray onto a square plate of agar or microtitre tray containing agar for culture. A modification of the method originally developed for sensitivity testing by breakpoint, it is a method which lends itself to full automation (Mastascan) or may be done manually.

A range of media should be used to optimize identification of mixed cultures.

5.2.4 Other methods

A semi-automated method for quantitative urine culture has been described (32) which uses a programmable diluter to obtain accurate and reproducible bacterial counts with relative ease of operation. Pour plates and dip-slides for urine culture have been used in certain circumstances but are not recommended for large volume work.

Protocol 5

Method for using filter paper strips (paper foot method)

Equipment and reagents

- CLED (cysteine lactose electrolyte-deficient) agar plate
- Sterile blotting paper (e.g. Bacteriuritest strip, Diamed Diagnostics Ltd.)
- Urine

Method

1 Mix the urine well.

2 Divide a square (120 mm) CLED plate into 36.

3 Dip a standard strip of sterile blotting paper (e.g. Bacteriuritest strip) into the urine up to the black line.

4 Remove excess urine by touching the strip against the side of the specimen container, and then bend the inoculated end of the strip and press flat against the agar for a few seconds.

5 Incubate the plates for 18 h in an aerobic atmosphere.

6 20–25 colonies indicate 10^5 to $>10^5$ cfu/ml.

5.3 Localization of site of infection

5.3.1 Lower versus upper urinary tract infection

The presence of bacteria in the urine does not define whether the bacteria are confined to the bladder (lower urinary tract) or if the kidney (upper urinary tract) is also involved. The antibody-coated bacteria (ACB) assay was first described in 1974 (33) and appeared to show good discrimination between upper and lower urinary tract infection in adults, the presence of ACB being associated with the former. Subsequent studies have given more variable results and the test is not used in routine practice in the UK. The presence of serum antibodies to urinary pathogens have also been postulated as being indicative of upper renal tract infection, but again opinion has varied and testing for serum antibodies is rarely, if ever, used in clinical practice to determine the level of infection. Fairley *et al.* (34) applied a more invasive bladder washout test to determine the level of infection. An MSU is taken, followed by insertion of a catheter to perform a bladder washout, followed by a further three timed urine specimens. Sustained growth of >3000 cfu/ml in all specimens is considered indicative of renal infection. The benefit of differentiating between upper and lower urinary tract disease must be balanced against the practicality of performing the test.

5.3.2 Diagnosis of prostatitis and urethritis

i. Prostatitis

This is a difficult condition to diagnose, but about 50% of men will experience symptoms of prostatitis at some time during their lives (35,36). Acute bacterial prostatitis causes an intense illness with a tender prostate and frequently systemic symptoms. Chronic bacterial prostatitis is a more low-grade insidious disease with non-specific symptoms related to the pelvis and back, it may also result in recurrent urinary tract infections. Non-bacterial prostatis and chronic pelvic pain syndrome are more common than bacterial prostatitis which makes the diagnosis of infection important, as the treatment is clearly different. Laboratory diagnosis of bacterial prostatitis is done by examining prostatic secretions in combination with sequential urine samples (see Protocol 6). This test was described by Meares and Stamey in 1968 (37). Interpretation of the test results is given in Table 3. The test can be very uncomfortable for the patient and therefore very few clinicians perform the test.

Protocol 6

Localization test for prostatitis 'Stamey test' (37)

Equipment and reagents

- CLED agar plates
- Blood agar plates
- Urine

Method

1 Ensure the patient has a full bladder at the beginning of the test.
2 Retract the foreskin of uncircumcised men throughout the procedure.
3 Cleanse the glans penis with soap and water.
4 Collect the first 10 ml of voided urine (voided bladder 1; VB1).
5 Discard next 100 ml voided.
6 Collect 10 ml of midstream urine (VB2).
7 Massage the prostate collecting any expressed prostatic secretions.
8 Collect the first 10 ml of urine voided after the massage (VB3).
9 Transport the specimens to the laboratory immediately for quantitative culture.
10 Culture of the urine should be a surface viable count dilution of 10^{-1}.

Protocol 6 continued

11   Culture onto CLED and blood agar plates as well as agar to support the growth of fastidious and anaerobic organisms (e.g. chocolate agar, FAA).

12   Culture the prostatic fluid directly onto a similar range of agar plates. Incubate all plates for 48 h.

Table 3 Interpretation of results of the 'Stamey-localization test'

All specimens $<10^3$ cfu/ml = negative test.
VB3 and/or EPS yielding colony count of one or more logs greater than VB1 = chronic bacterial prostatitis.
VB1 colony count>all other specimens = urethritis or specimen contamination.
All specimens > 10^3 cfu/ml = uninterpretable.[a]

[a] Treat patient for two to three days with an antibiotic that doesn't penetrate the prostate then repeat the procedure.

ii. Urethritis/urethral syndrome

This is a common condition in both males and females. In males the condition is most commonly due to a sexually transmitted disease such as *Chlamydia trachomatis* or *Neisseria gonorrhoeae* and symptoms include urethral discharge (see Chapter 4). In females urethritis or the urethral syndrome is a rather more controversial diagnosis (38, 39). Commonly defined as a syndrome of frequency and dysuria in the absence of a significant bacteriuria with a conventional pathogen, many investigators have concentrated on finding other microbial causes for the syndrome. The sexually transmitted diseases, as above, certainly cause some cases of urethritis in women, but the numbers presenting with this syndrome are far greater than can be accounted for by sexually transmitted diseases. Maskell and colleagues (40) suggested that fastidious organisms such as lactobacilli, corynebacteria, and *Streptococcus milleri* were responsible for the urethral syndrome recommending prolonged culture of CLED plates and additional culture on chocolate agar to detect these fastidious organisms. Others (41, 42) have suggested that the urethral syndrome is due to low numbers of bacteria or that it is an early stage in the evolution of urinary tract infection. There are also a long list of non-infectious possible causes for the urethral syndrome including anatomical, gynaecological, allergic, mechanical, psychological, and oestrogen deficiency.

5.4 Culture of urine for *Mycobacterium tuberculosis*

This is indicated when there is a clinical suspicion of renal tuberculosis or there is a persistent unexplained sterile pyuria, particularly in an elderly patient. The method is given in Protocol 7.

Protocol 7

Culture for *M. tuberculosis*

Equipment and reagents

- Centrifuge
- Universal bottles
- Urine
- 4% (w/v) sulfuric acid
- Suitable media

Method

1 Spin the urine[a] at 1800 g for 30 min in sealed universal bottles and buckets.

2 After centrifugation open the buckets in a Class I safety cabinet.

3 Pour off supernatant and decontaminate the deposit by adding an equal volume of 4% (w/v) sulfuric acid and leave for 30 min. Then fill the container to the top with distilled water.

4 Centrifuge again as in step 1. Decant the supernatant and with a disposable pipette incubate 0.4 ml of the deposit onto suitable media.[b]

5 Incubate slopes horizontally at 37°C in air for one week then examine. If negative re-incubate standing vertically and examine weekly for up to eight weeks.

6 Confirm mycobacterial colonies by Ziehl–Neelson staining (see Appendix I).

[a] Three early morning specimens of urine should be submitted to increase the likelihood of detecting *M. tuberculosis*.

[b] Usually Lowenstein–Jensens's medium (i) with pyruvate (ii) with glycerol, as slopes in screw-capped bottles.

6 Interpretation of culture results

6.1 The concept of significant bacteriuria

In 1957, Kass (43) showed that a count of 100 000 colony-forming units (cfu) per ml or higher of a single species in a midstream specimen of urine was almost invariably indicative of bladder bacteriuria, when he compared colony counts of *E. coli* in cultures of bladder urine collected by catheter with those in midstream urines from the same women. It was following this work that the term 'significant bacteriuria' was defined as the presence of at least 100 000 cfu/ml in two fresh carefully collected midstream urine specimens. However, too strong an emphasis has been placed on these criteria; indeed Kass found that some women with counts of 10^4 cfu/ml and even less had bladder infections, although when the first early morning specimen was collected counts usually rose to 10^5 cfu/ml or higher. Actually, bacteriuria is usually characterized by counts well in excess of 10^6 cfu/ml.

It has been suggested that the presence of pyuria together with a count of $>10^2$ cfu/ml should be used as criteria for a diagnosis of urinary infection, particularly in women with the acute urethral syndrome (41). However, unless the laboratory can be sure that specimens have been collected and transported correctly, there is a great danger of over-diagnosis if these lower counts are accepted as being significant. Nevertheless, it is true that too rigid an adherence to Kass's criteria may lead to both over- and under-diagnosis. Factors which may cause the latter are the following.

(a) A rapid rate of flow of urine due to a high fluid intake and frequent bladder emptying can dilute the bacterial content at least ten-fold (44).

(b) If the site of infection is other than in the bladder, for example renal stones or prostate; in these cases counts may be less than 10^5 cfu/ml.

(c) Bacterial pathogens other than E. coli may have different growth rates (45).

(d) The pH of the urine or the presence of antibacterial agents may depress the counts.

On the other hand urinary infection may be over-diagnosed because in stale urine a high count may merely be the result of multiplication of organisms.

The interpretation of cultures of midstream urine is a problem because of potential contamination from periurethral tissues or from the urethra itself, or from the vagina or bowel. Clearly when urine is collected aseptically from the renal pelvis, ureters, or bladder, the diagnosis of significant bacteriuria can be made regardless of the number of organisms found. In the case of bladder urine this applies to specimens collected by catheter or from suprapubic aspirates. Interpretation and reporting of specimens is given in Table 4.

6.2 Interpretation and reporting of specimens from patients with indwelling catheters and ileal conduits

Cultures under these circumstances are often mixed and impossible to interpret unless something is known of the reasons for sending the specimen. If the patient has a pyrexia then any of the organisms cultured may be significant, and for this reason it is usually wise to perform sensitivities on organisms isolated from catheter specimens, but not to report them unless the patient has a pyrexia or other evidence of extension of infection to the kidneys or bloodstream (46). It has become common clinical practice for samples of urine to be sent for testing when a catheter is removed. This is not a worthwhile procedure unless the patient is symptomatic (47). The concept of significant bacteriuria does not apply to these specimens, and thus although many laboratories report the number of organisms per ml as a matter of convenience, no special significance can be assigned to this. Indeed, it has been found that counts of 10^2 cfu/ml or more is a more valid index of infection when patients are catheterized and have urinary tract symptoms, although these counts usually increase to at least 10^5 cfu/ml within a few days (48).

Table 4 Interpretation and reporting of results

A. Midstream urines

1. Count the number of colonies and multiply by the factor to establish cfu/ml urine, e.g. if a 2 µl standard loop was used, multiply by 500.

2. Establish whether or not the culture is pure by colonial morphology and if necessary Gram stain (see Appendix I) and identify bacteria (See Tables 5 and 6).

3. *Examples of reports*:
   With a pure culture (e.g. a lactose-fermenting coliform, such as *E. coli*)

(a) If $>10^5$ colonies/ml report: $>10^5$/ml coliforms (significant growth).[a]
   Perform and give results of antimicrobial sensitivities (for choice, see Table 7).
(b) If 10^4 to 10^5 colonies/ml report: 10^4 to 10^5/ml coliforms (equivocal result).[a]
   Comment: suggest a repeat specimen.[b]
   Perform sensitivities but withhold from clinician.
(c) If $<10^4$ colonies/ml report: $<10^4$/ml coliforms (of doubtful significance).[a]

   With a mixed culture

(a) $>10^5$ colonies/ml report: $>10^5$/ml mixed culture including......[c]
   Comment: indicates contamination.
   Suggest a repeat specimen.[d]
(b) If $<10^5$ colonies/ml report: $<10^5$/ml mixed culture, indicates contamination.

B. Urinary catheters and ileal conduit specimens

1. Report the number of cfu/ml in the specimen and the identity (See Tables 5 and 6) of the organisms in pure or mixed cultures (as above).

2. Perform sensitivities on isolates (for method see Chapter 7) or perform primary sensitivity on the urine, to give an overall picture if there is a mixed growth (Section 8.2).

3. Only report sensitivities if there is a history of pyrexia, otherwise withhold the information from the clinician.

4. If no history of pyrexia is given, comment on the inadvisability of giving antibiotics to apyrexial catheterized patients.

---

[a] These comments are optional and on occasions may be misleading.

[b] Unless pyuria present, in which case it may be significant and sensitivities should be performed and reported.

[c] Give predominant organism types.

[d] Only repeat if pyuria present.

6.3 Interpretation and reporting of suprapubic aspirate and ureteric catheter specimens

There should be no problem with contamination of these specimens and so the concept of significant bacteriuria does not apply and indeed low numbers of organisms may be present, e.g. 10^2 cfu/ml. In this case purity is more important than a high count of bacteria. A mixed growth, particularly of more than two species, is still suggestive of contamination, but sensitivities should be performed and reported on any growth from these specimens.

6.4 Asymptomatic bacteriuria of pregnancy

Between 30–40% of pregnant women who have untreated bacteriuria during pregnancy will go on to develop acute pyelonephritis (49). It is therefore common practice to screen pregnant women for bacteriuria. If bacteriuria is detected in a pregnant woman sensitivities should be performed and appropriate non-teratogenic antibiotics reported. A repeat specimen should be requested for confirmation and follow-up is usually necessary after treatment.

7 Identification of bacteria

Ideally all significant cultures should be identified to species level, as this will provide the most epidemiological information. Laboratories using automated multipoint inoculator technology are able to do this. Without that level of automation it is rarely practicable in a busy diagnostic laboratory to identify all isolates to species level.

However it is important to identify some organisms to species level in certain circumstances:

(a) To assess if recurrent infection is due to relapse or re-infection.

(b) To define an episode of cross-infection in hospital.

(c) To monitor the prevalence of species and their antimicrobial sensitivities.

(d) When an organism is particularly resistant.

(e) To match with a blood culture isolate from the same patient.

Tables 5 and 6 provide a short identification schedule for Gram-negatives and Gram-positives respectively. A recent development which may both simplify and increase the identification to species level of uropathogens even further is chromogenic media which allows direct identification of uropathogens from the colour of colonies on the agar (50).

7.1 Yeasts

Yeasts are readily recognized by Gram staining. A totally resistant picture on direct sensitivity testing should also alert you to the possibility of a yeast being present. Perform a germ-tube test to differentiate between *Candida albicans* and other germ-tube negative yeasts (see Protocol 8).

Frequently *Candida* spp. are present in urine as contaminants from the perineal area, particularly in females, or colonizing long-term catheters. However if the isolate is considered to be significant, e.g. isolated from a sick, immunosuppressed patient, full identification and sensitivity testing against fluconazole and flucytosine should be carried out.

7.2 Identification of difficult or 'fastidious' organisms

When a wider range of plates are used for urine specimens, such as suprapubic aspirates or ureteric urines, identification of the organisms will be more difficult

Table 5 Identification of Gram-negative bacilli

1. Look for colonies characteristic of Gram-negative bacilli; these will usually be larger and more translucent than colonies of Gram-positive cocci. If in doubt perform a Gram stain (Appendix I).

2. Differentiate between lactose-fermenting and lactose non-fermenting organisms. On CLED media containing bromothymol blue and acid fuchsin, lactose fermenters form red colonies. (Take care to check which indicator is incorporated in the agar as colonies will have different colours with different indicators.) On MacConkey agar also red colonies are formed by lactose fermenters.

3. In many laboratories lactose-fermenting Gram-negatives are given the general term 'coliforms'. Again take care as laboratory practices do differ and some may term all oxidase negative Gram-negatives as coliforms.

4. If lactose non-fermenting colonies are found perform a urease test (see Chapter 6). If urease positive in 2–4 h call the organism *Proteus* spp. (Note *Proteus* spp. also resistant to nitrofurantoin, check direct sensitivity to aid identification.)

5. A lactose non-fermenting organism which is resistant to most of the first-line antibiotics tested is probably a *Pseudomonas* spp. Perform an oxidase test (see Chapter 4). If oxidase positive call it *Pseudomonas* spp.

6. If the organism is both urease and oxidase negative perform slide agglutination tests with polyvalent 'O' and 'H' antisera to check if it is a salmonella (see Chapter 6).

7. If all the above tests are negative call the organism a lactose non-fermenting coliform or Gram-negative bacillus or proceed to full biochemical identification.

8. If the organism has an unusual sensitivity pattern, or is multi-resistant, including resistance to aminoglyosides[a] identify to species level. Similarly fully identify any organisms suspected of being involved in cross-infection.

[a] Usually a good marker of plasmid-associated resistance which may be transferable from one bacterium to another.

Table 6 Identification of Gram-positive cocci

1. Look for colonies characteristic of Gram-positive cocci. If in doubt perform a Gram stain (Chapter 5).

2. If Gram-positive organisms are present perform a catalase test to differentiate between staphylococci (positive) and streptococci (negative).

3. If the organism is catalase positive perform a slide coagulase test, or a Staphaurex test (Wellcome diagnostics) and a DNase test. If coagulase, Staphaurex, and DNase positive identify as *Staphylococcus aureus* (Chapter 5).

4. If the organism is coagulase, Staphaurex, and DNase negative check the novobiocin sensitivity. If sensitive to novobiocin call it *Staphylococcus epidermis*, if resistant call it *S. saprophyticus*.

5. If the organism is catalase negative it is a streptococcus. Perform a bile aesculin test.[a] If it hydrolyses bile aesculin the medium will turn black. Call the organism *Enterococcus faecalis*.

6. If bile aesculin negative determine the Lancefield group (Chapter 5). If it groups report as a β-haemolytic *streptococcus* with the group. Subculture to blood agar to confirm and for sensitivities.

7. If the organism is haemolytic or non-haemolytic (and not *E. faecalis*) report as such; it is not usually necessary to take identification any further.

[a] Prepared by dissolving 1 g aesculin, 0.5 g ferric citrate (filter sterilized) in 1000 ml of bile agar at 55 °C.

than most of the 'routine' urine cultures. Start with a Gram stain. If Gram-positive bacilli are seen, consider lactobacilli which are large Gram-positive bacilli or *Corynebacteria*, which are smaller and may take on the appearance of 'Chinese lettering'. *Lactobacilli* are capnophilic, catalase negative, vancomycin resistant. *Corynebacteria* are catalase positive.

If pleomorphic Gram-negative bacilli are seen consider *Haemophilus* spp. in which case perform an X and V test (Chapter 3, Protocol 9).

Occasionally, for example in patients with bladder tumours, anaerobes may be isolated which should be identified if possible using a biochemical kit such as Rapid ID 32 (Biomerieux).

Protocol 8

Germ-tube test

Equipment and reagents

- Water-bath
- Microscope slide and coverslip
- Rabbit plasma
- Yeast

Method

1 Incubate a sterile tube of rabbit plasma with a few colonies of the yeast to be identified.

2 Place in 37 °C water-bath.

3 Examine at 2 h and 4 h for the presence of germ-tubes by removing a drop of plasma onto a microscope slide and adding a coverslip.

4 Germ-tubes appear as cylindrical filaments originating from the yeast cell.

8 Sensitivity testing

Full methods for sensitivity testing are described in Chapter 7. In this section we shall describe some of the principles of antibiotic sensitivity testing of urinary isolates such as the choice of agents to be tested and the use of primary or direct sensitivity testing.

8.1 Choice of first-line and second-line agents for sensitivity testing

Antibiotics which are excreted in a microbiologically active form in the urine are required for the treatment of most infections of the urinary tract, especially those

21

Table 7 Selection of antimicrobial agents for testing

First line (select six from the following)[a]		Second line
Ampicillin	Cephalosporins:	Cefuroxime
Trimethoprim		Cefotaxime
Nitrofurantoin		Ceftazidime
Cephalexin/cephradine		Cefixime (oral)
Co-amoxiclav (augmentin)		
Ciprofloxacin	Aminoglycosides:	Gentamicin
Gentamicin[b]		Tobramycin
Nalidixic acid		Amikacin
Cefuroxime		
	Carbapenems:	Imipenem
		Meropenem
	Quinolones:	Norfloxacin
		Ciprofloxacin
		Levofloxacin
Pseudomonas spp.	**Staphylococci**	
Ciprofloxacin	Penicillin (2IU)	
Gentamicin	Novobiocin	
Ceftazidime	Oxacillin (for flucloxacillin)	
Piperacillin–tazobactam	Trimethoprim	
Imipenem/meropenem	Nitrofurantoin	
Amikacin/tobramycin	Ciprofloxacin	

[a] It may be appropriate to select one set of six antibiotics for GP specimens and a different first line six for hospital patients.

[b] Testing of this agent on specimens from hospitalized patients will identify gentamicin-resistant isolates associated with noscomial infection.

of the lower tract. The choice of agents will be governed by whether the patient requires oral or parenteral antibiotics. For example, patients in the community usually require oral agents because of the difficulties of administering drugs by other routes. On the other hand hospitalized patients, particularly those on surgical wards or in intensive care, may require parenteral antibiotics. In general, however, laboratories choose to test mainly oral agents as their first line and follow this with parenteral agents as the second line, if a lot of resistance is seen to the first-line antibiotics, i.e. an organism sensitive to less than two agents. The request form should always be read carefully to see if a particular antibiotic is intended for therapy so that if possible this may be included. When disc diffusion tests are performed, six agents are tested to a plate (see Table 7).

The testing of nalidixic acid and nitrofurantoin is a useful adjunct for identification. All Gram-positive bacteria are resistant to nalidixic acid, whereas most coliforms are sensitive, and so it can be used to help differentiate between, for example, *Enterococcus faecalis* and a coliform. Also, all *Proteus* spp. are usually resistant to nitrofurantoin, whereas most other coliforms are sensitive. The choice between agents grouped together in Table 7 will depend upon the antibiotic prescribing policy of the particular hospital.

If staphylococci are isolated test penicillin (2IU) rather than ampicillin. Test oxacillin at 30 °C to detect resistance to flucloxacillin and the cephalosporins. Novobiocin may be included on the plate to aid with identification (see Table 6).

If enterococci are isolated consider testing vancomycin (5), particularly from hospitalized patients as vancomycin-resistant enterococci are increasingly being detected.

8.2 Primary sensitivity testing

Urine may be used as the inoculum for a sensitivity test set up at the same time as the primary culture. For details of the method see Chapter 7. The major advantage of this is that the results can be reported the following day along with the culture result. Also, the sensitivity results are more representative because they are performed on what has grown from the urine and not from what has been selectively picked for subculture. However, the disadvantages are, first, that the inoculum is not controlled and thus may produce too heavy or light a growth; secondly, the culture may be mixed and greater caution must be exercised in reporting on mixed growths. Thus, although there are obvious advantages in performing primary sensitivities they do require the observer to be prepared to discard them if the inoculum is not right or they are mixed, and repeat the test on colonies picked from the primary culture plates. If these rules are adhered to then primary sensitivity testing is a reliable method and is widely used.

It is clearly unnecessarily expensive and time-consuming to perform primary sensitivities on all urines received, and most laboratories will use specific criteria for performing them. These will vary from one laboratory to another but include such things as significant pyuria and the presence of motile bacteria. Some specimens, such as bag urines, will not be used for primary sensitivity testing because contamination is very common. Whatever the criteria adopted there will always be occasions when secondary testing is required.

8.3 Reporting of sensitivities

Most laboratories perform a form of selective reporting of sensitivities as part of their antibiotic prescribing policy. For example, if ampicillin is considered the first-line β-lactam antibiotic for the treatment of urinary tract infection, and the organism is sensitive, then other β-lactams included in first-line testing, such as a cephalosporin or co-amoxiclav, may not be reported. Similarly, although gentamicin may be tested in the first-line group, it is unlikely to be reported for patients in the community. To some extent each report will be tailored to the information available.

Selective reporting is very desirable in certain circumstances, such as urinary infection in pregnancy, when certain agents are contraindicated. In this situation, β-lactams are the most appropriate agents. Selective reporting is not entirely aimed at restricting the use of antibiotics, although it may be used for this purpose, but rather to offer guidance to the clinicians to use the most appropriate agents. Various factors determine this, including proven safety of the agents and their cheapness.

9 Further tests

9.1 Detection of antimicrobial substances in urine (51)

Routine use of this test is the subject of some debate, but is essential when using agar plates for multipoint methods, as an antibiotic, if present, will diffuse through the agar affecting neighbouring specimen results. Otherwise it can be useful to clarify situations where culture is negative but a significant pyuria is seen. In some laboratories it has become routine practice to screen all urines for the presence of antimicrobial substances.

References

1. Lewis, J. (1998). *Paediatr. Nurs.*, **10**, 15.
2. Young, N., Ridgway, E. J., and Burke, D. (1999). Poster P68 at 6th Conference of the Federation of Infection Societies, 1–3rd December 1999.
3. Porter, I. A. and Brodie, J. (1969). *Br. Med. J.*, **ii**, 353.
4. Johnston, H., Moss, M. V., and Guthrie, G. A. (1978). In Public Health Laboratory Monograph Series. *The bacteriological examination of urine: Report of a workshop on needs and methods.* HMSO London, **10**, 22.
5. Mackay, J. P. and Sandys, G. M. (1965). *Br. Med. J.*, **ii**, 1286.
6. Woodward, M. N. and Griffiths, D. M. (1993). *Br. Med. J.*, **306**, 1512.
7. Fowlis, G. A., Waters, J., and Williams, G. (1994). *J. R. Soc. Med.*, **87**, 681.
8. Kusumi, R. K., Grover, P. J., and Kunin, C. M. (1981). *J. Am. Med. Assoc.*, **245**, 1653.
9. James, G. P., Paul, K. L., and Fuller, J. B. (1978). *Am. J. Clin. Pathol.*, **70**, 671.
10. Tincello, D. G. and Richmond, D. H. (1998). *Br. Med. J.*, **316**, 435.
11. Semeniuk, H. and Church, D. (1999). *J. Clin. Microbiol.*, **37**, 3051.
12. Buxtorf, K. and Bille, J. (1994). *Med. Microbiol. Lett.*, **3**, 401.
13. Joint working Group on Quality Assurance: Near to Patient or Point of Care Testing, c/o Diagnostic Services Ltd.; Mast House, Derby Road, Liverpool L20 1EA.
14. Nilson, G. R. F. (1964). *J. Clin. Pathol.*, **17**, 571.
15. Cardoso, C. L., Muraro, C. B., Sigueira, V. L., and Guilhermetti, M. (1998). *J. Clin. Microbiol.*, **36**, 820.
16. Rippen, K. P., Stinson, W. C., Eisenstadt, J., and Washington, J. A. (1995). *Am. J. Clin. Pathol.*, **103**, 316.
17. Olson, M. L., Stanholtzer, C. J., Willard, K. E., and Peterson, L. R. (1991). *Am. J. Clin. Pathol.*, **96**, 454.
18. Hoff, R. G., Newman, D. E., and Staneck, J. L. (1985). *J. Clin. Microbiol.*, **21**, 513.
19. Deindoerfer, F. M., Gangwer, J. R., Laird, C. W., and Ringdd, R. R. (1985). *Clin. Chem.*, **31**, 1491.
20. Fenili, D. and Pirovano, B. (1998). *Clin. Chem. Lab. Med.*, **36**, 909.
21. Stevens, M., Michell, C. J., Livsey, S. A., and MacDonald, C. A. (1993). *J. Clin. Pathol.*, **46**, 817.
22. Stager, C. E. and Davis, J. R. (1990). *Diagn. Microbiol. Infect. Dis.*, **13**, 289.
23. McWalter, P. W. and Sharp, C. A. (1982). *Eur. J. Clin. Microbiol.*, **1**, 22.
24. Little, P. J. A. (1964). *Br. J. Urol.*, **36**, 360.
25. Fassett, R. G., Hargon, B. A., and Mathew, T. M. (1982). *Lancet*, **i**, 1432.
26. Lippman, R. W. (1957). *Urine and the urinary sediment. A practical manual and atlas,* 2nd edn. Charles, C. Thomas, Springfield, Illinois.
27. Fogazzi, G. B., Grignani, S., and Colucci, P. (1998). *Clin. Chem. Lab. Med.*, **36**, 919.
28. Sandys, G. M. (1960). *J. Med. Lab. Technol.*, **17**, 224.

29. Stevens, M. (1989). *Med. Lab. Sci.*, **46**, 194.

30. Leigh, D. A. and Williams, J. D. (1964). *J. Clin. Pathol.*, **17**, 498.

31. Faiers, M., George, R., Jolly, J., and Wheat, P. (1991). In *Multipoint methods in the clinical laboratory PHLS British Society for Microbial Technology*, 75.

32. Edmondson, S. G. and Enright, L. J. (1984). *J. Clin. Pathol.*, **37**, 831.

33. Thomas, V., Shelokov, A., and Forland, M. (1974). *N. Engl. J. Med.*, **290**, 588.

34. Fairley, K. F., Grounds, A. D., Carson, N. E., Laird, E. C., *et al.* (1971). *Lancet*, **18**, 615.

35. Lipsky, B. A. (1999). *Am. J. Med.*, **106**, 327.

36. Leigh, D. A. (1993). *J. Antimicrob. Chemother.*, **32**, Suppl A, 1.

37. Meares, E. M. and Stamey, T. A. (1968). *Invest. Urol.*, **5**, 492.

38. Brumfitt, W. and Gillespie, W. A. (1991). *Br. Med. J.*, **303**, 1.

39. Brumfitt, W. (1998). In *Urinary tract infections* (ed. W. Brumfitt, J. M. T. Hamilton-Miller, and R. Bailey). Chapman & Hall, London.

40. Maskell, R., Pead, L., and Allan, J. (1979). *Lancet*, **ii** 1277.

41. Stamm, W. E., Counts, G. W., Running, K. R., Fihn, S., *et al.* (1982). *N. Engl. J. Med.*, **307**, 463.

42. Kunin, C. M. (1997). *Urinary tract infections: detection, prevention and management*, 5th edn. Williams & Wilkins, Baltimore, MD.

43. Kass, E. H. (1956). *Trans. Assoc. Am. Physicians*, **69**, 56.

44. Cattell, W. R., Kelsey Fry, I., Spiro, F. I., Sanderson, J. M., *et al.* (1970). *Br. J. Urol.*, **42**, 290.

45. Anderson, J. D., Eftekhar, F., Aird, M. Y., and Hammond, J. (1979). *J. Clin. Microbiol.*, **10**, 766.

46. Gillespie, W. A. (1986). *J. Antimicrob. Chemother.*, **18**, 149.

47. Davies, A. J. and Shroff, K. J. (1983). *J. Hosp. Infect.*, **4**, 177.

48. Stark, R. P. and Maki, D. G. (1984). *N. Eng. J. Med.*, **311**, 560.

49. Kass, E. H. (1960). *Arch. Intern. Med.*, **205**, 194.

50. Carricajo, A., Boiste, S., Thore, J., Aubert, G., *et al.* (1999). *Eur. J. Clin. Microbiol. Infect. Dis.*, **18**, 796.

51. Glaister, D. (1994). *Br. Soc. Microb. Tech. Newsl.*, **17**, 23.

Chapter 2

Bacteriology of normally sterile body fluids

Olive Murphy
Pathology Department, Bon Secour Hospital, College Road, Cork, Ireland.

Roger Freeman
Director, Newcastle Regional Public Health Laboratory, Westgate Road, Newcastle upon Tyne, NE4 6BE, UK.

1 Introduction

The detection of micro-organisms in a normally sterile body fluid has important diagnostic, therapeutic, and prognostic implications. Whilst culture of the infecting bacteria will allow identification and antibiotic sensitivity testing to be carried out, these infections are often serious and a rapid diagnosis is required to ensure correct chemotherapy. Various strategies have been adopted to accelerate the diagnosis with the development of rapid culture and non-culture techniques. The recovery of a bacterium from these specimens should always be considered significant until proven otherwise. Organisms should be identified to species level; not an arduous task as most infections are caused by a single species. This chapter describes current methods for the examination of the various categories of normally sterile body fluids and interpretation of these data.

2 Methods for the examination of blood

2.1 Principles of blood culture

2.1.1 Number and timing of blood cultures

The number and timing of blood cultures should take into consideration the likely underlying disease. The timing of blood cultures in the continuous bacteraemia of endocarditis is probably not important, but in most other conditions the bacteraemia is intermittent and related to the fevers and rigors which follow the appearance of organisms in the blood by 30–60 min (1). Unless the fevers and chills follow a regular pattern, blood cultures should be taken as near to the onset of a spike of fever as possible.

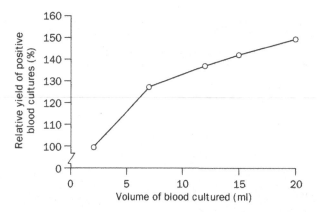

Figure 1 Relative yield of positive blood cultures with increasing volumes of blood cultured between 2 and 20 ml (after A. L. Bisno, *The diagnosis of infective endocarditis*).

In endocarditis, only a small number of samples are needed to isolate an organism, but three sets should be taken in order to help distinguish contamination from true infection (Figure 1). If the first few cultures are negative in suspected endocarditis, do not persist, since further samples are unlikely to be rewarding (2). In such cases consideration should be given to the reason for the negative cultures and investigations modified accordingly.

The diagnosis of other conditions may be helped by repeated cultures, although more than six sets are unnecessary. Three sets, taken not less than one hour apart, will give a success rate of 99%, compared with 80% for one set (3). Thereafter the success rate will not improve. Single sets may be adequate in neonates, in whom the density of bacteraemia is higher (4). The sending of large numbers of repeat blood cultures from the same patient, whether positive or negative, should be avoided since they simply waste laboratory time.

2.1.2 Collection of the sample

Appropriate training of ward-based staff should be undertaken on a regular basis to ensure the optimum quality specimen is received in the laboratory (Protocol 1).

Protocol 1

Taking a blood culture

Equipment and reagents

- Blood culture bottles
- Ethanol/propanol

- Iodine-containing agent

Protocol 1 continued

Method

1 Ensure that the blood culture bottles have attained ambient temperature.

2 Select the venepuncture site and clean it with ethanol/propanol, followed by an iodine-containing agent.

3 Allow time for drying and do not touch the cleaned area except with sterile gloves.

4 Wipe the penetrable diaphragm with antiseptic, again allowing time for drying (or follow manufacturer's instructions on removing any seal).

5 Perform the venepuncture and inoculate an adequate amount of blood (see Section 2.1.3) into each bottle. If it proves impossible to obtain an adequate sample, inoculate fewer bottles.

6 Where blood is taken at the same venesection for other tests (e.g. haemoglobin, white blood cell count) insist that the blood culture bottles are inoculated first to avoid bacterial contamination from anticoagulants.

7 Mix the contents of the bottles gently after inoculation.

2.1.3 Size of the sample

The volume of blood withdrawn is the single most important factor in isolating bacteria and fungi (5, 6). The number of bacteria present in the blood of bacteraemic patients is often less than 1 cfu/ml. Figure 2 shows the relative increase in yield of positive blood cultures per ml of blood cultured in a series of over

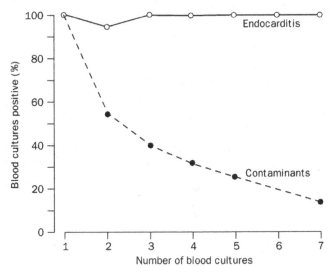

Figure 2 Demonstration of the value of multiple independent blood cultures in distinguishing between contamination and the bacteraemia of infective endocarditis (after A. L. Bisno, *The diagnosis of infective endocarditis*).

1000 cases of sepsis in one centre and suggests that at least 10 ml of blood must be taken in an adult patient. Increasing the volume to 20 ml per venesection may produce a further modest yield and should be encouraged. The majority of modern blood culture systems accept inocula of up to 10 ml allowing appropriate inoculation of each bottle if 20 ml blood is collected.

In infants, and in particular neonates, a denser bacteraemia is experienced and adequate results may be obtained from much smaller volumes (4).

2.1.4 Recovering organisms from the blood sample

The various methods, which have been devised, for the recovery of organisms from blood samples all attempt to satisfy four essential aims:

(a) The creation of the richest possible culture medium to allow the recovery of very small numbers of even fastidious bacteria.

(b) The removal, or neutralization, of any substances inimical to bacterial growth, including both natural components of blood and extraneous tractors, such as antibiotics.

(c) The minimizing of both ward-based and laboratory-based contamination.

(d) The earliest possible detection of the presence of bacteria in the system.

The methods available for detecting micro-organisms in blood have developed rapidly over the last ten years. The conventional broth culture technique has been replaced in many laboratories by semi-automated or automated commercial systems (7). The diversity of available units has ensured that automated systems are an option in smaller laboratories (8).

2.2 Principles of blood culture methods

2.2.1 Choice of media

The theoretical range of bacteria to be recovered from the blood is unending and no single medium will isolate all bacteria. The principles are the same, regardless of the system used, but in laboratories using commercial systems the media is part of the package. Most systems in common use employ separate media for the isolation of aerobic and anaerobic bacteria.

(a) *Blood to broth ratio.* In conventional broth culture systems the relative volumes of blood sample and medium should be arranged such that a dilution of at least 1 in 5, and preferably 1 in 10, is achieved. A dilution factor of at least 1 in 15–30 is necessary to remove the antibacterial effects of normal human blood (9). The addition of sodium polyethanolsulfonate (SPS, Liquoid®) allows the more modest dilution to produce the same effect.

(b) *Media for aerobic bacteria.* Aerobic bottles are available with all current commercial systems and vary in their broth base and additives. In conventional broth culture the systems use nutrient broth or glucose broth as the basis of the medium. The addition of the sample will convert this medium into 'human blood broth' which is very rich, capable of supporting the growth of many fastidious aerobes and facultative anaerobes. The choice of nutrient broth varies, but good examples are Nutrient Broth No. 2 (Oxoid) or Columbia Broth.

(c) *Media for anaerobic bacteria.* The frequency of anaerobic bacteraemia appears to be decreasing (10). In addition many anaerobes can be isolated in the aerobic bottles of currently marketed systems and although the speed of isolation may be reduced, the routine use of an anaerobic bottle may not be cost-effective. Some centres now use two aerobic bottles routinely with selective use of anaerobic blood cultures. Anaerobic bottles are available with all current commercial systems.

In the case of conventional systems, it is necessary to add substances capable of producing a reducing atmosphere. The addition of thioglycollate salts achieves this, but different thioglycollate preparations produce variable results.

(d) *Specialist media.* Certain unusual and extremely fastidious bacteria demand specialized media, which should be considered when specific conditions are clinically suspected. Although the available commercial systems have a range of media available, some directed at the isolation of more fastidious bacteria and fungi, it is worthwhile critically assessing the situation and considering other avenues in difficult cases. The principal special medium encountered until now has been that for the isolation of brucellae. A diphasic system (called by many 'Castenada's medium') is used in which the broth and slope consist of serum dextrose medium (11). This is incubated at 37 °C in an atmosphere containing 10% CO_2 for up to six weeks, inoculating the slope within the bottle regularly by tipping of the container, the fluid being allowed to flood the slope. This system has the advantage that containment is provided by the diphasic bottles. All subcultures and subsequent procedures must be performed within a safety cabinet.

(e) *Antimicrobial agents in blood cultures.* Many methods for the neutralization or removal of antibiotics have been devised. Dilution of antibiotics when the sample is added to the blood culture medium will usually render them non-inhibitory. In addition most commercial systems contain SPS at a concentration that inhibits aminoglycosides and polymyxins. Some systems use products that inactivate or remove antimicrobial products. These include, the Antibiotic Removal Device (ARD) (12), the resins found in BACTEC blood culture bottles (13), and the BacT/Alert FAN blood culture bottles (14). These systems accrue an additional cost and further clinical trials are necessary to establish their cost-effectiveness.

2.2.2 Duration of incubation

Complete clinical information will have an influence on the length of incubation. All the common pathogens, such as staphylococci, coliforms, etc., will be isolated within the first two to three days. Data available for most commercial systems support incubating bottles for five to seven days (8).

If endocarditis is suspected, the period should be prolonged although the length of incubation necessary is debated, a compromise of 12 days has been suggested.

2.2.3 Detection of a positive blood culture

(a) The conventional broth system relies on three methods, which must be combined.

    i. Inspect the undisturbed bottles daily. Note the appearance of turbidity, gas production, and look for the development of 'colonies' on the sedimented blood layer, or in the case of diphasic bottles on the agar surface.

    ii. Gram stain any suspicious looking bottles. Inform the ward or, better, go and see the patient.

    iii. A programme of routine subculturing must be undertaken. Subcultures performed within 12–18 h of receipt will detect 50–60% of all positives, but subcultures performed within 6 h of receipt are probably not worthwhile, detecting only 30% (15).

(b) The method of detection in automated and semi-automated systems varies (see Sections 2.3.4 and 2.3.5). The operator is alerted to the presence of a positive bottle in the system.

2.2.4 Processing of positive blood cultures

Once a bottle has been identified as positive, a Gram stain is performed and processed using a standard protocol based on the Gram result. Such a system is outlined in Protocol 2. In order to provide a rapid result a 'direct' sensitivity test should be performed using the blood culture broth as the inoculum. The test can be repeated with a carefully standardized inoculum the following day if necessary. Sensitivity testing also serves as a useful adjunct to identification.

Protocol 2

Summary of blood culture subculture plate procedures for positive cultures based on Gram stain

Gram morphology	Subcultured on to	Atmosphere of incubation
Gram-positive		
Cocci or bacilli	Blood agar	Air + 5–10% CO_2
	Blood agar	Hydrogen + 10% CO_2
	Neomycin–blood agar	Hydrogen + 10% CO_2
Gram-negative		
Cocci	Blood agar	Air + 5–10% CO_2
	Chocolate agar	Air + 5–10% CO_2

Protocol 2 continued		
	Blood agar	Hydrogen + 10% CO_2
	Neomycin–blood agar	Hydrogen + 10% CO_2
Bacilli	As above+	
	MacConkey's agar	Air
Fungal elements		
	Blood agar	Air + 5–10% CO_2
	Chocolate agar	Air + 5–10% CO_2
	Fungal medium	Air (30 °C)
	e.g. Sabaroud's dextrose agar	
Gram-stain negative		
	Blood agar	Air + 5–10% CO_2
	Blood agar	Hydrogen + 10% CO_2

Note: all plates should be incubated for at least 48 h and seven days in the case of those from neutropenic immunocompromised patients.

2.2.5 Characterization of isolates

All significant blood culture isolates should be identified to species level. Whilst a number of commercial identification kits exist (API 20E, API Staph, etc.) and automated sensitivity/identification systems (Vitek, ATB, etc.) it is important to carry out basic tests such as the Gram stain, oxidase, and catalase tests before proceeding to these specialized identification systems. This is particularly important as most systems offer a computer database to provide a 'best fit' identification which may be erroneous without this simple preparatory information, or, embarrassingly wrong if incorrect assumptions have been made at this preliminary stage. Some organisms isolated will not be suited to a commercial identification kit, and reference should be made to a standard work on the identification of clinically important bacteria (16, 17). Although not used presently because of cost, the direct sequencing of 16S rRNA genes from blood culture isolates is not only feasible but enables the easy identification of unusual organisms using the Micro Seq 500 kit (PE Biosystems) (18). A check should always be made that Gram-negative bacilli isolated from blood cultures do not slide agglutinate with polyvalent salmonella 'O' antisera prior to formal identification.

2.2.6 Contamination

Contamination arises in three distinct ways. The first two mechanisms are ward-based and not directly controlled by the laboratory. However, it is important that a quality assurance mechanism is in place to address the problem of excessive contamination. The regular presence of a microbiologist on the wards will help minimize these.

(a) *Cross-contamination.* Blood culture bottles may become cross-contaminated with saprophytic bacteria (e.g. *Stenotrophomonas maltophilia* and *Flavobacterium* spp.) from non-sterile containers for other (non-microbiological) tests (19), leading to a problem which has been called 'pseudobacteraemia'. Blood cultures should either be performed as a separate procedure, or the bottles inoculated before other containers.

(b) *Skin organisms*. Contamination may arise from the skin organisms of the patient and should be suspected when typical organisms (coagulase negative staphylococci and/or diphtheroids) are isolated within one to three days from one set of cultures but not all. However, it is important to remember that the pathogens *Streptococcus mutans* and *Listeria monocytogenes* may exhibit diphtheroid morphology and that some coryneforms can cause serious disease in compromised patients. The isolation from blood cultures of skin type organisms is not uncommon, and their significance must be assessed (Protocol 3). Occasionally bacteria other than those commonly associated with skin contamination appear in blood cultures, e.g. *Clostridium perfringens*. The likely source of these is the patient's skin; it is claimed that these spores are found more commonly on the skin of patients than on the skin of healthy people (20).

(c) *Laboratory-based contamination*. This is less of a problem with automated systems but has been reported. The range and types of bacteria isolated usually suggest this source and the isolation of the same organism from patients with widely varying clinical conditions should alert the microbiologist.

Protocol 3

Procedure for the assessment of blood culture isolates thought to be contaminants

1 Visit the patient. Patients with septicaemia are ill; those in whom the positive culture results from contamination are often well and lack other markers of serious sepsis, both clinical (e.g. fever, rigors) and laboratory (e.g. leukocytosis, raised CRP).

2 If in doubt, request further cultures, stressing the need to take them from different sites.

3 Ensure that the ward staff are not taking blood for culture via an indwelling intravenous line or similar device.

4 If a series of well taken cultures continues to yield a possible contaminant, consider the possibility that the infection is genuine. Obtain additional evidence that this may be the case by trying to prove that the isolates are identical. Various methods exist for typing such isolates (see Chapter 11).

2.2.7 Troubleshooting blood culture systems

Occasionally bacteria are seen in the Gram film, or in conventional systems a bottle is turbid, but the subcultures fail to yield an organism.

(a) Consider whether or not the full range of subculture media and atmospheric conditions have been used.

(b) If no inadvertent omissions have occurred, plan a strategy for the isolation of more fastidious bacteria. The most common problem is that Gram-positive cocci can be seen in films from the bottles but without growth on subculture. This is strongly suggestive of a nutritional variant streptococcus (NVS). Such strains often require supplementation of subculture media with one or more vitamins, most commonly pyridoxal and L-cysteine (21). A simple method of isolating the organism by providing a large range of extra nutrients is to cross-streak the media with *Staphylococcus aureus* following inoculation with the broth. NVS will grow as satellite growths near the streak. It is possible to supplement chemically defined media with a range of individual vitamins and other growth factors to define the dependence more precisely (22).

(c) In the absence of any bacteria being seen in the Gram stain but where the bottle appears to be positive, consider other possibilities. These include *Legionella* spp., *Campylobacter* spp., and mycoplasmata (particularly *Mycoplasma hominis*). Make subcultures onto the specialized media and incubate taking care to observe unusual atmospheric or temperature requirement.

(d) Remember that weakly Gram-positive rods may be mycobacteria or other actinomycetes, including *Nocardia* spp. Performing full or modified acid-fast staining may resolve this problem.

2.3 Blood culture methods

2.3.1 Conventional broth blood cultures

This is now the most labour-intensive method. The principles of this system have already been outlined.

2.3.2 Diphasic method

A variation on the aerobic broth medium is the diphasic medium in which a nutrient agar slope is incorporated into the bottle in addition to the broth (23). Frequent tipping of the bottle so that the broth phase regularly re-inoculates the agar slope obviates the need for subculture. This technique is often recommended for culture of potentially dangerous organisms (e.g. *Brucella* spp.) since it offers containment and may also reduce laboratory-introduced contamination. Several commercial systems are available such as the Septicheck (Roche) and HyFlask® (Lab M).

2.3.3 Lysis–centrifugation methods

This system was initially developed in the early 20th Century and was adapted in the 1970s. The Isolator blood culture system and Isostat sytems are commercially available (24). The isolator tube contains Saponin as a lysing agent, polypropylene glycol as an antifoaming agent, SPS and EDTA as anticoagulants, and an inert fluorochemical liquid. Although this method is quick, it is labour-intensive and contamination is one of the major disadvantages. The system has been found to be better that conventional and radiometric methods for the isolation of fungi and mycobacteria. Results are probably comparable to the newer automated systems.

2.3.4 Semi-automated systems

(a) *Manometric method.* The Signal system uses a gas capture device, which is connected to the culture bottle on receipt in the laboratory. It gives similar results to the radiometric methods but may miss some fastidious organisms and is not generally used (25).

(b) *BACTEC® radiometric and non-radiometric (NR) systems.* The BACTEC® radiometric system was the first semi-automated system developed but is now rarely used for routine bacteriology because of the problem with the disposal of radioactive material (26). It is still used for mycobacterial culture. The method involves the detection of radioactive CO_2 produced by the growing culture from ^{14}C-labelled substrates in the broth medium. The instrument samples gas from the headspace in the bottle, and when a predetermined CO_2 concentration is reached (the 'growth index') the bottle is identified as provisionally positive.

The NR version of the machine uses infrared detection of CO_2, eliminating the problem of radiation exposure (27). Bottles are incubated independently of the instrument and the system is an automated substitute for the daily visual inspection used with conventional systems. Semi-automated systems have the disadvantage that the incubators and the reading device are separate. Thus staff need to move the bottles to conduct the readings and are not alerted to a positive bottle by the system itself.

2.3.5 Continuous-monitoring systems

These systems automatically detect growth and signal the operator, they are now very widely used. The systems usually comprise a growth indicator, detection mechanism, and signalling system. The units vary in their methodologies, bottle capacity, measurement frequency, types of media and supplements, blood to broth volume, and inoculation volume.

The detection unit is usually a self-contained unit with an incubator, agitator, and detector. It interfaces with a computer system with the necessary software (Figure 3). Such software allows the development of growth detection algorithms to monitor bottles for rates of change and absolute change. These systems offer the advantage of reduced laboratory workload, reduced contamination levels, increased speed of detection and, therefore, increased speed of microbial recovery.

Improvements in design, detection methods, and media formulation continue to be made. When choosing a system each laboratory must critically assess their needs and then look at the functions offered by the various systems.

(a) BacT/Alert (Organon Teknika Corporation, Durham, NC) uses colorimetry to detect the production of CO_2 in bottles (28). Two unit sizes (120 and 240) are available. Bottles are agitated at a rate of 70 cycles/min. Each bottle is scanned

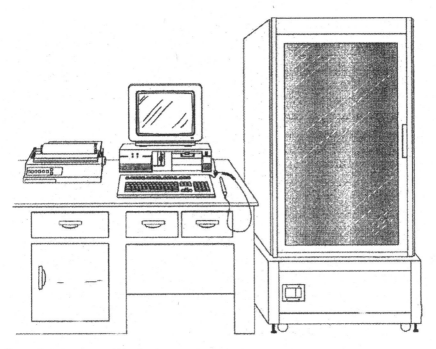

Figure 3 An automated blood culture system.

by the unit every 10 min. A variety of media are available including standard aerobic and anaerobic, paediatric bottle, and FAN formulation. This is an adsorbent charcoal-containing material which has been found to improve recovery of some pathogens.

(b) BACTEC 9000 series (Becton Dickinson Microbiology Systems, Sparks, MD) use a fluorescent indicator to detect CO_2 (29). Three unit sizes (50, 120, and 240) are available. Bottles are agitated at a rate of 30 cycles/min. Each bottle is monitored every 10 min. A variety of media are available including standard aerobic, anaerobic, paediatric bottle, and bottles for more fastidious organisms.

(c) DIFCO Extra Sensing Power (ESP) System (Difco Laboratories, Detroit, MI) detects pressure changes in the headspace of blood culture bottles secondary to microbial gas production and/or consumption (30). Three unit sizes (128, 256, and 384) are available. Bottles are agitated at a rate of 160 cycles/min. Aerobic bottles are monitored every 12 min and anaerobic bottles every 24 min. A variety of media are available.

(d) Vital Blood Culture System (Biomerieux, Marcy, l'Etoile, France). This system incorporates a fluorescent indicator which detects changes in redox potential, pH, or CO_2 (31). Three unit sizes (200, 300, and 400) are available. Bottles are agitated at a rate of 150 cycles/min. The bottles are monitored every 15 min. Aerobic and anaerobic media are available.

37

2.4 Blood culture diagnosis of catheter-related sepsis

The diagnosis of central venous catheter (CVC)-related sepsis relies on clinical features (which are inadequate on their own) and culture of the catheter tip after removal. Only 15–25% of central venous catheters (CVC) removed are found to be infected following removal resulting in the loss of a large number of otherwise uninfected lines (32).

2.4.1 Differential blood culture techniques

Differential quantitative blood cultures of samples taken simultaneously from the catheter and a peripheral vein have been found to have a sensitivity of the order of 80% in the presence of bacteraemia for the detection of CVC-related sepsis (32). The need for the presence of bacteraemia together with the complexity of the method has meant it has had a low take up. Because continuous monitoring blood culture systems detect changes in bacterial load it has been reported that time to positivity correlated closely with the size of the initial inoculum when using the BACT/Alert system (33). This preliminary study has been validated and extended. If a cut off for the differential positivity time (difference in minutes between the peripheral and central line culture) of +120 min was used 100% specificity and 96.4% sensitivity was obtained (34).

2.4.2 Direct staining of blood

An alternative approach for the diagnosis of CVC-related sepsis is the direct straining of blood drawn from the catheter (Protocol 4). A positive cytospin smear is shown in Figure 4. The technique was applied to 50 cases of CVC-related sepsis

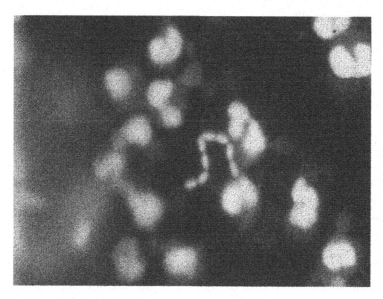

Figure 4 Acridine orange stained polymorphs in the blood film of patient with septicaemia, a chain of eight streptococci can clearly be seen.

and found to have a sensitivity of 96% and specificity of 92%, the Maki tip roll method had figures of 90% and 55%, respectively (35).

Protocol 4

Gram and acridine orange leukocyte cytospin test for CVC sepsis diagnosis (35)

Equipment and reagents

- Cytocentrifuge (Cytospin4® Thermo Shandon Inc.)
- Bench centrifuge
- Hot plate
- UV/light microscope with oil immersion ×90 or ×100 objective
- 12 mm × 75 mm polystyrene capped tubes (Sarstedt, Leicester, UK)
- Microscope slides
- 10% (v/v) formol saline (0.025 mol/litre NaCl)
- 0.19 mol/litre NaCl solution
- 10 mg/ml acridine orange solution
- Gram stain reagents

Method

1 Two 50 µl aliquots of blood anticoagulated with EDTA are each placed into polystyrene tubes.

2 Add 1.2 ml of formol saline to each tube, mix gently, and leave for 2 min at room temperature.

3 Add 2.8 ml of 0.19 mol/litre NaCl solution, mix.

4 Centrifuge at 350 g for 5 min and decant off the supernatant.

5 Emulsify the deposit by vortexing for 5 sec.

6 Transfer the cellular deposit to a cytocentrifuge cupule with a microscope slide (a pair are used) and spin at 150 g for 5 min.

7 The monolayer of cells is stained with acridine orange on one slide for 30 sec then washed with sterile distilled water; the other slide is stained with Gram stain.

8 Examine at least 100 high power fields (HPF) for the presence of micro-organisms (bacteria and fungi should be clearly visible) and report the morphology of any micro-organisms. If at least 100 HPF are negative the sample should be reported as negative.

2.5 Alternative methods to broth cultures

2.5.1 Detection of bacterial antigen/chemical markers

Although there have been several attempts to replace blood cultures by the detection of bacterial antigens or chemical markers in blood, these have remained experimental and unhelpful. Examples include the Limulus lysate test for endotoxin, gas–liquid chromatography for volatile products of certain bacteria, and counterimmune electrophoresis for capsular antigens. Apart from technical limitations, which are considerable, none of these methods achieves the recovery of the live bacteria to determine antibiotic sensitivity patterns and subtype to identify nosocomial cross-infection.

2.5.2 Molecular technology

Polymerase chain reaction (PCR) of blood can be used to detect microbial DNA in patients with septicaemia (36). Primers are now available for the common pathogens, however the technique is not routinely used at present. The considerable costs of these methods are likely to limit their use to carefully defined situations in which the clinical advantages of this approach (principally, speed) clearly outweighs the cost. One application in which the balance appears to be in favour of molecular technology is the rapid detection of bacteraemia caused by MRSA. An assay using real-time fluorescence PCR has shown to have a specificity 100% and sensitivity of 96% for the detection of S. aureus in 50 positive blood cultures. With the addition of primers/probe for the mecA gene the specificity was 100% for the detection of MRSA (37). An alternative assay using three multiplexed primers (mecA, 16S rRNA for the identification of the genus Staphylococcus, and nuc identifies S. aureus) has also been shown to be valuable (38).

Because of the relatively higher density of bacteraemia in neonates, direct detection of bacteraemia in neonates is another alternative area of application for molecular technology. Using a 5 h pre-enrichment culture step amplification of 200–500 μl of blood in 4 ml of typtic soy broth, followed by PCR amplification of a 380 bp fragment of the 16S rRNA gene revealed a sensitivity, specificity, positive, and negative predictive value of 96.0, 99.4, 88.9, and 99.8% compared to culture in a BACTEC 9240 system (39).

3 Methods for the examination of cerebrospinal fluid

3.1 Introduction

The correct examination of cerebrospinal fluid (CSF) is an essential task in all laboratories. Some of the 'bacteriological' results, especially the cell count (both red and white) and the identification of xanthochromia will conform non-bacteriological diagnoses and are thus as important as the bacteriology investigations.

3.2 Bacteriological aspects of specimen collection

CSF must be collected under sterile conditions. Separate specimens are preferable for biochemical and bacteriological analyses to avoid inadvertent contamination of the sample. CSF should be taken into sterile 'one use' containers since recycled containers may harbour debris from previous samples which can cause confusion in stained smears.

3.3 Microscopy

Prior to microscopy the macroscopic appearance of the specimen should be noted, looking for turbidity, blood staining, and xanthochromia, then the procedure described in Protocols 5 and 6 should be followed.

Protocol 5

Procedure for microscopy of CSF, the total cell count

Equipment and reagents

- Fuchs–Rosenthal counting chamber
- Coverslip
- Glass Pasteur pipette
- CSF
- Lytic staining fluid: 100 mg crystal violet, 1 ml glacial acetic acid, 50 ml water, and 40 µl of 15% (w/v) phenol

Method

Perform a total cell count on uncentrifuged fluid using a Fuchs–Rosenthal counting chamber as follows.

1. Using a sterile glass Pasteur pipette add one drop of lytic staining fluid to 10 drops of CSF, and mix well.
2. Place a drop in the counting chamber and apply the coverslip, pressing firmly either side until an interference pattern appears.
3. Count the number of cells in the entire ruled area and divide this total by three to obtain the number of cells/mm^3 of diluted CSF (Figure 5). The slight error introduced by this approximation is small compared to dilution errors.
4. If the CSF sample appears blood stained, or if the clinician indicates a suspicion of intracerebral haemorrhage, repeat the count on unstained CSF in order to count the number of red cells. In obviously blood stained CSF it may be useful to ask the haematology staff to examine the specimen on a Coulter counter to count the red cells.
5. Note the apparent presence of any bacteria in the counting chamber, but be wary of attaching too much significance to any suspicious particles seen. Small particles undergoing Brownian movement can look very similar. Note also any debris in the specimen. The presence of starch granules from gloves may indicate contamination.

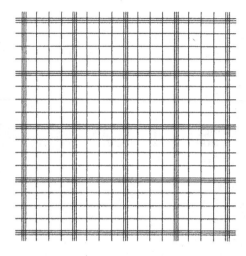

Figure 5 The ruled area of the Fuchs–Rosenthal counting chamber. The depth is 0.2 mm and the entire ruled area is 16 mm^2, the volume therefore being 3.2 mm^3.

Protocol 6

Procedure for microscopy and culture of CSF, Gram stain, and differential count

Equipment and reagents

- Sterile centrifuge tube or universal container
- Centrifuge or cytocentrifuge
- Glass slides
- Microscope

- Gram stain
- 1% carbol fuchsin
- Blood agar
- Chocolate agar
- Giemsa's stain

Method

1. Place a small amount of the CSF into a sterile centrifuge tube or universal container and centrifuge (or cytocentrifuge if available) at 1800 g for 10 min. Observe the appearance of the supernatant fluid before discarding. Xanthochromia is easily seen.

2. Use the sediment to make smears on three sterile, new glass slides. Never use cleaned old glass slides since it is possible that previous material may still adhere. Several drops of sediment should be placed on one spot on the slide, each being allowed to dry before the next is added, thus concentrating any bacteria present.

3. Gram stain the first slide, using 1% carbol fuchsin as the counterstain (Appendix I); this increases the chances of staining small numbers of Gram-negative bacteria. Examine carefully using a ×40 and ×90 oil immersion objective for at least 5 min.

4 Use the remainder of the centrifuged deposit to inoculate the following media:

   (a) Blood agar incubated aerobically at 37 °C for 48 h and inspected daily.

   (b) Chocolate agar plate incubated in 5–10% CO_2 at 37 °C for 48 h and inspected daily.

   (c) Blood agar incubated anaerobically at 37 °C for 48 h and inspected daily.

   (d) In patients with a pleocytosis, prosthetic material, an anatomical defect, or when unusual organisms are suspected place a few drops of the deposit into an enrichment broth and incubate for 48 h, performing subcultures onto the range of media described above at 24 h and 48 h.

5 Stain the second smear with Giemsa's stain and examine, noting the distribution of the different white blood cell types. Although this slide cannot be used to enumerate these cells, identification of the types is easy and the percentage distribution can be applied to the total count (from the counting chamber). If in doubt about the identity of the white blood cells have it examined by a haematologist or cytologist. Leukaemic meningitis may present with all the clinical appearances of bacterial meningitis. The demonstration of lymphoblasts in the CSF may be the initial diagnostic clue.

6 Use the third smear to perform a stain for acid-fast bacilli (Appendix I). Again, be prepared to spend 5 min searching the slide before declaring the examination negative.

3.4 Culture

Neisseria meningitidis and *Streptococcus pneumoniae* remain the commonest pathogens isolated (40). Although the incidence of *Haemophilus influenzae* meningitis has declined with the advent of vaccination this organism should still be sought. In infants, especially neonates, coliform bacilli and Lancefield group B streptococci can cause infection. Following neurosurgical operations, a wide range of organisms may be isolated, including *Staphylococcus aureus*, coagulase negative staphylococci (CNS), coliforms, and fungi.

Although contaminants are possible, most commonly from the skin or laboratory plate contaminants, all isolates should be thoroughly investigated and fully identified before making a final report. Two particular traps are the following.

(a) Coagulase negative staphylococci (CNS) isolated from CSF should always lead to an appraisal of the patient and the clinical information. In children and adults with CSF shunt devices, CNS are the commonest infecting organisms. Do not be put off by the relative paucity of white cells in such CSF samples, which is typical (41).

(b) Never dismiss a coryneform rod in CSF as a 'diphtheroid' contaminant. *Listeria monocytogenes* can look very similar to a diphtheroid in Gram films and in culture on certain media, and all such bacteria should be checked. Simple tests such as the presence of β-haemolysis and ability to grow on Tellurite agar, together with 'tumbling motility' at room temperature should alert laboratory staff to this organism.

3.5 Additional tests

3.5.1 Tests on bacterial isolates

Each isolate should be identified and typed as completely as possible. This is particularly important for isolates of N. meningitidis, in which the serogroup determination will guide vaccination responses, but also applies to the other pathogens, e.g. S. pneumoniae and H. influenzae. In addition to routine methods for identification and sensitivity testing, preliminary data on typing of N. meningitidis and H. influenzae can be obtained from commercially available latex agglutination kits. Further information can then be obtained by sending isolates to a reference laboratory.

3.5.2 Tests on CSF

The detection of bacterial antigens in CSF has become an important part of a diagnostic strategy. At least three different methods have been devised: counter-immune electrophoresis (CIE), co-agglutination (Phadebact® CSF Test; Pharmacia Diagnostics AB), and passive agglutination of latex particles sensitized with high titre antiserum to capsular antigens. The latter two methods are much quicker than CIE and more convenient since they require little equipment. Several systems are available for the detection of polysaccharide capsular antigens of H. influenzae, S. pneumoniae, N. meningitidis, and group B streptococci in CSF. These tests have been shown to be sensitive and specific in patients with clinical bacterial meningitis. It is important that they are used appropriately and the results are interpreted in the light of the clinical history and other CSF findings. However, it has been estimated (for pneumococci, at least) that capsular antigen detection systems have a sensitivity of between 10^6 and 10^7 cfu/ml, although antigen may remain detectable when viable organisms can no longer be detected (42). Hence, negative capsular antigen tests cannot be taken to exclude the diagnosis. Recently, molecular biological techniques, especially PCR, have been pursued as a means of devising yet more sensitive methods for the detection of microbial pathogens in CSF (43, 44). As yet, the diagnostic use of molecular techniques on CSF has been primarily targeted on viral infections (enterovirus, herpesvirus) and tuberculous meningitis (see Section 3.7), when the considerable cost is more easily offset against the benefits. Primers are now available for the common bacterial pathogens, and a set of multiplexed primers used in a real-time PCR format for the three most common pathogens were able to identify a significant number of 'missed' cases of N. meningitidis disease as well as potentially providing a robust tool for the early diagnosis (45). The technique is not routinely used except in the case of meningococcal infection in which the PCR used will identify the serogroup and, thus, guide local vaccination strategy.

Table 1 Expected results of basic tests on CSF in the common forms of meningitis

Type of meningitis	Cell count	CSF glucose	CSF protein
Bacterial	High, almost all polymorphs	Very low	Increased
Viral	Raised, almost all lymphocytes except first 24 h	Normal	Normal or slightly raised
Tuberculous	Raised, almost all lymphocytes	Low	Increased

3.6 Interpretation of results

It frequently falls to the bacteriologist to collate the immediate results on CSF samples and to make an initial judgement on the likelihood of meningitis. The classical interpretations of the three 'simple' tests, cell count, glucose concentration, and protein, are shown in Table 1. It is important to bear in mind that these categories are but guidelines and that certain caveats must be applied.

3.6.1 Cell count

Whilst numerous polymorphs are usually observed in bacterial meningitis, infection of shunt devises with CNS does not always follow this pattern. The classical lymphocytosis is not always present in viral meningitis. In the first 24 h of viral meningitis, polymorphs may be present, or the first CSF sample may contain no cells at all. Subsequent samples later in the illness will show the typical lymphocytosis.

3.6.2 Glucose concentration

The microbiologist should insist on knowing the blood glucose level of the patient at, or near, the time of lumbar puncture before making any assessment of the CSF glucose concentration. A CSF glucose level within the 'normal' range may be very abnormal in a patient with hyperglycaemia or hypoglycaemia. Occasionally, slightly low CSF glucose concentrations occur in severe viral meningitis, due often to Coxsackie virus infections.

3.6.3 Traumatic taps

Sometimes the CSF sample is contaminated with a small amount of blood because the operator has damaged a tiny blood vessel during the puncture. There are two ways of resolving this problem. If possible, the operator can take two or three sequential samples. The later samples will contain less and less blood and the cell count can be performed on the second or third sample although small variations in count should be ignored as the counting technique is relatively inaccurate. If however only one (blood contaminated) sample is available, proceed as follows. Perform a red cell count on the sample and then, using the lytic staining fluid (Section 3.3), count the white cells. Allow one white cell for an appropriate number of red cells, based on the peripheral blood count at the time. Subtract the 'allowed' number of white cells, approximately one per 500 red cells; if a significant excess of white cells remains, report that there is a pleocytosis in the CSF.

Note that in very small children the density of bacteraemia may be very high and the contamination of CSF samples with a small amount of peripheral blood may give rise to a positive CSF culture in the absence of true meningitis.

3.7 Tuberculous meningitis (TBM)

Clinicians periodically make enquiries to the laboratory about the diagnosis of TBM. They are, quite rightly, very concerned to exclude this life-threatening but treatable condition. However, the limitations in the laboratory diagnosis of this condition must be accepted (Protocol 7). The absence of acid-fast bacilli in a Zichl–Neelsen smear of the centrifuged CSF deposit (or in a smear stained with auramine phenol and examined under UV light) does not exclude the diagnosis. Culture by one of the several Continuous Automated Mycobacterial Liquid Culture, or CAMLiC, systems (46) remains the most sensitive diagnostic test, outstripping both acid-fast staining and even PCR (see Chapter 3).

Protocol 7

Procedure for the diagnosis of tuberculous meningitis

Equipment and reagents

- Centrifuge
- Auramine phenol or ZN stain
- TB culture media
- H_2SO_4

Method

1 Centrifuge the sample at $1800\,g$ for $20\,min$ and make auramine phenol or ZN stained films (Appendix I). Examine the film for a least $5\,min$ before reporting it as negative.[a]

2 Use the remainder of the deposit to inoculate liquid medium Lowenstein–Jensen's medium and pyruvate egg medium. Increasingly often the culture is now performed in a CAMLiC system, which can be expected to grow M. *tuberculosis* much more quickly than conventional solid culture and is more sensitive than solid culture.

3 CSF normally does not require any prior treatment before culture for TB. In those rare cases in which TB culture is justified in the presence of other organisms in the CSF, add $20\,\mu l$ of 5% (w/v) H_2SO_4 to the deposit before inoculating the TB culture media. Allow $15–20\,min$ for the H_2SO_4 to work.

4 It is common in patients undergoing anti-tuberculous therapy for TBM to have CSF collected several times during the course of treatment. Do not be alarmed to find that the lymophocytosis does not immediately resolve. It may rise in the first few days or weeks, although over a long period the pleocytosis does resolve with further fluctuations.

[a] Very unusually, on standing, the CSF from cases of TBM may form a very fine clot ('spider web coagulum'); use it after careful removal for the staining procedures.

Whilst more sophisticated tests (PCR, CAMLiC) can now be brought to bear on each individual sample of CSF examined for *M. tuberculosis*, it is important to remember that all tests for the diagnosis of TBM, be they conventional or new, are more likely to be positive with larger volumes of CSF and/or when repeated on several samples taken on different days.

4 Methods for the examination of peritoneal dialysis effluents

Continuous ambulatory peritoneal dialysis (CAPD) is an important therapy for end stage renal failure. Its major complication, and the one most likely to limit its usefulness, is peritonitis (47). Similar techniques can be applied to specimens received from patients undergoing intermittent peritoneal dialysis (IPD) for acute renal failure.

4.1 Definition of CAPD peritonitis

Peritonitis in CAPD is defined as:

(a) The presence of cloudy effluent with more than 100 white blood cells/mm^3, whether clinical symptoms (usually fever and/or abdominal pain) are present or not (48).

(b) The presence of organisms in the fluid together with abdominal pain (49).

In CAPD peritonitis the commonest finding is cloudy effluent (99%), then abdominal pain (96%). Systemic abnormalities are less common (fever 35%, leukocytosis 25%).

Only specimens taken from patients with either cloudy effluent or abdominal pain should be examined in the laboratory. Occasionally peritoneal dialysis effluents (PDE) samples will be cloudy due to fibrin or chyle (50), but in general a visually cloudy effluent is a good indication that excess white blood cells will be found on laboratory examination.

4.2 Sampling PDE

It is important to obtain an adequate sample. Ideally the whole bag should be examined, but this usually proves impracticable. A sample from the bag is obtained as follows:

(a) Disinfect the port of the bag with alcohol, and allow the alcohol to dry for 2 min.

(b) Collect at least 30 ml of fluid using a needle and syringe, placing the sample into sterile containers with a careful aseptic 'no touch' technique.

(c) In the event of any delay before the sample is sent to the laboratory, hold it at 4 °C, but try to avoid the need for this.

4.2.1 Cell counts and culture

Enumeration of the white blood cells will help to confirm a diagnosis of peritonitis. On a stained preparation a differential count is performed so that the presence of large numbers of eosinophils can be detected when present. Gram stains will be positive in only 25–30% of PDE samples from which organisms are subsequently isolated.

As the number of bacteria may be as low as cfu/ml techniques such as centrifugation, filtration, broth enrichment, and pour plates will be required to maximize the detection rate (51). Unfortunately such methods involve extra manipulations and greatly increase the risks of contamination and false positive cultures. Inoculation into an automated blood culture system is practised in some laboratories (52).

A routine scheme for the examination of PDE samples is set out in Protocol 8. Using such a system the rate of positive cultures should approach 90%, although this figure will apply only to correctly taken and appropriate samples. Repeat samples taken during therapy of CAPD peritonitis should be discouraged unless there is clearly no clinical response to treatment or the effluent remains cloudy after 48–72 h of therapy.

Protocol 8

Routine bacteriological examination of PDE sample

Equipment and reagents

- See Protocol 5
- Centrifuge
- Blood agar plates
- Bacteriological filter (0.45 μm, Millipore Corporation)
- Gram stain
- Giemsa stain
- Blood culture broths

Method

1 Using an identical method to that in Protocol 5 for CSF samples, perform a white blood cell count on the uncentrifuged sample.

2 From the original sample of 30 ml take 20 ml and centrifuge at 1800 g for 10 min. From the spun deposit prepare two fixed smears. Perform a Gram stain on one and a differential white cell stain on the other using Giemsa stain (Appendix I).

3 Using the remainder of the centrifuged deposit inoculate two blood agar plates. Incubate one plate aerobically at 37 °C for 72 h, examining it for growth at intervals. Incubate the second plate under anaerobic conditions examining at similar intervals.

4 An alternative method to step 3 is to use filtration.

Protocol 8 continued

(a) Filter the 20 ml of PD effluent through a 0.45 μm bacteriological filter.

(b) Cut the filter into two halves using sterile scissors.

(c) Place one-half of the filter on a blood agar plate for aerobic culture and the other half on blood agar plate for anaerobic culture as in step 3.

5 Inoculate the remaining 10 ml of PDE into two blood culture broths (aerobic and anaerobic and 5 ml/bottle) and incubate at 37 °C for five to seven days.

4.2.2 Additional techniques

Several studies have suggested that although the viable count of organisms in PDE fluid is very low, substantial numbers of bacteria may be present within the polymorphs. Logically, lysis of the white blood cells might be expected to release these organisms, increase the viable count, detect additional organisms and, occasionally, lead to bacteria being detected when conventional methods are completely negative. At least two studies suggest that this is so (53, 54). Lytic agents employed include Triton X and Saponin, both methods resulting in improved results; however increased contamination may occur.

Acridine orange staining of films may detect intracellular bacteria when the conventional Gram film does not (55). Unfortunately, if subsequent culture cannot confirm the presence of the intracellular bacteria, the information may be of only limited value.

4.3 Interpretation of culture results

Gram-positive organisms (*Staphylococcus aureus*, CNS, and occasionally, diphtheroids predominate. Gram-negative bacilli ('coliforms') account for up to 25–30% of infections.

Expect very little return on the anaerobic cultures but be assiduous in testing for these organisms. On the very rare occasions when faecal anaerobes, especially *Bacteroides* spp., are isolated, suspect perforation of the bowel, either by catheter trauma or as a consequence of intra-abdominal disease.

4.4 Identification and sensitivity testing

Isolates should be identified to species level. Occasionally it may be necessary to subtype staphylococci (phage or PFGE) when attempting to differentiate between relapse and recurrences of infection. A limited range of intraperitoneal antibiotics including vancomycin, gentamicin, netilmicin, and cefuroxime are used in most units.

4.5 Culture negative peritonitis

Certain possibilities should always be considered when a cloudy PDE is culture negative.

(a) Early morning effluents often have an increased white cell count (due to the longer overnight dwell time) in the absence of infection.

(b) Intra-abdominal conditions such as cholecystitis, appendicitis, diverticulitis, and genital infections may produce an increased white cell count in the effluent.

(c) Menstruation and ovulation may occasionally change the appearance of the effluent, usually due to bleeding.

(d) Eosinophilic peritonitis is thought to be due to a hypersensitivity reaction to some component of the dialysis system. Suspect this when differential stain shows greater than 15% eosinophils. This condition is not an infection.

If despite all this there is genuine peritonitis but cultures remain negative, consider setting up cultures for unusual organisms. Atypical mycobacteria, *Mycobacterium tuberculosis*, fungi, and parasites have all, rarely, been implicated in CAPD peritonitis. It is most likely, however, that culture negative CAPD peritonitis is a case of infection with a common organism where the viable count is so low that the culture technique is inadequate (56). Empirical treatment based on this assumption is usually successful.

5 Methods for the examination of serous fluids

Microbiology departments occasionally receive samples of serous fluid from a range of body sites. Common examples are ascitic, hydrocoele, pleural, pericardial, and synovial fluids. If serous cavities are obviously infected, the specimen received is almost always frank pus which should be investigated as outlined in Chapter 5. What follows is a system for the examination of fluid from serous cavities which is not pus.

5.1 Examination of non-purulent serous fluids

The scheme set out in Protocol 9 can be used for all fluids.

Protocol 9

Routine bacteriological examination of non-purulent serous fluids

Equipment and reagents

- See Protocol 5
- See Protocol 7
- Centrifuge
- Sterile isotonic saline
- Gram stain
- Chocolate agar plates
- Liquid enrichment medium

Method

1. Using an identical method to that used for CSF (Protocol 5) perform a white blood cell count on the uncentrifuged sample. Since some fluids (particularly synovial fluid) can be very viscous, it may be necessary to make a preliminary 1 in 10 dilution in sterile isotonic saline and then multiply the observed count by 10.

2. Centrifuge the remainder at 2000 g for 15 min and use the spun deposit.

3. Prepare two fixed smears for Gram stain and differential white cell stain.

4. Inoculate three chocolate agar plates. Incubate one aerobically, one anaerobically, and the third in an atmosphere containing 5–10% CO_2, all at 37 °C. It may be helpful to inoculate a MacConkey's plate and incubate it aerobically at 37 °C. Observe the plates for growth at intervals over 48 h.

5. Using the remainder of the deposit, inoculate a liquid enrichment medium such as Robertson's cooked meat broth, and incubate it at 37 °C. Observe for turbidity, subculturing on to the media described in step 4 and routinely at 48 h before discarding. In some laboratories this practice has been replaced by inoculating the fluid into a blood culture bottle in a continuously monitored system (57).

6. If tuberculosis is suspected, prepare an additional smear to be stained for acid-fast bacilli and use some of the centrifuged deposit to inoculate the range of media described for the diagnosis of tuberculous meningitis (Protocol 7). It is unnecessary to decontaminate clear serous samples prior to examination for acid-fast bacilli.

5.1.1 Pleural fluid

Absolute numbers of white blood cells/mm^3 are not a particularly valuable diagnostic parameter in clear pleural fluid, but the differential stain may yield useful information. Lymphocytes and, occasionally, eosinophils suggest tuberculous effusions. It is not uncommon for smears from such conditions to be negative in these circumstances since they most commonly occur in primary tuberculosis. Pleural biopsy material may be more useful.

Detection of any unclassifiable or bizarre cell types should always suggest the possibility of malignancy and lead to the specimen being referred to a cytologist.

Very rarely an apparently hazy pleural fluid proves to contain chyle on microscopy (usually suspected in 'wet preparations') and should be referred for biochemical analysis.

5.1.2 Pericardial fluid

The same caveat regarding tuberculosis should be observed, and tissue from the pericardium is often necessary to adequately investigate suspected tuberculous pericarditis.

5.1.3 Synovial fluid

Although pyogenic infection of a joint almost inevitably produces a fluid of such purulence that formal cell counts are unnecessary, it is important to realize that many non-infective conditions (for instance, rheumatoid arthritis, crystal synovitis) will often produce cell counts in synovial fluid to 50 000/mm^3 or more (58). Intra-articular injections may also lead to high white cell counts in synovial fluid in the absence of infection.

References

1. Bennett, I. L. and Beeson, P. B. (1954). *Yale J. Biol. Med.*, **26**, 241.

2. Werner, A. S., Cobbs, C. G., Kaye, D., and Hook, E. W. (1967). *J. Am. Med. Assoc.*, **202**, 199.

3. Crowley, N. (1970). *J. Clin. Pathol.*, **23**, 166.

4. Minkus, R. and Moffet, H. L. (1971). *Appl. Microbiol.*, **22**, 805.

5. Hall, M. M., Ilstrup, D. M., and Washington, J. A. (1976). *J. Clin. Microbiol.*, **3**, 643.

6. Ilstrup, D. M. and Washington, J. A. (1983). *Diagn. Microbiol. Infect. Dis.*, **1**, 107.

7. Wilson, M. I. (1994). *Clin. Lab. Med.*, **14**, 1.

8. Wilson, M. I., Weinstein, M. P., and Reller, L. B. (1994). *Clin. Lab. Med.*, **14**, 149.

9. Salventi, J. F., Davies, T. A., Randall, E. L., Whitaker, S., *et al.* (1979). *J. Clin. Microbiol.*, **9**, 248.

10. Sharp, S. E. (1992). *Clin. Microbiol. Newsl.*, **13**, 179.

11. Casteneda, M. R. (1947). *Proc. Soc. Exp. Biol. Med.*, **64**, 114.

12. Appleman, M. D., Swinney, R. S., and Heseltine, P. N. R. (1982). *J. Clin. Microbiol.*, **15**, 278.

13. Cregan, P., Fiss, E. H., Sullivan, A., Brooks, G. F., *et al.* (1993). *Diagn. Microbiol. Infect. Dis.*, **17**, 569.

14. McDonald, L. C., Fune, J., Gaido, L. B., Weinstein, M. P., *et al.* (1996). *J. Clin. Microbiol.*, **34**, 2180.

15. Ganguli, L. A., Keaney, M. G. L., Hyde, W. A., and Fraser, S. B. (1985). *J. Clin. Pathol.*, **38**, 1146.

16. Murray, P. R. (1999). *Manual of clinical microbiology*, 7th edn. American Society for Microbiology, Washington.

17. Cowan, S. T. (1993). *Cowan and Steel's manual for the identification of medical bacteria*, 3rd edn. Cambridge University Press, Cambridge.

18. Qian, Q., Tang, W-H., Kolbert, C. P., Torgerson, C. A., *et al.* (2001). *J. Clin. Microbiol.*, **39**, 3578.

19. Gould, J. C. and Duerden, B. I. (1983). *J. Clin. Pathol.*, **36**, 963.

20. Watt, B. (1983). *J. Clin. Pathol.*, **36**, 968.

21. Roberts, R. B., Krieger, A. G., Schiller, N. L., and Gross, K. C. (1979). *Rev. Infect. Dis.*, **1**, 955.

22. Bouvet, A., Van de Rijn, I., and McCarty, M. (1981). *J. Bacteriol.*, **146**, 1075.

23. Bradley, S. F., Wilson, K. H., Roslonicc, M. A., and Kauffman, C. A. (1987). *Infect. Control*, **8**, 281.

24. Bille, J., Edson, R. S., and Roberts, G. D. (1983). *J. Clin. Microbiol.*, **19**, 126.

25. Robner, P. and Aukenthaler, R. (1989). *Eur. J. Clin. Microbiol. Infect. Dis.*, **8**, 150.

26. Weinstein, M. P., Mirret, S., Reimer, L. G., and Reller, L. B. (1989). *J. Clin. Microbiol.*, **27**, 427.

27. Jungkind, D., Millan, J., Allen, S., Dyke, J., *et al.* (1986). *J. Clin. Microbiol.*, **23**, 262.

28. Thorpe, T. C., Wilson, M. I., Turner, J. E., DiGuiseppi, J. L., Willert, M., Mirret, S., *et al.* (1990). *J. Clin. Microbiol.*, **28**, 1608.

29. Nolte, F. S., Williams, J. M., Jerris, R. C., Morello, J. A., *et al.* (1993). *J. Clin. Microbiol.*, **31**, 552.

30. Zwadyk, P., Pierson, C. L., and Young, C. (1994). *J. Clin. Microbiol.*, **32**, 1273.

31. Wilson, M. L., Mirret, S., McDonald, L. C., Weinstein, M. P., *et al.* (1999). *J. Clin. Microbiol.*, **37**, 1709.

32. Bouza, E., Burilla, A., and Munuoz, P. (2002). *Clin. Microbiol. Infect.*, **8**, 265.

33. Rodgers, M. S. and Oppenheim, B. A. (1998). *J. Clin. Pathol.*, **8**, 635.

34. Blot, F., Schmidt, E., Nitenberg, G., Tancrede, C., *et al.* (1998). *J. Clin. Microbiol.*, **36**, 105.

35. Kit, P., Dobbins, B. M., Wilcox, M. H., and McMahon, M. J. (1999). *Lancet*, **354**, 1504.

36. Heininger, A., Binder, M., Schmidt, S., Unertl, K., *et al.* (1999). *J. Clin. Microbiol.*, **37**, 2479.

37. Tan, T. Y., Corden, S., Barnes, R., and Cookson, B. (2001). *J. Clin. Microbiol.*, **39**, 4529.

38. Maes, N., Magdalena, J., Rottiers, S., De Gheldre, Y., *et al.* (2002). *J. Clin. Microbiol.*, **40**, 1514.

39. Jordan, J. A. and Durso, M. B. (2000). *J. Clin. Microbiol.*, **38**, 2574.

40. Kaplan, S. L. (1999). *Infect. Dis. Clin. North Am.*, **13**, 579.

41. Cohen, S. J. and Callaghan, R. P. (1961). *Br. Med. J.*, **2**, 677.

42. Holloway, Y., Boersma, W. G., Kuttschutter, H., and Snijder, J. A. (1992). *J. Clin. Microbiol.*, **30**, 517.

43. Read, S. J. and Kurtz, J. B. (1999). *J. Clin. Microbiol.*, **37**, 1352.

44. Bonington, A., Strang, J. I., Klapper, P. E., Hood, S. V., *et al.* (2000). *Tuber. Lung Dis.*, **80**, 191.

45. Corless, C. E., Guiver, M., Borrow, R., Edwards-Jones, V., *et al.* (2001). *J. Clin. Microbiol.*, **39**, 1553.

46. Magee, J. G., Freeman, R., and Barrett, A. (1998). *J. Med. Microbiol.*, **47**, 547.

47. von Graevenitz, A. and Amsterdam, D. (1992). *Clin. Microbiol. Rev.*, **5**, 36.

48. Gokal, R., Ramos, J. M., and Francis, D. A. (1982). *Lancet*, **ii**, 1388.

49. Pierratos, A. (1984). *Perit. Dialysis Bull.*, **4**, 2.

50. Prowant, B. F. and Nolph, K. D. (1981). In *Peritoneal dialysis*, p. 257. Churchill Livingstone, Edinburgh.

51. Ludlam, H., Dickens, A., Simpson, A., and Phillips, I. (1990). *J. Hosp. Infect.*, **16**, 263.

52. Catchpole, C. R., Macrae, F., Brown, J. D., Palmer, M., *et al.* (1997). *J. Clin. Pathol.*, **50**, 241.

53. Gould, I. M. and Casewell, M. W. (1986). *J. Hosp. Infect.*, **7**, 155.

54. Law, D., Freeman, R., and Tapson, J. (1987). *J. Clin. Pathol.*, **40**, 1267.

55. Beardsworth, S. F., Goldsmith, H. J., and Whitfield, E. (1983). *Lancet*, **i**, 348.

56. Spencer, R. C. and Fenton, D. A. (1984). *J. Hosp. Infect.*, **5**, 233.

57. Bourbeau, P., Riley, J., Heiter, B. J., Master, R., *et al.* (1998). *J. Clin. Microbiol.*, **36**, 3273.

58. Ward, J., Cohen, A. S., and Bauer, W. (1960). *Arthritis Rheum.*, **3**, 522.

Chapter 3

Bacteriology of the respiratory tract

Steve O'Hara and J. Andrew Lowes
Health Protection Agency Laboratory, General Hospital,
Southampton SO9 4XY, UK.

Grace Smith
Birmingham Laboratory, Health Protection Agency, Birmingham
Heartlands Hospital, Birmingham B5 5SS, UK.

1 Introduction

The isolation and detection of potential pathogens of the respiratory tract in disease is often complicated by the presence of commensal flora in the upper tract. Unless specialized specimen collection techniques are used most respiratory tract specimens sent to a diagnostic laboratory are contaminated with commensal flora. Reporting of all isolates present with their antibiotic sensitivities is inappropriate and may be misleading. Microscopy and cultural findings must be interpreted taking into account the quality of the specimen, the expected commensal flora of a given site through which the specimen was collected, the relative amounts of potential pathogens, and the clinical history of the patient including antimicrobial treatment.

2 Upper respiratory tract

2.1 The nose

The commonest bacterial lesion of the anterior nares is a boil and microbiological sampling of this is rarely necessary. Swabs from the anterior nares are most often taken to detect carriage of certain organisms, often for control of infection purposes, such as:

(a) Methicillin-resistant *Staphylococcus aureus* (MRSA) when it has been detected in a patient or group of patients.

(b) *S. aureus* in a patient or family suffering from repeated staphylococcal infections, or when there is a clustering of staphylococcal wound infections.

(c) β-haemolytic streptococcus, Lancefield group A, when there is an outbreak of infection, for example on a maternity unit. In the case of Lancefield group A throat swabs will also be taken.

(d) *Corynebacterium diphtheriae* when it has been isolated from a throat or other swab from a patient. In these circumstances it is necessary to swab an individual patient with disease and individuals who have had close contact with the patient.

Nasal swabs are occasionally included in surveillance screens performed in special 'at risk' groups, such as the immunocompromised, but rarely contribute to patient management. The value of MRSA screening arouses much debate.

A number of international studies have shown that screening to ascertain possible sources and spread may aid in the control of MRSA spread (1). The sensitivity of detection of MRSA carriage during screening depends on many factors, particularly the laboratory methods used to detect MRSA. Culture techniques may involve the use of a salt enrichment broth or direct plating of samples on to a solid culture medium. Broth enrichment allows detection of small numbers of MRSA enhancing the sensitivity of detection (1) but has the disadvantage of requiring an extra 24 hours incubation. Whether inoculated directly or following broth enrichment the choice of solid culture medium is critical to the rapid and reliable detection of 'presumptive MRSA'. Molecular techniques which detect the presence of the *mecA* gene may offer some hope for the future but culture methods are, and are likely to remain the mainstay of MRSA screening in most routine diagnostic laboratories.

Protocol 1 gives the methods of screening for carriage of MRSA. For the method of phage typing of staphylococci, see Chapter 11.

Protocol 1

Method of screening for nasal carriage of methicillin-resistant S. *aureus*

Equipment and reagents

- Cotton bud swab
- Blood agar plate
- Commercial agglutinating kit
- Selective medium
- 7% NaCl nutrient broth
- Selective agar

Method

1 Using a cotton bud swab collect a sample by rubbing the swab against the anterior nares, rotating the swab as this is done.

2 Plate out the swab on to an appropriate selective medium, such as mannitol salt agar (MSA)[a] containing 2 mg/litre oxacillin.

3 Where increased sensitivity is required, after inoculating the plates place the swab into 7% NaCl nutrient broth.

4 Incubate for 18–24 h at 30 °C. Subculture the enrichment broth on to an appropriate selective agar and incubate at 30 °C for a further 24 h.

5 Incubate the enrichment broth for 18–24 h at 37 °C and subculture on to blood agar plate, incubating this for 18–24 h and 48 h at 37 °C.

6 Examine plates and test presumptive staphylococcal colonies using a rapid screening test such as commercial agglutinating kits. Confirm presumptive MRSA colonies with a tube-coagulase or DNase test (see Chapter 5).

7 Test colonies for methicillin sensitivity (see Chapter 7).

[a] *S. aureus* colonies on MSA are bright yellow on the pink medium because of the fermentation of mannitol.

2.2 The nasopharynx

2.2.1 Collection of specimens

Three types of specimen are taken from the nasopharynx.

(a) Post-nasal swabs obtained by inserting a cotton wool swab through the mouth to the posterior wall, behind the uvula, and rubbing the swab against posterior wall. This is often used for assessing carriage of meningococci for which the swab should be plated on to a selective medium used *for Neisseria gonorrhoeae* (see Chapter 4). For the identification of neisseria, including meningo-cocci, see Chapter 4. Tests include a Gram stain, oxidase test, carbohydrate utilization, and an agglutination test to exclude *N. gonorrhoeae*.

(b) Pernasal swabs are used for the isolation of *Bordetella pertussis* the cause of whooping cough (see Figure 1). The specimen should be plated out immedi-ately although charcoal containing transport media improves the organisms short-term viability.

(c) Nasopharyngeal aspirates, which are obtained via the nose using a fine-bore catheter attached to a sputum trap, to which suction is applied. These are usually used for the diagnosis of viral infections such as those caused by the respiratory syncytial viruses, but can also be used for isolation of *Bordetella* spp.

2.2.2 Laboratory diagnosis of *B. pertussis* and *B. parapertussis*

The diagnosis of whooping cough is usually made clinically. Negative bacteri-ology, particularly from a specimen taken late in the illness, does not exclude the diagnosis. The best chance of isolating *B. pertussis* or *B. parapertussis* is during the early catarrhal stage of the illness. Traditionally, the culture medium used

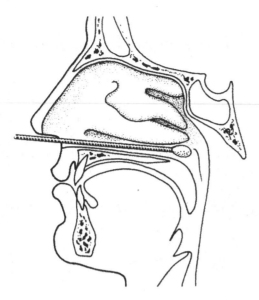

Figure 1 Collection of pernasal swab for isolation of *Bordetella* spp. Guide the swab on a flexible wire horizontally to the back of the nose. If obstruction is encountered, withdraw the swab and reinsert through the other nostril.

was Bordet–Gengou or a modification of it. Plates have a limited shelf-life (about five days) and so the medium may be impractical for laboratories handling only small numbers of specimens or where media is not prepared on site. For practical reasons most laboratories now use charcoal cephalexin blood agar which has a shelf-life of about six weeks. The method for culture and identification of *B. pertussis* or *B. parapertussis* is given in Protocol 2. There are three types of *B. pertussis* that can cause human disease: 1,2, 1,3 and 1,2,3. Presumptive isolates or paired sera for serodiagnosis should be referred to a reference laboratory. PCR methods are now used at reference laboratories, offering speed and higher sensitivity over culture, and are particularly useful for diagnosis of infection in infants (2). For those in older age groups with prolonged cough (two to three weeks) serology is particularly useful (3). Disc sensitivity testing is not performed routinely because slow growth of the organisms makes it difficult to perform accurately. Erythromycin and co-trimoxazole may be used to decrease the infectivity of clinical cases and for prophylaxis of unimmunized contacts.

Protocol 2

Method for culture and identification of *B. pertussis* or *B. parapertussis*

Equipment and reagents

- Charcoal cephalexin blood agar plates
- *B. pertussis* and *B. parapertussis* antisera (Division of Microbiological Reagents and Quality Control, PHLS)
- Gram stain
- Saline

Method

1 Plate the swab on to charcoal cephalexin blood agar, streaking out the first two quadrants with a swab and the later quadrants with a loop.[a]

2 Incubate in a moist atmosphere (e.g. inside pierced plastic bag) at 35–37 °C in air.

3 Examine the plates for characteristic pearly colonies after 48 h and then daily for a total of five days.

4 Gram stain suspicious oxidase positive 'pearly' colonies (round, smooth, shiny, and domed) and examine under the microscope.

5 Further identify small Gram-negative rods or coccobacilli by making agglutination reactions as follows:

   (a) Place a drop of saline on a microscope slide.

   (b) Pick a colony from the plate with a wire loop and emulsify it in a drop of saline to produce a cloudy suspension. Then add a drop of appropriate antiserum. Mix well and look for clumping (agglutination).[b,c]

[a] This is advised for improved sensitivity given the reduced surface area of the pernasal swab compared with a standard rigid swab.

[b] Agglutination with one specific antiserum and no agglutination with saline indicates a positive result.

[c] Occasionally auto-agglutination may occur or equivocal reactions may be seen. Subculturing on to antibiotic-free media may be helpful and encourage strains to become smooth. Growth on nutrient agar may help in differentiating B. parapertussis from B. pertussis which does not grow on nutrient agar.

2.3 The throat

Infections of the throat may be bacterial or, more commonly, viral in aetiology. The commonest bacterial cause is Lancefield group A haemolytic streptococcus (S. pyogenes), although groups C and G can also cause pharyngitis. β-haemolytic streptococci will grow readily on blood agar but their presence may be masked by oral commensal flora. Detection can be enhanced by culturing under anaerobic conditions using 48 h rather than 24 h incubation and by the use of selective media (e.g. gentian violet, nalidixic acid, or colistin oxolinic acid blood agars) (see Chapter 11).

Other bacterial pathogens of the throat include C. diphtheriae, C. ulcerans, and Arcanobacterium haemolyticum. Corynebacteria are Gram-positive, catalase positive bacilli which can be detected by their ability to convert tellurite to tellurium (C. diphtheriae) producing black or grey/black colonies on Hoyles tellurite agar. Only C. diphtheriae and C. ulcerans produce diphtheria exotoxin giving rise to diphtheria, or a diphtheria-like illness. Non-toxigenic C. diphtheriae strains may cause severe or recurrent sore throats.

Table 1 Choice of media for culture of throat swabs

Medium	Organism	Atmosphere	Length of incubation
Blood agar (selective/ non-selective)	β-haemolytic streptococci *Arcanobacterium haemolyticum* *C. diphtheriae, C. ulcerans*	Anaerobic	24–48 h
Tellurite		Aerobic	24–48 h

Arcanobacterium haemolyticum (previously *C. haemolyticum*) has been implicated as the cause of recurrent sore throats, particularly in young adults. The organism looks like a haemolytic streptococcus on blood agar but is a catalase negative, Gram-positive rod which leaves a small indentation in the media when the colony is moved. All β-haemolytic colonies isolated from throat swabs which do not agglutinate with Lancefields grouping antisera should be Gram stained to rule out the presence of this organism.

Haemophilus influenzae Pitman type b is a cause of acute epiglottitis. There is usually a concomitant bacteraemia and blood cultures should also be taken. For identification of *Haemophilus influenzae*, see Section 3.2.4.

Neisseria gonorrhoeae may be found in the throat. Usually the patient is asymptomatic but pharyngitis can occur. Screening of throat swabs for gonococci is best confined to specimens from a genitourinary medicine clinic, unless specifically requested by the clinician. For methodology see Chapter 4.

2.3.1 Specimen collection and culture of throat swabs

Throat swabs are collected as follows:

(a) Take a cotton wool swab and, depressing the tongue with a spatula, direct the swab to the back of the throat with the other hand and swab the tonsillar area on both sides, rotating the swab as this is done.

(b) Place the swab in bacterial transport medium if it is not be to plated out immediately. Choice of media for routine culture of throat swabs is given in Table 1.

The methods for culture of throat swabs for β-haemolytic streptococci and *C. diphtheriae* are given in Protocols 3 and 4, respectively.

Protocol 3

Culture and identification of β-haemolytic streptococci

Equipment and reagents

- Throat swab
- Blood agar plate
- Selective medium

Method

1 Inoculate a blood agar plate and selective medium, if chosen, with the throat swab ensuring all parts of the swab tip touch the media by rotating the swab as this is done.

2 Incubate anaerobically overnight. A further 24 h incubation gives a slightly higher yield and may be appropriate in some circumstances (e.g. recurrent pharyngitis).

3 Look for colonies surrounded by complete clearing of the blood agar (i.e. β-haemolytic). β-haemolytic streptococci are catalase negative, Gram-positive cocci often occurring in chains.

4 If there is sufficient growth, perform direct grouping by latex agglutination (see Chapter 5) at this stage, otherwise pick a single colony and spread out over a fresh blood agar plate.

5 Perform a sensitivity test as described in (Chapter 7), including penicillin, erythromycin, and tetracycline. Incubate this plate and the subculture plate aerobically.

6 Read and report penicillin and erythromycin sensitivity results.[a]

[a] Tetracycline should not be reported for children and pregnant women.

There are three main methods of testing for the exotoxin of *C. diphtheriae*: guinea pig inoculation, the Elek plate, and PCR directed at the A subunit of the *tox* gene, the structural gene for diphtheria toxin. The first and third are performed only by reference laboratories in the UK and it is becoming increasingly difficult to justify Elek testing in routine diagnostic laboratories. Laboratory-acquired *C. diphtheriae* is a rare but potentially serious infection. Laboratories continuing to perform Elek test should perform a risk assessment to determine whether continuing proficiency in the performance and interpretation of tests for toxin production, which requires periodic handling of known toxigenic strains, is justified when specialized reference services may be able to offer a faster, quality assured, service.

Generally, most diagnostic laboratories perform four provisional tests: catalase, urease, pyrazinamidase, and nitrate reduction (Table 2) in addition to colonial morphology and the Gram stain for a presumptive identification of *C. diphtheriae* within four hours. If *C. diphtheriae* or *C. ulcerans* is suspected a reference laboratory should be involved immediately. PCR is rapid and can be completed within three to four hours of strains being received within a reference facility. Not all strains of *C. diphtheriae* produce toxin, and laboratory efforts should be directed towards detecting toxin-producing organisms in the shortest possible time.

A throat swab is the normal specimen received in a laboratory, but specimens from the nose, pharynx, or larynx may be taken. Nose and throat swabs are sent from contacts in an outbreak. Cutaneous diphtheria occurs, especially in the tropics.

Protocol 4

Culture and identification of *Corynebacterium diphtheriae*

Equipment and reagents

- Swab
- Blood agar and tellurite medium
- Gram stain
- Commercial identification test strips

Method

1. Plate out the swab on to blood agar (to check quality of specimen collection) and tellurite medium and incubate overnight aerobically.

2. Examine plates and Gram stain any black or grey/black colonies on the tellurite medium. Re-incubate negative plates for a further 24 h.[a,b]

3. Suspect colonies should be tested for catalase, urease,[c] pyrazinamidase activity, and nitrate reduction. Many of these tests are now available on commercial identification strips and these should be used according to the manufacturer's instructions.

[a] Coryenebacteria are Gram-positive, pleomorphic rods and are often arranged in pairs giving a 'V' or Chinese lettering formation.

[b] All work on suspected *C. diphtheriae* isolates which is likely to generate aerosols must be performed in a Class 1 safety cabinet.

[c] Urea slopes are generally safer than urea broths.

Those responsible for Communicable Disease Control should be informed immediately of any presumptive identification of *C. diphtheriae* and the culture referred immediately to a reference facility for toxin testing, confirmation of identification, and sensitivity testing.

2.3.2 Identification of organisms causing Vincent's angina

Vincent's angina is an uncommon bacterial infection affecting the mouth as well as the throat. It is a rapidly spreading, indurated cellulitis without abscess formation or lymphatic involvement, which begins in the floor of the mouth, and involves the submandibular and sublingual spaces bilaterally. The infection is caused by spirochaetes (*Borrelia vincenti*) and anaerobic fusiforms, is characterized

Table 2 Presumptive identification of *Corynebacterium diphtheriae*

	Catalase	Urease	Pyrazinamidase	Nitrate
C. diphtheriae	+	−	−	+
Biotype *C. belfanti*	+	−	−	−
C. ulcerans	+	+	−	−

by ulceration of the pharynx or gums, and occurs in adults with poor mouth hygiene or serious systemic disease. Identification is made as follows:

(a) Make a smear from a lesion on a microscope slide and stain for 2 min with carbol fuchsin or neutral red.

(b) Examine the slide under the microscope and look for large numbers of fusiforms, red tightly coiled spirochaetes, and many pus cells.

2.4 The ear

Ear swabs are amongst the least rewarding specimens microbiologically. This is partly because patients are often treated with numerous courses of systemic and local antibiotics before the swab is taken, making it impossible to interpret the results because of the growth of organisms which would normally be considered secondary colonizers. Ear infections fall into three categories: those of the outer ear (otitis externa), those of the middle ear (otitis media), and those of the mastoid. In practice in the laboratory, all these specimens are handled in much the same way, often because the category is not obvious on the request form.

2.4.1 Specimens for otitis externa

The following organisms may be pathogens in acute and chronic otitis externa: β-haemolytic streptococci, *Staphylococcus aureus*, and *Pseudomonas aeruginosa*. The last is particularly important in malignant otitis externa, an invasive and necrotizing infection which may be fatal if not treated properly with antibiotics and sometimes surgery as well. It occurs usually in elderly diabetic patients. Milder infections are seen in swimmers, divers, and users of whirlpool spas. The role of coliforms in chronic otitis externa is not at all clear, as they are usually present as secondary colonizers, particularly after antibiotics have been given. Otomycosis, commonly caused by *Apsergillus niger*, result in the characteristic 'wet newspaper' appearance inside the auditory canal. A method for culture of ear swabs is given in Protocol 5. Otitis externa or dermatitis of the outer ear may respond to local toilet and control of inflammation with topical steroids.

2.4.2 Specimens from the middle ear and mastoid space following mastoidectomy

Middle ear contents are only accessible in the event of spontaneous perforation of the ear-drum or myringotomy. Rarely, middle ear fluid may be aspirated through the ear-drum by tympanocentesis. In the absence of microbiological specimens, as is usually the case in acute otitis media, antibiotics are given on the basis of a knowledge of the common pathogens, which include *Streptococcus pneumoniae*, *Haemophilus influenzae*, *Staphylococcus aureus*, and less commonly β-haemolytic streptococci and *Branhamella catarrhalis*. The management of the chronically discharging ear can be a difficult problem requiring local toilet, antibiotics, or surgery.

Protocol 5

Method for culture of ear swabs

Equipment and reagents

- Suitable selective agar plates
- Swab

Method

1. Inoculate a chocolate agar, blood agar, CLED plate, and a selective anaerobic (e.g. neomycin 75 mg/litre) and non-selective (e.g. fastidious anaerobe agar) with the swab and incubate at 37 °C aerobically overnight.[a]

2. Incubate the chocolate agar plate in CO_2, and the blood agar and CLED agar in air or CO_2. Examine the plates at 24 h and 48 h. Leave the anaerobic cultures undisturbed and examine at 48 h.

3. Identify the colonies resembling β-haemolytic streptococci (Protocol 3), pneumococci (Protocol 8), haemophili (Protocol 9), staphylococci (Chapter 5), and branhamellae (Chapter 4).[b]

4. Perform sensitivity tests as described in Chapter 7.[c]

5. Report the organisms grown and their relative amounts.[d]

[a] A Sabouraud plate may be inoculated for yeasts and moulds, although many will appear on a blood agar plate re-incubated for 24 h.

[b] It may not be necessary to identify coliforms, pseudomonads, and anaerobes unless the clinical information suggests that these may be important.

[c] Topical sensitivities are often performed on all ear specimens, with antibiotics being chosen which are available as ear drops or ointments, e.g. chloramphenicol, tetracycline (broad spectrum antibiotic but not appropriate for *Pseudomonas* spp.), gentamicin, polymyxin (suitable for *Pseudomonas* spp.), neomycin (suitable for staphylococci), and bacitracin (suitable for some streptococci and staphylococci). It is sometimes prudent to perform topical sensitivities on coliforms but to withhold this information from the clinician unless it is obviously of relevance.

[d] Sensitivities of the organisms to systemic antibiotics are required for acute otitis media. For chronic infections topicals are frequently used (although aural toilet and microscopic examination of the ear-drum if the discharge recurs is often more appropriate). The exact choice of topicals reported is best agreed locally after discussion with ENT surgeons, particularly as patterns of usage vary considerably. If organisms such as β-haemolytic streptococci, pneumococci, *H. influenzae* are cultured from an ear with evidence of acute inflammation, systemic antibiotics should be used.

2.5 The maxillary sinuses

Nose swabs are unsuitable for the investigation of sinus infections. Maxillary antrum wash-out specimens are sometimes received and should be centrifuged, Gram stained, and cultured as for middle ear specimens. Commonly isolated pathogens are pneumococci, *H. influenzae*, *S. aureus*, *B. catarrhalis*, anaerobes, and an increasing number of fungal species.

3 Lower respiratory tract (LRT)

3.1 Specimen collection

3.1.1 Non-invasive methods

Examination of expectorated sputum is the only non-invasive method of sampling lower respiratory tract secretions in disease. It is the sample most commonly sent to the laboratory but it is most important that the quality is good. Sputum should be collected under supervision before starting or changing antibiotics, and ideally with the help of a physiotherapist. Patients with exacerbations of chronic obstructive airways disease with excessive secretion of mucus can usually produce a sputum sample representative of lower respiratory tract secretions. Patients presenting in the early stages of pneumonia may not be able to produce a sputum sample and blood cultures should be taken from these patients.

3.1.2 Invasive methods

Transtracheal aspiration has been advocated in the USA but is rarely performed in the UK. Although often helpful in establishing a microbiological diagnosis, effective clinical management is usually possible without this investigation, which may have serious complications in unskilled hands. The method involves inserting a cannula through the cricothyroid membrane into the trachea bypassing the upper respiratory tract. Research comparing the results of microscopy and semi-quantitative culture of transtracheal aspirates and sputum collected at the same time has allowed the development of interpretative criteria for potentially contaminated sputum microscopy and culture (4).

Biopsies, brushings, and lavage specimens taken during bronchoscopy are usually contaminated by upper respiratory secretions carried into the lower tract by the bronchoscope. Local anaesthetic solutions are used to desensitize the airways and may constitute a large proportion of any aspirate. A bronchial brush enclosed within telescoping inner and outer catheters, the inner of which is plugged, is available for semi-quantitative culture of bronchial secretions. This technique largely overcomes the problems of contamination with upper respiratory secretions if used by a skilled operator (MediTech contamination-free microbiology specimen brush BFW 1.07090, KeyMed UK, Ltd.).

Ventilator-associated infection of the lower respiratory tract is the commonest infective complication occurring in intubated patients in critical care units. Endotracheal aspirates may be taken to detect likely causative pathogens in patients who are deteriorating with features consistent with a ventilator associated LRTI. They may also be taken as part of a surveillance programme to detect colonization by potential pathogens such as *Staph. aureus* (including MRSA), *Ps. aeruginosa*, coliforms, *Acinetobacter* spp., and *Stenotrophomonas maltophilia*, or in anticipation of clinically apparent infections so that treatment can be directed to include potential pathogens known to be colonizing the lower airways.

The investigation of ventilator-associated lower respiratory tract infections has been the subject of a great deal of work and controversy, leading to a wide range of methods of collecting, processing, and interpreting results from specimens from the lower airways. Currently there is a good case for using the simplest and least expensive techniques (5).

3.2 Routine microscopy and culture

Some laboratories will discard specimens which are mucoid on naked eye examination, but this may be unreliable and those for examination for mycobacteria should be processed (6). Most laboratories discard specimens which appear to be only saliva and request a further sample. There is great variation in the method of processing sputum and, because there is no clear consensus, the main methods are detailed below. Specimens should be processed as soon as possible after collection or refrigerated and processed later on the same day. All manipulations on lower respiratory tract specimens, because of the possibility of occult tuberculosis, should be performed in a Class 1 exhaust protective cabinet ideally in a containment level 3 laboratory.

3.2.1 Specimen preparation

Homogenization to reduce within-specimen sampling error is widely practised but some laboratories feel the extra labour is unjustified and it is better to pick purulent flecks of sputum. Both methods are given below. A method using N-acetyl-L-cysteine for homogenization is an alternative to the Sputasol method.

i. Homogenization
    (a) Add an equal volume of Sputasol (Oxoid Ltd.) at working dilution to the specimen and mix.
    (b) Shake the mixture well and place in a 37 °C water-bath. Incubate with periodic shaking until liquefaction is complete.
    (c) Plate out sample (Protocol 7) and make a thin smear on a microscope slide.
ii. Direct sampling
    (a) Select a purulent fleck and tease out in sputum pot with a sterile swab.
    (b) Inoculate plates (Protocol 7) and make a thin smear on a microscope slide.

3.2.2 Microscopy

A method for microscopy of sputum is given in Protocol 6. Comparisons have been made between cultures of transtracheal aspirates and expectorated sputum, and on the basis of these it has been suggested that specimens with many squamous epithelial cells are heavily contaminated by oropharyngeal secretions.

Protocol 6

Method for microscopy of sputum

Equipment

- Microscope
- Microscope slides

Method

1 Make a thin film on a microscope slide, allow to dry in air, and heat-fix on an electric hot plate in a Class 1 cabinet before staining by Gram's method (see Appendix I).

2 Examine the film using ×100 magnification (×10 eyepiece, ×10 objective). Assess the number of squamous epithelial cells and polymorphonuclear leukocytes per low power field in at least five representative fields and then take the average.

3 Record the quantity of squamous epithelial cells and polymorphs as follows: <10 = +/−, 10 − 25 = +, >25 = ++.

4 Examine with high power oil immersion objective and concentrating on purulent areas of the slide. Report the abundance and different morphological types of organisms seen (i.e. +/−, +, ++, etc.).

Criteria such as >25 or >10 squamous epithelial cells per low power field of a film prepared from neat sputum have been proposed as a basis for discarding such specimens without culture although not for mycobacterial examination (7, 8). It has been argued that if microscopic criteria are to be used for rejection of specimens, then those with <25 leukocytes per low power field should be discarded because they are unrepresentative of infected parts of the lower respiratory tract (9). However, there should be caution in introducing such a policy because specimens from some patients, such as those with neutropaenia, may not have pus cells and it is not always possible to obtain further specimens in a hurry from a severely ill patient. In order for this kind of policy to be effective, there needs to be good collaboration between clinicians and microbiologists. An alternative method using only the proportions of pus cells to epithelial cells in the sample rather than concentration and proportions together has been described to overcome the problem associated with the thickness of the Gram film examined.

3.2.3 Specimen culture

After preparation of the sample either by homogenization or direct sampling of purulent material (Section 3.2.1), the specimen is plated out on appropriate media:

(a) Blood agar for pneumococci, moraxella, staphylococci, and other Gram-negative bacteria.

(b) Chocolate agar for *H. influenzae*.

Some laboratories will prefer to supplement the agar above with antibiotics, to increase the selectivity of culture, e.g. chocolate agar with 100–300 mg/litre bacitracin for *H. influenzae*. Some laboratories use MacConkey agar to facilitate the recognition of Enterobacteriaceae, rare but important causes of pneumonia, most commonly hospital-acquired. Methods for sputum culture, which can also be used for endotracheal aspirates, are given in Protocol 7. Transtracheal aspirates can be cultured similarly, but anaerobic culture should be performed as well. Any anaerobes grown will usually be relevant because contamination with upper respiratory tract anaerobes is avoided, unless the catheter is dislodged into the oropharynx (which can happen when coughing is induced).

Semi-quantitative culture results have been used as one measure of response to treatment of patients with chronic suppurative chest infections (such as cystic fibrosis), along with clinical parameters like temperature, weight gain, and decrease in sputum volume. This is particularly relevant when eradication of infection is not a realistic objective, but a decrease in the microbial load may slow further deterioration of lung function.

3.2.4 Recognition and identification of isolates

The main pathogens in lower respiratory tract infections are *Streptococcus pneumoniae*, *Haemophilus influenzae*, *Moraxella catarrhalis*, and rarely *S. aureus*. Members of the Enterobacteriaceae, notably *Klebsiella pneumoniae* and also *Pseudomonas aeruginosa*, can be respiratory pathogens. The recognition and identification of these is dealt with in Chapter 6. The recognition and identification of *S. aureus* is dealt with in Chapter 5 and thus the other three will be described here.

Streptococcus pneumoniae cultured on blood agar in 5% CO_2 overnight produces 0.5 mm round translucent or mucoid colonies with an entire edge, which are initially domed but later partially collapse (due to autolysis) to form the characteristic draughtsman-shaped colony, surrounded by a zone of alpha-haemolysis (greening of the agar surrounding the colony). Some strains are very mucoid, particularly capsular serotype 3. On microscopy Gram-positive lanceolate diplococci are seen which may be capsulated. The identity of such colonies is confirmed by an optochin sensitivity or a bile solubility test, as shown in Protocol 8.

Protocol 7

Methods for sputum culture

Equipment and reagents

- Sterile loop
- Optochin identification disc
- Bacitracin disc
- Appropriate media
- Blood agar and chocolate blood agar plates
- Phosphate-buffered saline

A. General method

1   Inoculate appropriate media with a purulent portion of sputum using a swab or with a sterile standard loopful of homogenate (see Section 3.2.1). Using a sterile loop,

streak out in three further areas, using a previously uncontaminated part of the loop to streak into each area, and using the whole plate in a uniform manner to allow relatively standardized reporting.

2 Place an optochin identification disc (which causes autolysis of pneumococci and aids in their identification) at the junction of the initial inoculum and the first set of streaks on the blood agar plate.

3 Similarly place a bacitracin disc (8 U) on the surface of a chocolate blood agar plate (if a selective medium for haemophilus is not used) to inhibit the growth of Gram-positive organisms.

4 Incubate the plates overnight in CO_2. Re-incubate if there is no growth. Note the quantity of suspect colonies, i.e. pneumococci, haemophili, and moraxella.

B. Semi-quantitative method[a]

1 Plate out a 10 μl loopful (standard loop) of homogenized sputum specimen on one-half of a blood agar and chocolate blood agar plate. Mix another 10 μl with 10 ml of phosphate-buffered saline. Mix on a vortex mixer and plate out a 10 μl loopful on the other half of each plate.

2 Incubate overnight in CO_2, and read the plate the next day. Re-incubate for a further 24 h and re-examine the next day if no growth has occurred, the patient is on antibiotics, or organisms seen on the Gram film have not grown.

3 500 colonies from the 10 μl loopful of homogenate (i.e. initial dilution) correspond to 10^5 cfu/ml in the original specimen. 500 colonies from the 10 μl of diluted homogenate corresponds to 10^2 cfu/ml in the original specimen.

4 Note quantity of suspect pathogens on the report form. (See Section 3.26)

[a] This is also appropriate for specimens collected using a microbiological specimen brush at bronchoscopy (Section 3.1.2).

Haemophilus spp. on Gram staining are pleomorphic fine Gram-negative rods. They have requirements for growth, called X (haemin) and V factors (NAD). Depending on the species, the requirement is for one or other of these factors or both, as in H. influenzae. X factor is contained in blood and V factor is released from red cells when blood is heated in the production of chocolate agar. V factor is also produced by S. aureus.

Haemophilus spp. may be provisionally identified by enhanced growth on chocolate blood agar. It is, however, a variable phenomenon depending upon the blood agar used. H. influenzae on chocolate blood agar after 24 h incubation forms 1–2 mm greyish smooth semi-opaque flat convex round colonies with an entire edge and a characteristic smell.

Protocol 8

Methods for the identification of *Streptococcus pneumoniae*[a]

Equipment and reagents

- Optochin identification disc
- Blood agar plate
- Sodium deoxycholate

A. Optochin sensitivity test

1 If a disc method of sensitivity testing for pneumococci is being used, place an optochin identification disc on the sensitivity plate.

2 Incubate in CO_2.

3 A zone of growth inhibition of diameter >16 mm confirms the identification of a pneumococcus; strains with smaller zones should only be identified as pneumococci if bile soluble.

B. Rapid bile solubility test for presumptive identification

1 Touch a loop charged with 10% solution of sodium deoxycholate pH 7.0 on to a suspect colony on a blood agar plate.

2 Incubate the plate at 37 °C for 15 min.

3 Observe lysis of the colony if it is a pneumococcus, leaving a zone of alpha-haemolysis at the site of the colony.

[a] For these tests use *S. pneumoniae* as a positive control and *S. faecalis* as a negative control.

Protocol 9

Method for identification of *Haemophilus* spp.[a]

Equipment and reagents

- Nutrient agar plate
- Discs containing X factor and V factor

Method

1 Inoculate evenly one or two colonies of the strain to be identified with a swab over half the surface of a plate of a nutrient agar plate, turn through 90°, inoculate over half the plate again until the whole plate is covered.

2 Apply discs containing X factor alone, V factor alone, and X and V factor together to the surface, about 1 cm in from the edge, and equally spaced at 4, 8, and 12 o'clock.

Protocol 9 continued

3 Incubate overnight at 37 °C in CO_2, for up to 48 h if necessary.

4 Record the growth around the discs. *H. influenzae* is both X- and V-dependent and grows only around the combined XV disc. *Haemophilus* spp. growing around the combined XV disc and the V disc require V factor and include *H. parainfluenzae*.

[a] Commercial strips are now available.

Confirmation of identity of *Haemophilus* spp. in the routine laboratory is most usually performed by testing for X and V factor dependence. The method is given in Protocol 9.

Nutrient agar base used for identifying *Haemophilus* spp. varies in its X and V content and also the growth factors can diffuse widely in the agar which can cause erroneous results, for instance *H. influenzae* may be misidentified as *H. parainfluenzae*. The latter problem can be overcome partially by cutting ditches in the agar between the discs, and the former by quality controlling each batch of medium and sets of discs used with known strains. Tests for the lack of ability to utilize 6-aminolaevulinic acid for porphobilinogen synthesis (X factor dependence), and an absolute need for V factor tested by detecting growth around a V factor disc on blood agar chocolated by autoclaving to remove all V factor from the medium are recommended for definitive identification (10).

Moraxella catarrhalis is a Gram-negative diplococcus. Unlike *Neisseria* spp., it will grow on basal media such as nutrient agar. Colonies are non-haemolytic on blood agar, 0.5–1.0 mm diameter, grey, opaque, and smooth. Basic tests for confirmation that should be performed are Gram stain, oxidase, growth on nutrient agar at 35 °C, and a tributyrin test (butyrate esterase) (11), see Chapter 4.

3.2.5 Antimicrobial sensitivity testing

Direct (primary) sensitivity testing on sputum specimens is generally not recommended because it is difficult to control the inoculum.

The following scheme of sensitivity testing is suggested.

(a) *Streptococcus pneumoniae*: benzylpenicillin, ampicillin, erythromycin, cefotaxime, and tetracycline.

(b) *Haemophilus influenzae*: ampicillin, co-amoxiclav, trimethoprim, tetracycline, a fluoroquinolone, cefotaxime, and test for β-lactamase production by nitrocefin test or equivalent (see Chapter 7).

(c) *Moraxella catarrhalis*: ampicillin, erythromycin, tetracycline, a fluoroquinolone, and test for β-lactamase production by nitrocefin test or equivalent (see Chapter 7).

If more than one of these organisms are isolated from the same patient with chronic obstructive airways disease, it is sensible to perform and report the same sensitivities for each, testing additional agents if necessary.

Other organisms that may require sensitivity testing, although their isolation is not necessarily significant, are S. aureus, coliforms, and *Pseudomonas aeruginosa*. These may be tested for susceptibility to the following antimicrobials.

(a) Coliforms: cefuroxime, cefotaxime, gentamicin, ampicillin, and a fluoro-quinolone.

(b) *P. aeruginosa*: gentamicin, piperacillin-tazobactam, ceftazidime, and cipro-floxacin.

(c) *S. aureus* (see Chapter 5).

If it is decided to test for co-amoxiclav and a disc test is used, a low content disc (3 µg) should be selected, to detect *H. influenzae*, which will not respond to conventional doses of amoxycillin-clavulanate, but will appear falsely sensitive if a high content disc (10 or 25 µg) is used.

3.2.6 Interpretation and reporting

If media are inoculated and plated as described in Section 3.2.3, reporting for sputum specimens can be standardized as follows.

(a) Disregard growth of a potential pathogen in the first and second quadrants.

(b) Report growths of five or more colonies of potential pathogens in the third quadrant as +++.

(c) Report growths of five or more colonies of potential pathogens in the fourth quadrant as ++++. However, a flexible approach is essential, and on occasions low numbers of organisms may be reported. If the specimen was cultured semi-quantitatively, report all potential pathogens present in concentrations of 10^5 orgs/ml or greater and their approximate numbers per ml.

(d) Report no growth if there is no bacterial growth.

The main pathogens in non-intubated patients are *Streptococcus pneumoniae* and *H. influenzae*, and sensitivities of these should be reported if they are present in significant numbers. Growths of *S. aureus*, β-haemolytic streptococci (with their Lancefield group, see Chapter 5), coliforms, and *Pseudomonas aeruginosa* in 'significant' numbers may be reported. Predominant growths of *Moraxella catarrhalis*, if found in conjunction with intracellular Gram-negative diplococci in pus cells on microscopy, should be reported with antibiotic sensitivities. The significance of these isolates will vary and is more likely to be important if they are grown from uncontaminated specimens (see Section 3.2.2). Antibiotic sensitivities should be performed. Report all isolates of potential pathogens with appropriate sensitivities in intubated patients.

Fungi, such as *Aspergillus* spp. and *Candida* spp., may cause lower respiratory tract infections, almost always in immunocompromised or ventilated patients.

3.3 Special microscopy and culture

3.3.1 Culture of specimens from patients with cystic fibrosis

The major pathogens associated with pulmonary infection in cystic fibrosis are *S. aureus*, *Haemophilus influenzae*, *Pseudomonas aeruginosa* (particularly mucoid strains), and in late stages of the disease *Burkholderia cepacia*. *Aspergillus fumigatus*, atypical *Mycobacteria* species, and *Stenotrophomonas maltophilia* may also be recovered from the respiratory tract and play a role in disease.

The microbiological challenge of culturing respiratory specimens from cystic fibrosis patients arises from the difficulty of detecting the major respiratory pathogens amongst contaminating oropharyngeal flora, particularly *Ps. aeruginosa* masking the presence of *H. influenzae*. Most laboratories attempt to overcome these problems in one, or a combination of the following ways:

(a) Liquefaction and dilution of the sputum specimen to dilute out the presence of oropharyngeal flora leaving the respiratory pathogens which are normally present in higher numbers.

(b) The use of highly selective and differential culture media to suppress the growth of oropharyngeal flora enabling the detection and presumptive identification of respiratory pathogens. Suitable media are commercially available for the detection of *Pseudomonas aeruginosa*, *Burkholderia cepacia*, *S. aureus*, and *Haemophilus influenzae*.

All pathogens should be identified to species level and be accompanied by appropriate antimicrobial susceptibility test results that may assist organism identification as well as aiding treatment regimens. For example, *Burkholderia cepacia* is invariably resistant to colomycin whilst *Pseudomonas aeruginosa* is generally sensitive.

All isolates of *Pseudomonas aeruginosa* should be reported as 'mucoid' or 'non-mucoid' as alginate production, which leads to mucoid colonies, is an important virulence factor (12). It is important to report initial isolates of *P. aeruginosa* as eradication therapy may delay chronic colonisation by months or years. *B. cepacia* should be reported provisionally to allow appropriate infection control measures, and it should always be confirmed.

3.3.2 Microscopy and culture for mycobacterial infections

Diagnosis of pulmonary tuberculosis has important public health implications as well as affecting care of the individual patient. In the world-wide effort to control tuberculosis rapid detection of infectious cases—principally pulmonary tuberculosis—is recognized as a critical control point in management and prevention of spread. It is of great importance that diagnosis on the basis of clinical and radiological findings should be supported by a vigorous effort to isolate the causative organism using sensitive and rapid techniques. There have been important advances in laboratory methods for isolation, identification, and antibiotic susceptibility testing for mycobacteria in the last decade. American guidelines published by the Centre for Disease Control in 1993 (13) set criteria relating to turnaround time for all these elements.

1 A smear for detection of acid-fast bacilli should be performed within 24 hours of specimen collection.

2 Results of identification to the level of *Mycobacterium tuberculosis* complex should be available within 10–14 days.

3 Results of drug susceptibility testing to first-line antibiotics should be available within 30 days.

These criteria cannot be met without the employment of automated liquid-based culture techniques and sensitivity testing, which will be described below alongside conventional techniques.

Human tuberculosis is caused by *Mycobacterium tuberculosis* or, very infrequently, by *Mycobacterium bovis*. In addition, there are many species of mycobacteria which normally exist in the environment that occasionally cause disease in humans, particularly where there is pre-existing lung disease or severe immune suppression. These are referred to as atypical, opportunistic, or mycobacteria other than tubercle (MOTT) and include *Mycobacterium avium intra-acellulare* group, *Mycobacterium malmoense*, *Mycobacterium kansasii*, *Mycobacterium xenopi*. Infection with atypical mycobacteria may cause clinical confusion as microscopy of respiratory samples will be positive for acid-fast bacilli. Patients may be notified as cases of tuberculosis and commenced on conventional treatment, unless mycobacterial culture is performed to allow differentiation of species by identification and susceptibility testing. Although the proportion of drug-resistant tuberculosis cases appears to be stable in the UK at present, more than 1 in 20 patients has drug-resistant disease at diagnosis and more than 1 in 100 has multi-drug resistant disease. Efforts to minimize the emergence of drug resistance include rapid diagnosis and rapid identification of drug resistance as well as supervised treatment and the maintenance of comprehensive surveillance (14).

i. Mycobacterium avium intracellulare (MAI)

Pulmonary infection due to MAI usually occurs in association with existing lung disease—silicosis, chronic bronchitis, emphysema, healed tuberculosis, or bronchiectasis. MAI may also cause cervical lymphadenopathy in children and disseminated infection in patients with HIV/AIDS.

In non-sterile samples such as sputum samples, the isolation of MAI from a single sample is not definite evidence of infection. Two or more specimens of sputum or bronchial washings should be confirmed positive before a confident diagnosis can be made. Blood cultures should be taken in appropriate media for culture of mycobacteria from patients with HIV/AIDS who are pyrexial.

ii. Mycobacterium kansasii

Pulmonary infection, most often in patients with a pre-existing chronic lung disease or pneumoconiosis, is the most common form of disease caused by

M. kansasii. Consequently, miners, welders, sandblasters, and painters are at highest risk of development of disease. Symptoms are similar to TB, although generally milder, and dissemination is uncommon even in immunocompromised hosts. Diagnosis of *M. kansasii* infection is by AAFB smear and culture of sputum samples with at least two specimens of sputum or bronchial washings confirmed positive before a confident diagnosis is made.

iii. Mycobacterium malmoense

M. malmoense causes pulmonary disease in adult patients typically presenting with a chronic pulmonary infection with pre-existing pneumoconiosis. Diagnosis of *M. malmoense* infection is as for *M. kansasii*, although incubation times on conventional solid media may need to be as long as 12 weeks before colonies become visible.

iv. Mycobacterium xenopi

Most infections with this organism occur in males aged 45 years and over and resemble pulmonary TB. Diagnosis of *M. xenopi* infection is as for *M. malmoense* with incubation times on conventional media at 37 °C as long as 12 weeks. Incubating at its optimal temperature of 42–43 °C can reduce incubation times, but this is not always practical in a routine diagnostic laboratory.

v. Mycobacterium fortuitum, Mycobacterium chelonae

The lungs are normally the commonest site of colonization for both of these organisms. *M. chelonae* may contaminate tap-water and has been associated with false positive diagnoses and pseudo outbreaks involving flexible bronchoscopy. *M. fortuitum* or *M. chelonae* grow rapidly on conventional media.

vi. Safety

Mycobacterium tuberculosis is classed as a Category 3 organism. Considerable care is required when working with clinical material likely to contain mycobacteria, and specimens should be handled in containment level 3 accommodation. Every laboratory should issue clear instructions for the safe testing of specimens. Precautions should be taken, which include the following:

(a) All testing must be performed in an approved Class 1 safety cabinet in level 3 containment.

(b) Disposable loops should be used to avoid spluttering of aerosols created by flaming a loop.

(c) Bunsen burners should not be used, unless shielded because they disturb the pattern of air circulation through the cabinet.

(d) Sealed bucket centrifuges should be used and the sealed buckets containing the specimens opened inside the safety cabinet.

vii. Specimen collection

Sputum is the specimen most often sent from the respiratory tract for mycobacterial examination. Early morning specimens are the best because secretions which have pooled overnight in the bronchi are likely to yield the greatest number of bacteria. These techniques should be performed in negative pressure ventilated facilities whenever drug resistance is expected or where other patients may be immunocompromised. If the patient is unable to produce sputum, specimens may be collected by bronchoalveolar lavage using a bronchoscope. Pleural fluid, pleural biopsies, and tissue biopsies from the respiratory tract may also be obtained. Gastric aspirate, collected in the morning before breakfast on three consecutive days, is usually used for children who are unable to produce sputum. Urine is a useful non-invasive specimen for the investigation of miliary tuberculosis as well as urinary tract disease. The methods for preparation of specimens for microscopy is given in Protocol 10.

The microscopic examination of stained smears from samples for acid-fast bacilli (AFB) is still one of the most useful tests for the initial diagnosis of TB. Although direct microscopy is less sensitive and specific than culture, sensitivity is improved by using auramine–phenol instead of Ziehl–Neelsen. It is estimated that 5000-10 000 acid-fast bacilli/ml of sample are required for detection by microscopy, whereas culture may detect as few as 10 viable cells of *Mycobacterium* species.

Protocol 10

Preparation of specimens for microscopy for acid-fast bacilli (AFB)

Equipment and reagents

- Centrifuge
- Tissue grinder
- Hot plate
- Saline

Method

1 If the specimen is sputum, use a neat or homogenized sample (Section 3.2.1).[a]

2 If pleural fluid, centrifuge at 2000 g for 30 min and examine the deposit.[b]

3 If tissue, either homogenize tissues in sterile distilled water or saline with a sterile tissue grinder (Griffiths tube or preferably unbreakable alternative) or by agitating with glass beads over a vortex mixer.

4 Prepare smears in the usual fashion, heat-fix[c] on a hot plate, preferably inside the cabinet.

[a] Centrifugation at 3200 r.p.m. for 15 min and using the deposit to make the smear improves the quality and sensitivity of the smear.

[b] The container must be sealed. Do not allow fluid to swirl up to the top of the container. Wait before opening the specimen in a safety cabinet so that aerosolized particles may settle first.

[c] Heat fixing does not kill all *Mycobacterium* species. Slides should be handled carefully.

Slides may then be subjected to staining by the auramine or the Ziehl–Neelsen method (ZN—see Appendix I). Both utilize the fact that mycobacteria resist decolorization after staining with an arylmethane dye. Auramine staining is recommended for testing large numbers of specimens because a low power objective is used and this permits a larger field of the slide to be examined in the same period of time. Over-staining with Ziehl–Neelsen and examining under oil immersion is not recommended, as it is a less sensitive technique and so is unsuitable to confirm positive smears. The species cannot be determined reliably from the morphological appearance as seen on the examination of primary specimens. Positive control slides should be included for all methods.

The detection of single bacilli needs very careful consideration. Repeat smears should be prepared and additional specimens obtained if possible.

It should be noted that environmental mycobacteria may be present if a specimen container has been washed with tap-water or if tap-water is used to make up stains.

With carbol fuchsin-based stains, acid alcohol-fast bacilli (AAFB) appear red against a blue, turquoise, or green background, depending on the counterstain. Acid alcohol-fast bacilli seen should be reported with an index of quantitation. A variety of grading systems may be used. The requesting clinician should be made aware of positive smear results on new patients as should those responsible for public health control measures, including infection control teams, if the patient is in hospital or is a health care worker.

viii. Culture

When culturing for mycobacteria, it is necessary to minimize overgrowth by contaminants, as mycobacteria are slow growing. Contaminated specimens such as sputa require a digestion-decontamination step followed by concentration before culture to maximize the yield of mycobacteria. Non-contaminated specimens, such as pleural fluids, generally do not require a digestion-decontamination step, but may require concentration prior to culture. As there are several digestion-decontamination procedures available using sodium hydroxide, oxalic acid, or sulfuric acid the mildest procedure appropriate to the specimen should be employed. Contamination rates should be monitored within each laboratory. Rates below 2% indicate over-harsh decontamination whereas rates above 5% suggest inadequate decontamination. Both would reduce the sensitivity of the culture method.

ix. Culture media

The media most often used for mycobacterial work are egg-based, e.g. Löwenstein Jensen (LJ) for the Zaher and Marks' modification, acid egg medium (15) in which phosphate and malachite green concentrations have been changed. Penicillin may be added if the decontamination procedure has not been successful. Some mycobacteria can be inhibited by glycerol, and for M. bovis isolation, media should be formulated without glycerol but with added pyruvate. The media are poured as slopes in universal bottles with screw caps to prevent desiccation. A liquid medium (Kirshner's) is available but semi-automated and continuous automated mycobacterial liquid culture systems are more sensitive and rapid than conventional culture for *M. tuberculosis* and most significant atypical mycobacteria.

Nucleic acid amplification techniques have been developed for detecting *M. tuberculosis* in clinical specimens. Currently two commercial amplification methods are licensed by the American Food and Drugs Administration. Sensitivity is less than that for culture, on all tissues and specimens, and the methods should not be used to exclude the diagnosis of tuberculosis. Sensitivity and specificity is robust for smear-positive respiratory samples, is useful for rapid confirmation of suspected pulmonary tuberculosis, and is required to precede molecular tests for rifampicin resistance (16).

Semi-automated, and more recently continuous monitoring systems, using liquid culture have been developed specifically for the isolation of *Mycobacterium* species and are proving increasingly useful for all types of specimen. The driving force for the introduction of these systems arises from the Centers for Disease Control (CDC) criteria (13) for a modern mycobacteria service. The standard set by CDC is the detection and identification of all *M tuberculosis* within 14–21 days of specimen collection. With the hopes of molecular biology as the 'modern smear' yet to be realized (17) many diagnostic laboratories are turning to continuous automated mycobacterial liquid culture (CAMLiC) systems which have three essential elements:

(a) A suitable liquid medium (usually a variant of Middlebrook 7H9).

(b) A formalin-resistant incubation cabinet.

(c) A sensing system enclosed in the incubation cabinet which detects growth.

All the commercial systems currently available employ slightly different variations on the same theme. All are more sensitive than conventional culture with reduced time to detection, and the potential for rapid sensitivity testing, enabling laboratories which employ the technology and adopt new work patterns to achieve the CDC standard.

Protocol 11

Method of sputum culture for mycobacteria using conventional medium

Equipment and reagents

- Mechanical agitator
- 4% NaOH
- Acid egg slopes
- Pyruvate
- Ziehl–Neelsen stain

Method

1 Add an equal volume of 4% NaOH to the specimen and mix at least twice (or continuously on a mechanical agitator) for 20 min[a].

Protocol 11 continued

2 Inoculate 0.2 ml on to two acid egg slopes (4.5 ml of medium per slope) with and without pyruvate and incubate at 37 °C.

3 Examine all cultures weekly. Discard any overgrown with contaminants and set up repeat cultures if possible. Send a report to the clinician requesting further specimens if no clinical material was stored.

4 If there is a positive culture,[b] record whether growth occurs differentially on pyruvate- and non-pyruvate-containing media, the period of incubation, and pigmentation, if any.

5 Perform a Ziehl–Neelsen stain, noting if colonies are difficult to emulsify, which is characteristic of M. tuberculosis.[c]

6 If any acid-fast bacilli are demonstrated send out a report but do *not* specify M. tuberculosis, even if morphology, etc. is typical.[d]

7 Extend the incubation period if no growth is apparent at ten weeks but acid-fast bacilli were seen in the smear from the original specimen (M. *malmoense* may take up to 12 weeks to grow), or if the patient is being treated on clinical grounds for a mycobacterial infection.

8 Subculture any positive isolates on to neutral slopes and send cultures to the local reference laboratory, where molecular probes will be applied to identify cultures as 'M. tuberculosis complex' within one working day.

[a] Colonies of M. tuberculosis are not likely to be visible for two weeks and may take up to 10 weeks or so to appear. They are typically buff-coloured, dry, and may resemble breadcrumbs.

[b] M. tuberculosis typically are evenly stained bacilli, regular in length, and may be arranged as serpentine cords.

[c] It is important to notify all culture positive isolates by telephone and to enquire whether there are risk factors for drug resistance, such as previous treatment, probable drug-resistant source, or acquisition in an area of high incidence of drug resistance.

[d] It is important to avoid cross contamination between specimens by using individual, sterile aliquots of NaOH or other reagents, and disposable pipettes for each specimen.

All specimens, such as tissue, which are difficult to obtain, should be cultured by automated liquid techniques (CAMLiC), in addition to using conventional media, as sensitivity is improved and such specimens usually contain low numbers of mycobacteria.

Protocol 12

Method of culture for acid-fast bacilli of tissue, pleural fluid, swabs, and pus

Equipment and reagents

- See Protocol 13
- Neutral LJ slopes (with and without pyruvate)

Protocol 12 continued

Method

1 Take tissue and fluid specimens as prepared for microscopy, i.e. homogenized tissue or centrifuged deposit from a fluid. Immerse swabs in 5 ml of 2% NaOH in a universal container for 20 min and treat 'contaminated' pus specimens as for sputum.

2 Inoculate 0.2 ml of alkalinized specimens on to slopes (4.5 ml of medium per slope) as for sputum. Rub treated swabs over acid slopes ensuring a generous inoculum, as a volume of 0.2 ml is optimal to give correct neutralization.

3 If bacterial contamination is unlikely, as in fresh tissue and pleural fluids, inoculate a pair of neutral LJ slopes (with and without pyruvate) using approx. 0.2 ml.

4 If the specimen is large, store a small portion at −20 °C so that repeat cultures can be set up in the event of contamination of the original cultures.

5 Incubate all cultures as for sputum and examine in the same way (see Protocol 11).

The method for sputum culture is given in Protocol 11 and for other respiratory specimens in Protocol 12.

Due to the difficulty in performing identification and sensitivity tests on mycobacteria all isolates should be referred to designated reference laboratories. The identity of *M. tuberculosis* is confirmed by a lack of pigment production, failure to grow at 25 °C, and sensitivity to *p*-nitrobenzoic acid. DNA probes are used for species determination for *M. tuberculosis* complex which includes *M. tuberculosis* and *M. bovis*. Sensitivity testing for slow-growing organisms requires special methodology which has evolved differently in different countries. The method used in the UK is a modification of the resistance ratio method in which the 'mode' resistance of a number of wild strains is regularly determined. The behaviour of the test strain is then interpreted in relation to this mode. This has been validated by the correlation between *in vitro* results and *in vivo* therapeutic response. Molecular methods are used for rapid detection of mutations confirming rifampicin resistance, which is a good proxy for multiple drug resistance. Molecular methods are available for detecting resistance to other anti-tuberculous drugs but a substantial proportion of strains are not detected.

3.3.3 Special culture for actinomyces and nocardia

Actinomyces israelii may cause a chronic pulmonary infection which can present like malignancy or tuberculosis with cavitation. The diagnosis is often unsuspected until sinus formation occurs (see Chapter 5). *Nocardia asteroides* may also cause chronic pulmonary infection or, occasionally in immunocompromised patients, an acute infection with rapid dissemination to other organs. For a culture method, see Protocol 15.

3.3.4 Special microscopy and culture for *Legionella* spp.

Legionella pneumophila is the cause of between 1% and 15% of pneumonia (18). The standard method of diagnosis in most laboratories has been the indirect immunofluorescent antibody test on paired sera, but this by its nature leads to a retrospective diagnosis. Direct immunofluorescent examination of respiratory tract specimens is less often performed. Non-cultural methods are discussed in Section 3.4 and are widely used for rapid diagnosis.

Protocol 13

Method of microscopy and culture for *Nocardia* spp.

Equipment and reagents

- Plate microscope
- Blood agar plates
- Sabouraud dextrose plates
- Gram stain
- Ziehl–Neelsen stain

Method

1 Perform a Gram stain on the specimen and look for branching Gram-positive rods.

2 Culture on to blood agar aerobically and a Sabouraud dextrose plate (without antibiotics), which is particularly suitable for studying the colonial morphology.

3 Examine the plates after three days with a plate microscope and then at intervals for 10 days. Nocardia colonies range from white to yellow/ochre, orange, and pink and their surfaces are usually folded into convoluted patterns (resembling a star, hence *N. asteroides*). Look for aerial mycelia that may give a chalky or downy appearance to the colony macroscopically.

4 Check any suspect colonies with a Gram stain and perform a modified Ziehl–Neelsen stain for acid-fast bacilli (see Appendix I).

5 Report aerobic Gram-positive acid-fast rods as presumptive *Nocardia* spp.[a]

[a] Further confirmatory tests for *N. asteroides* include growth at 46 °C, positive urease and nitrate reduction, and aesculin hydrolysis. Definitive identification is best performed by laboratories with a special interest in *Nocardia* spp.

Legionella culture is performed more commonly now because of improvements in media composition and selectivity, and all laboratories should have the ability to culture this genus. Culture offers a definitive diagnosis of legionnaires' disease and enables speciation and serogrouping to be performed, which is important in determining the source of an outbreak. Culture is more sensitive than immunofluorescence techniques and highly specific, but at least three days are required for growth to be apparent. Negative DFA does not always exclude legionella, and false positives may occur.

Sputum may be cultured and improvements in media have resulted in increased isolation rates. As only about 50% of patients with legionnaires' disease have a productive cough, other specimens may have to be cultured, including transtracheal aspirates, broncho-alveolar washings, blood, pleural fluid, and transbronchial lung biopsies. A detailed account of laboratory methods will be found elsewhere (19).

Infrequently legionellae may be seen on conventional Gram stain, but prolonged counterstaining with carbol fuchsin is recommended. It has been suggested that the appearance on Gram stain of pale, small, pleomorphic Gram-negative rods, followed by no bacterial growth after conventional overnight culture should prompt consideration of legionella (20). Culture for legionellae is most appropriate for patients with suspected atypical pneumonia, those with pneumonia who fail to respond to antibiotics, or who are immunocompromised. Heat or acid treatment of contaminated specimens followed by plating on to selective media helps avoid overgrowth of cultures by contaminants. Various legionella culture media have been devised. The most successful is buffered charcoal yeast extract agar with alpha ketoglutarate (BCYE) (Oxoid Ltd.). Selective BCYE plates containing vancomycin, polymyxin, and cyclohexamide should be used, particularly for heavily contaminated specimens, together with a non-selective plate. Ten days incubation is required for some species of legionella associated with pneumonia (e.g. *L. bozemanii, L. dumoffii, L. gormanii,* and *L. micdadei,* although *L. pneumophila* usually grows in three to five days).

For the method for *Legionella* culture, see Protocol 14.

Protocol 14

Method of culture for *Legionella* spp.

Equipment and reagents

- Plastic beads
- Centrifuge
- Selective and non-selective BCYE

Method

1. The various specimen types should be treated as follows:
   (a) *Sputum:* homogenize by shaking with plastic beads.[a] If a Gram stain shows heavy bacterial contamination, the specimen may also be vortex-mixed with an equal quantity of distilled water and then diluted 1 in 100. Heat-treat the homogenized specimen and dilutions if made, by incubating in a water-bath at 50 °C for 30 min.
   (b) *Pleural fluid:* centrifuge at 2000 g for 30 min and culture the deposit.
   (c) *Bronchial washings:* no preparation needed.
   (d) *Biopsies/tissues:* grind up specimen in a minimum of distilled water.
   (e) *Transtracheal aspirate:* examine a Gram stain and heat-treat specimen, as for sputum, if many organisms are present.
2. Plate the prepared specimen on to selective and non-selective BCYE.

3 Incubate at 35–37 °C in humidified air.

4 Examine plates after two days and at intervals until 10 days incubation is completed.[b]

5 Subculture likely colonies on to BCYE and BCYE without L-cysteine.[c]

6 Identify the isolate further by agglutination reactions or direct immunofluorescence, and send to a reference laboratory for confirmation.

[a] It has been found that sodium ions frequently leach from soda glass beads and this inhibits legionellae.

[b] Suspect colonies have a characteristic cut-glass appearance when viewed with a plate microscope. They are 1–2 mm in diameter, flat or convex with complete edges, and vary in colour from white to bluish/white.

[c] Colonies growing only on the complete BCYE can be identified presumptively as *Legionella* spp., owing to their dependence on L-cysteine.

3.4 Non-cultural methods of diagnosis

3.4.1 Antigen detection in body tissues and fluids

Some patients in the early phase of pneumococcal pneumonia, particularly those without pre-existing chronic obstructive airways disease, do not produce sputum, and many patients are treated with antibiotics by their general practitioner before being referred to hospital. Blood cultures should always be taken from patients in hospital with pneumonia, but again only a small proportion are positive. Attempts to detect pneumococcal antigen in sputum, blood, and urine may help, and a variety of methods have been used, such as counterimmune electrophoresis (CIE), and agglutination of latex particles or red cells coated with specific antibody (see Chapter 2, Section 3.5.2). Urine specimens can be concentrated before examination using a Minicon BIS concentrator (Amicon Corp.) which concentrates the specimen up to 50-fold (21). Sometimes false positive results are obtained.

In legionella infections, the detection of urinary antigen using commercial kits is becoming an increasingly common technique in the routine clinical diagnostic laboratory's repertoire. It increases the speed of diagnosis and also allows diagnosis after commencement of antibiotics. Commercial ELISA kits are readily available with excellent sensitivity and specificity. The disadvantage of the test is that only *L. pneumophila* serogroup 1 can be detected reliably.

Chlamydia trachomatis (serotypes D–K) are associated with sexually transmitted genital tract infections. Neonates may acquire chlamydial infection following passage through an infected birth canal, resulting in inclusion conjunctivitis and, less commonly, an interstitial pneumonia. Approximately half the neonates with chlamydial pneumonia have a history of conjunctivitis. *C. trachomatis* can be grown from nasopharyngeal secretions and conjunctival smears of concurrent conjunctivitis. Commercial systems based on monoclonal antibodies are available for the detection of elementary bodies by immunofluorescence, or for antigen detection by other methods such as ELISA, facilitating rapid laboratory diagnosis (see Chapter 4).

3.4.2 Detection of antibody response in serum

This has been the mainstay for the diagnosis of atypical pneumonia caused by *Mycoplasma pneumonia*, *Chlamydia psittaci*, *Chlamydia pneumoniae*, and *Coxiella burnetii* (Q fever).

Protocol 15

Titration of complement and haemolytic serum

The haemolytic titre of each new batch of complement must be determined by 'chessboard' titration against each new batch of lysin.

Equipment and reagents

- Pipette dropper
- U-bottomed microtitre plate
- Hot-plate
- Ca–Mg buffered diluent (Oxoid Ltd.)

- Preserved complement
- Haemolytic serum
- 4% washed sheep red blood cells

Method

1 With a pipette dropper add 2 vols of 25 μg diluent to each well of a U-bottomed microtitre plate. This represents one volume of serum and one volume of nobreak antigen in the CFT. Add a third volume of diluent to the control column in place of complement.

2 Prepare in tubes dilutions of complement with a 20% difference in concentration between each, as follows:

   (a) Set out a row of tubes to cover a series of dilutions from 1 in 30 to 1 in 179.

   (b) Into the second and each subsequent tube pipette 2 ml diluent. In the first tube make 12 ml of 1 in 30 dilution of complement by adding 0.5 ml preserved complement to 3.5 ml water and then adding 8 ml diluent.

   (c) From the first tube transfer 8 ml of diluted complement to the second tube; wash the pipette with diluent; mix the contents of the second tube and transfer 8 ml to the third, and so on, to the end of the row, washing out the pipette between each dilution.

3 Add 25 μl of each complement dilution into the appropriate column of the plate.

4 Wrap the plate securely in foil to prevent evaporation and stand at 4 °C overnight. Next morning prepare in 1 ml amounts a series of doubling dilutions of haemolytic serum from 1 in 25 to 1 in 800 plus one tube containing 1 ml diluent as a control.

Protocol 15 continued

    Mix each dilution with an equal volume of 4% washed sheep red blood cells, and sensitize for 10 min in a water-bath at 37 °C or at room temperature for at least 30 min.

5 Remove plates from refrigerator and warm on a 37 °C hot-plate for 20 min.

6 Pipette 25 μl volumes of sensitized cells into appropriate row of wells, starting with the control cells without haemolysin and continuing with the highest dilution of haemolysin. Seal with tape and place in incubator room on a hot-plate for 40 min at 37 °C, shaking on a microshaker after about 15 min, 30 min, and again on removal from incubator.

7 Place plates in refrigerator overnight or for several hours at room temperature until cells have settled and then read.

    0 = no cells remaining, i.e. complete lysis to approx. 10% cells remaining.

    1 = approx. 25% cells remaining.

    2 = approx. 50% cells remaining.

    3 = approx. 75% cells remaining.

    4 = approx. 100% cells remaining.

Note: The optimal sensitizing concentration (OSC) of the haemolytic serum is the dilution giving most lysis with the highest dilution of complement. One unit of complement (HC_{50}) is the dilution which gives 50% lysis at the optimal sensitizing concentration of the haemolytic serum. In the test proper, 4 units are used ($4HC_{50}$).

Protocol 16

Titration of antigen and positive control standard antiserum

It is necessary to obtain the optimal dilution of each antigen and the titre of the corresponding standard antiserum. It is carried out as a 'chessboard' titration in U-bottomed microtitre plates.

Equipment and reagents

- See Protocol 15
- 1 ml automatic pipette
- Antigen
- Antiserum

Method

1 Using a 1 ml automatic pipette, prepare in tubes serial doubling dilutions of (a) antigen and (b) antiserum (inactivated at 56 °C for 30 min). If antigen and antiserum have not been tested previously, dilutions should range from 1 in 2 for antigen and

Protocol 16 continued

    1 in 8 for antiserum, otherwise from four times previous optimal dilution and titre respectively.

2 Put 1 vol. (25 μl) diluent into control wells (antiserum row and antigen column controls).

3 Add 1 vol. of each of the antiserum dilutions to each well of the appropriate row, starting at the highest dilution.

4 Add 1 vol. of each of the antigen dilutions to each well of the appropriate column.

5 Add 1 vol. of complement ($4HC_{50}$) to each well.

6 Put respectively 2, 2, 2, 2, and 3 vol. diluent in five wells for complement controls at 4, 2, 1, 0.5, and 0 (cell control) $\times HC_{50}$. Add indicated dose of complement.

7 Leave plate overnight at 4 °C. Next morning warm the plate on 37 °C hot-plate for 20 min.

8 Pipette 1 vol. of sensitized red cells to each well on the plate. Seal with tape and continue as in Protocol 15.

9 Reading: The optimal dilution of antigen (OPD) is that which gives most fixation with the highest dilution of serum. This is the dilution to be used in tests with unknown sera. The titre of serum is that dilution which gives a reading[a] of 2 with the optimal dilution of antigen.

[a] A reading of 2 is expected at the titre of the standard serum, but because here the cells are most sensitive to differences in complement concentration, a reading from trace to 3 is acceptable. At twice the titre (i.e. in the preceding well) there should be a reading of 4, and at half the titre (i.e. the well following) there should be a reading of 0–1.

Cultivation of *M. pneumoniae* can be attempted on suitable media but it is rarely performed in the UK. The organism takes approximately 10 days to grow, and overgrowth by contaminants is a problem. For a full account of isolation and identification the reader is referred elsewhere (22). The main test for laboratory diagnosis is the complement fixation test (CFT) to detect a rising antibody titre to *M. pneumoniae* seen between an acute and convalescent sample. The general principle of the CFT is as follows. The patient's serum is mixed with complement and antigen. If an antigen–antibody reaction takes place, complement is fixed. This is demonstrated by testing for residual complement. Sheep red cells, sensitized with anti-sheep haemolytic serum, are added. If lysis does not occur, complement has been fixed in the first reaction and the test is positive. If there is lysis, free complement is available and the test is negative. A general CFT method which can be applied to the detection of antibodies to atypical pathogens causing pneumonia is given in Protocol 17. An agglutination test detecting IgM and IgG can be used to confirm high CFT titres (Serodia, Mast

Diagnostics). IgM tests have been described (e.g. using ELISA or immunofluorescence) but are only performed by specialist laboratories. A DNA probe directed against RNA from *M. pneumoniae* is now available (Gen-Probe Inc.), but it is expensive.

Protocol 17

Complement fixation test

All sera are stored at $-20\,°C$ to prevent them from becoming anti-complementary.

Equipment and reagents

- See Protocol 16
- Reagent dispenser
- Serum
- Complement
- Antigen

Method

1   Heat 1 in 5 serum dilutions (0.2 ml serum, 0.8 ml diluent) at $56\,°C$ for 30 min to inactivate complement.

2   Titrate the acute and convalescent stage sera in parallel with one row for each antigen to be tested.

3   With the reagent dispenser put 1 vol. of diluent into wells 2–12 for each test serum and for each specific reagent control. (It is best to put these controls together on a separate plate when several antigens are being tested.)

4   With the pipette dropper add diluent to five complement control wells: 2, 2, 2, 2, and 3 vol. respectively for complement at 4, 2, 1, 0.5, and 0 $\times HC_{50}$ (cell control).

5   Using the automatic pipette, with a separate tip for each serum place 0.1 ml of each test serum into the master well (well 1 of each row).

6   Make doubling dilutions with diluters by transferring 25 µl from wells 1–2 and so on to 8; mix well at each transfer by rotating the diluters four times. Blot diluters dry after removal from well 8. Make three further transfers of sera from well 1 for (a) non-specific reactivity (with doubling dilutions from wells 9–10), and (b) serum controls (1 in 10 dilutions in wells 1, 1, and 12). Blot diluters between (a) and (b) and clean by flaming, cooling in deionized water, and blotting dry.

7   Make doubling dilutions of standard sera from 4 × test titre (4T) to 0.25 test titre (T/4); include serum controls (at 4T in wells 1, 1, and 12).

8   Add 1 vol. complement ($4HC_{50}$) to wells 2–11 in test rows and to wells 2–7, 9, and 11 in control wells. Add 1 vol. complement at $2HC_{50}$ to well 12 of test rows and wells 8, 10, and 12 of control rows; for complement controls add 1 vol. of 4, 2, 1, and 0.5 $\times HC_{50}$ respectively.

9   Add 1 vol. of antigen at OPD to test serum dilutions (wells 2–8) and then to specific reagent row (wells 2–8).

10 Add appropriate negative antigen control (same dilution as the antigen) to wells 9–10, and to control negative antigen control (wells 9–10) of specific reagent control.

11 Add 1 vol. of diluent to wells 1, 1, and 12 to make up 3 vol.

12 Wrap plates in foil and stand overnight[a] at 4 °C. Continue as in Protocol 18, except add 1 vol. of 2% sensitized sheep red cells to each well.

13 Readings:

    (a) *Test*: The highest dilution of serum giving a reading of 4 or 3 is taken as the titre.

    (b) *Controls*: Negative antigen control—complete haemolysis. Serum control—complete haemolysis.

14 Layout for plates.

    (a) Plate with serum dilutions for CF test:

        Well 1 = master dilution of test serum.

        Well 2–8 = serum dilutions.

        Well 9–10 = negative antigen control (for non-specific reactions).

        Well 11–12 = serum control (for anti-complementary activity).

    (b) Plate with reagent controls:

        Well 1 = master dilution of specific antiserum.

        Well 2–6 = specific serum dilutions.

        Well 7–8 = antigen control.

        Well 9–10 = negative antigen control.

        Well 11–12 = serum control.

[a] The technique of short fixation CFT is the same as the long, except that to allow fixation of complement the tests are incubated for 1.5 h at 37 °C instead of overnight at 4 °C. The required concentrations of reagents for use may differ and all agents must be standardized under similar conditions to those chosen for performing the diagnostic tests.

Chlamydia psittaci (a Category 3 pathogen) isolation is hazardous for the laboratory worker and is not performed outside high containment laboratories. *C. psittaci* and *C. pneumoniae* are initially diagnosed by CFT which detects group antigen. Immunofluorescence is performed by specialist laboratories to confirm the diagnosis.

Coxiella burnetii belongs to the *Rickettsiaceae*. Infection is diagnosed by CFT, and phase variation of the CF antigen is unique in *C. burnetii*. The pattern of antibody response to phase 1 and 2 antigens in conjunction with the clinical findings permits serological recognition of acute or chronic infection and endocarditis. During acute disease, antibody to phase 2 antigens increases, while anti-phase 1 antibodies remain at low levels. In chronic disease, anti-phase 1 antibodies equal or exceed the titre of anti-phase 2 antibodies. Diagnosis is confirmed by immunofluorescence or PCR at reference laboratories.

Protocol 18

Method for serological detection of *Legionella pneumophila* infection using an indirect fluorescent antibody test (IFAT)

Equipment and reagents

- Fluorescent microscope
- PTFE-coated microscope slide
- Formalized yolk sac antigen
- Acetone
- PBS
- Fluorescein isothiocyanate-labelled conjugate

Method

1 Apply 5 µl of formalized yolk sac antigen to each 3 mm well of a PTFE-coated microscope slide (Chapter 4, Section 5.1.3). Allow the spots to dry for 20 min in a 37 °C incubator. Fix in acetone for 15 min at room temperature.

2 Make 1 in 16 and 1 in 32 dilutions in PBS of patients' sera. Use a positive control serum diluted 1 in 128 and apply 10 µl of each dilution to an antigen-coated well.

3 Incubate slides in a moist chamber at 37 °C for 30 min.

4 Wash twice in PBS for 10 min and quickly rinse with distilled water. Dry at 37 °C.

5 Add to each well 5 µl of a 1 in 40 dilution of fluorescein isothiocyanate-labelled conjugate (sheep anti-human whole globulin).

6 Incubate slides and wash and dry as before.

7 Examine under a fluorescent microscope and score the intensity of the bacterial fluorescence from − to +/−, +, ++, +++.

8 Titrate further sera showing any fluorescence at a dilution of 1 in 32. The titre of serum is the reciprocal of the highest dilution at which + fluorescence is seen, providing that the positive control gives a result of 1 in 128. If the positive control is reading high or low, adjust the test sera results accordingly.

9 Interpret as follows: a titre of >1 in 16 against serogroup 1 antigen in a patient with pneumonia should alert the clinician to the likelihood of legionnaires' disease. To confirm the diagnosis a four-fold rise in paired sera to a titre of at least 1 in 64 or a single titre of >1 in 128 with a relevant clinical history is required.

Legionella pneumophila infection is most commonly diagnosed by antibody detection (18), although culture, and more recently urinary antigen detection is becoming more popular. Around 25% of patients may have detectable antibody within two days of admission to hospital (23), although in some cases up to six weeks may be required for seroconversion. Commonly used methods include a

Table 3 Principles of some enzyme immunoassay systems

All tests require the use of appropriate positive and negative controls.

A.   Non-competitive assays

1 *Direct method* (e.g. antigen detection)
   (a) Unlabelled antibody is bound to solid phase support (plastic microtitre plates, tubes, beads, or cuvettes).
   (b) After adsorption, unbound antibody is removed and untreated binding sites are blocked by certain agents (e.g. bovine serum albumin, gelatin, non-ionic detergent).
   (c) Test serum is added, incubated, and unreacted components are removed by washing.
   (d) Enzyme-conjugated specific antibody is added. Enzyme labelled antibody binds to antigen captured by the first antibody.
   (e) Unreacted conjugate is removed by washing and enzyme substrate added.
   (f) Enzymic activity is measured by hydrolysis or oxidation of the substrate to develop a coloured reaction product.
   (g) Amount of substrate product is judged visually or measured spectrophotometrically or fluorimetrically.
   (h) Reaction product is directly related to concentration of antigen in sample.

2 *Indirect method*
   Advantages: conjugate does not have to be prepared for each antigen being assayed. Greater sensitivity than direct method.
   As (a)–(c) above, then:
   i.   Unlabelled viral antibody, prepared in an animal species different from that used for the production of the viral antibody bound to the solid phase, is added.
   ii. Unreacted components are removed by washing, and enzyme labelled anti-species gamma globulin against the second antibody is added.
   iii. Unreacted conjugate is removed and substrate added. Then as (f) and (g) above.

3 *Antibody 'capture' method for class-specific antibodies*
   Problems in assay of IgM are mainly due to presence and competition of large amounts of IgG in test sera.
   (a) Chain-specific anti-human IgM is adsorbed to the solid phase to 'capture' IgM.
   (b) Test serum is added and IgM content is bound to the solid phase.
   (c) Antigen is added, and antigen bound to specific IgM is detected by enzyme-conjugated specific antibody or in two steps by specific antibody and then enzyme labelled anti-species gamma globulin.
   Positive tests of IgM antibody tests should always be interpreted with caution because of the potential for rheumatoid factor to give false positives.

B.   Competitive assays (e.g. antibody detection)
   (a) Unlabelled antibody is bound to solid phase and antigen is captured onto this.
   (b) Test serum is added together with enzyme-conjugated specific antibody. Competition for binding to immobilized antigen occurs between specific antibody in the test serum and conjugated antibody.
   (c) Unreacted components are removed by washing and enzyme substrate is added.
   (d) Enzymic activity is measured and is inversely related to the concentration of specific antibody in the test serum.

---

latex agglutination screening test, an indirect fluorescent antibody test (IFAT), using a formalized yolk sac antigen prepared from *L. pneumophila* serogroups 1–6 (DMRQC), and a rapid microagglutination technique (24). The IFAT method is given in Protocol 20.

As a general point, ELISA methods are becoming increasingly popular as a means of non-cultural diagnosis. They are often commercially produced and come with manufacturer's instructions, but they do vary in their basic principles and some examples of these are given in Table 3.

References

1. Combined Working Party Report. (1998). *J. Hosp. Infect.*, **39**, 253.
2. Reischl, U., Lehn, N., Sanden, G. N., and Loeffelholz, M. J. (2001). *J. Clin. Microbiol.*, **39**, 1963.
3. Miller, E., Fleming, D. M., Ashworth, L. A. E., Mabbett, D. A., *et al.* (2000). *Commun. Dis. Public Health*, **3**, 132.
4. James, L. and Hoppe-Bauer, J. E. (1994). In *Clinical microbiology procedures handbook* (ed Isenberg) Vol. 1 ASM, Washington DC.
5. Consensus statement (1995). *Am. J. Respir. Crit. Care Med.*, **153**, 1711.
6. Flournoy, D. J. and Davidson, L. J. (1993). *Am. J. Infect. Control*, **21**, 64.
7. Wong, L. K., Barry, A. L., and Horgan, S. M. (1982). *J. Clin. Microbiol.*, **16**, 627.
8. Bartlett, J. G., Ryan, K. J., Smith, T. F., and Wilson, W. R. (1987). *Cumitech 7A, Laboratory diagnosis of lower tract respiratory infections.* American Society for Microbiology, Washington DC.
9. Van Scoy, R. E. (1977). *Mayo Clin. Proc.*, **52**, 39.
10. Kilian, M. (1985). In *Manual of clinical microbiology*, (ed. E. H. Lennette, A. Balows, W. J. Hausler Jr, and H. J. Shadomy), 4th edn, p. 390. American Society for Microbiology, Washington DC.
11. Christensen, J. J., Gadeberg, O., and Bruun, B. (1986). *Acta Pathol. Microbiol. Immunol. Scand. Sect. B*, **94**, 89.
12. Stenvange, S., Hoiby, N., Espersen, F., and Koch, C. (1992). *Thorax*, **47**, 6.
13. Tenover, F. C., Crawford, J. T., Huebner, R. E., Geiter, L. J., *et al.* (1993). *J. Clin. Microbiol.*, **31**, 767.
14. Djuretic, T., Herbert, J., Drobniewski, F., Yates, M., Smith, E. G., Magee, J. G., Williams, R., Flanagan, P., Walt, B., Rayner, A., Crowe, M., Chadwick, M. V., Middleton A. M., Watson, J. M. (2002). *Thorax*, **57**, 477.
15. Zaher, F. and Marks, J. (1977). *Tubercle*, **58**, 143.
16. Soini, H. and Musser, J. M. (2001). *Clin. Chem.*, **47**, 809.
17. Vuorines, P., Miettinen, A., Vuento, R., *et al.* (1995). *J. Clin. Microbiol.*, **33**, 1856.
18. MacFarlane, J. T., Ward, M. J., Finch, R. G., and Macrae, A. D. (1982). *Lancet*, **ii**, 255.
19. Dournon, E. (1988). A *laboratory manual for Legionella* (ed. T. G. Harrison). John Wiley.
20. Fallon, R. J. (1986). *Med. Lab. Sci.*, **43**, 64.
21. Ramsey, B. W., Marcuse, E. K., Foy, H. M., Cooney, M. K., *et al.* (1986). *Pediatrics*, **78**, 1.
22. Edelstein, P. H. and Meyer, R. D. (1984). *Chest*, **85**, 114.
23. Harrison, T. G. and Taylor, A. G. (1982). *J. Clin. Pathol.*, **35**, 211.
24. Holliday, M. G. (1990). *J. Clin. Pathol.*, **43**, 860.

Chapter 4

Bacteriology of the genital tract

Catherine A. Ison
Department of Infectious Diseases and Microbiology, Imperial College London, St. Mary's Campus, London W2 1PG, UK.

Alun J. Davies
Sandwell District General Hospital, Lyndon, West Bromwich, West Midlands B71 4HJ, UK.

Peter M. Hawkey
Health Protection Agency, Birmingham Heartlands Hospital, Birmingham B9 5SS, UK
and
University of Birmingham, Birmingham B15 2TT, UK.

1 Introduction

Whilst the diagnosis of genital infections by means of bacteriological examination is straightforward in those infections where an organism has a clear pathogenic role, such as is the case in gonorrhoea and syphilis, other infections are encountered where the contribution of diagnostic bacteriology is less clear. Culture of specimens from patients with genital infections may yield organisms such as *Gardnerella* spp., *Listeria* spp., and anaerobic bacteria, which, although capable of causing infections under suitable conditions, do not do so invariably. Unless an organism is generally recognized as a pathogen, its presence in large numbers does not provide evidence of pathogenicity.

Detection of infection in the female genital tract is complicated by the normal microbial vaginal flora and the changes in vaginal flora that occur throughout a woman's life. The laboratory examination of specimens from the genital tract is heavily influenced by the clinical details supplied and the department from which the specimen was sent, so that only organisms relevant to the presenting complaint are sought.

1.1 Normal vaginal flora

(a) *Pre-pubertal.* Immediately post-delivery, circulating maternal oestrogen may result in a microbial flora in babies similar to that in adults. This changes in approximately two weeks as the oestrogens are metabolized, so that throughout childhood the vaginal epithelium lacks glycogen, and so carries a scanty background flora of skin organisms and upper respiratory tract commensals.

(b) *Post-pubertal.* The vaginal epithelium has a high glycogen concentration due to the influence of circulating oestrogens. This is metabolized by lactobacilli to lactic acid, producing a low pH. The vaginal flora may superficially resemble faecal flora due to transient perineal contamination, but many organisms have a very close association with the lower genital tract, e.g. *Prevotella bivia*, *Gardnerella vaginalis*, and *Mycoplasma hominis* (1). In vaginal secretions, anaerobic bacteria outnumber aerobic at 10^9 to 10^8 cfu/ml. The commonest anaerobes found are anaerobic or facultatively anaerobic lactobacilli, *Prevotella* spp., and anaerobic Gram-positive cocci, Diphtheroids and coagulase negative staphylococci are the commonest aerobic bacteria (2, 3). Pregnancy has little effect on this flora, but the number of aerobic bacteria drops in the premenstrual week. Cultures from the cervix yield fewer organisms than from the vagina, due to the different epithelia and pH values of the two sites.

One further difficulty in correlating routine laboratory work with the results of carefully controlled studies of the vaginal flora is the problem of sampling. A high vaginal swab (HVS) is the usual specimen received by a routine laboratory, but most studies have used vaginal secretions collected with a calibrated loop or pipette. There is not always a precise correlation between the numbers of bacteria isolated by these more exact techniques with the flora detected by an ordinary swab, so that interpretation of results depends very much on previous experience and knowledge of the likely flora.

(c) *Post-menstrual women.* The microbial flora alters again at the menopause, with skin and perineal organisms predominating in vaginal culture. Vaginal discharge due to bacterial overgrowth in later life usually responds to local or systematic oestrogen therapy, which alters the pH of the vaginal environment.

1.2 Changes in normal vaginal flora

Vaginal discharge can be physiological or pathological, and there may be fluctuations of a 'normal' discharge associated with ovulation or the use of an intrauterine device. In assessing the microbiology of vaginal discharge it is simplest to consider:

(a) Organisms normally present in low numbers which can cause symptoms when found as the predominant isolate.

(b) Organisms not normally isolated, whose presence is usually associated with disease.

The bacteria encountered, together with comments on their significance, are listed in Table 1. Note that whilst the yeast *Candida albicans* does not fall within

Table 1 Bacteria found in specimens from the vaginal tract

Organism	Significance and comments
(a) Normally present in low numbers, may cause symptoms when dominant isolate	
Staphylococcus aureus	Uncommon pathogen, sometimes cause of purulent post-delivery/surgery discharge or the watery discharge of the toxic shock syndrome.
Streptococcus pyogenes Lancefield gp A β.H.S.)	Classical cause of puerperal fever, normally present in large numbers if (causing disease). Presence of this bacterium or *Staphylococcus aureus* may indicate nosocomial infection.
Streptococcus agalactiae (Lanceficid gp B β.H.S.)	Commonly a neonatal pathogen but can cause infection in mothers and atrophic vaginitis in older women.
Escherichia coli and other 'coliforms'	Difficult to interpret as colonization with these bacteria can follow antibiotic administration. Large numbers of *E. coli* may accompany anaerobes in post-surgical infections. Heavy introital carriage of *E. coli* has been associated with persistent urinary tract infections.
Listeria monocytogenes	Similar pathogenic role to *Streptococcus agalactiae*, presence in specimens may be significant but must be assessed clinically. Pregnant women more susceptible, outbreaks resulting from contaminated dairy products reported (5).
Clostridium perfringens	Large number isolated following delivery/surgery usually significant (see Chapter 5, Section 3.2.3).
Actinomyces spp.	Associated with IUCD-related infections (see Chapter 5, Section 6.3).
Gardnerella vaginalis	Part of the normal flora, but in association with anaerobic, curved rod-shaped bacteria such as *Mobiluncus curtissii* and *M. mulieris* may cause 'bacterial vaginosis' (previously called non-specific vaginitis) (6, 7).
Mycoplasma hominis	A cause of pelvic inflammatory disease and post-partum fever when it may be isolated from blood cultures (8). Can be found in asymptomatic individuals, so positive culture results may be difficult to assess. Few laboratories carry out culture or serological tests for this organism.
Ureaplasma urealyticum	Similar constraints to interpretation of positive cultures as *Mycoplasma*. Associated with 'non-gonococcal urethritis' but not routinely cultured.
(b) Bacteria not normally isolated, substantial pathogenic role	
Neisseria gonorrhoeae	Presence always indicates disease which may be disseminated. Very occasionally *N. meningitidis* and *N. lactamica* may be isolated from the genital tract of symptomatic patients, careful clinical assessment needed.
Chlamydia trachomatis	Various serotypes: A–C cause trachoma, L1–3 lymphogranulonia vencreum, and D–K genitourinary infections in adults and pneumonial conjunctivitis in children.
Treponema pallidum	Causative agent of syphilis, non-culturable. Diagnosis by direct microscopy of lesions (rarely practised) or serology. Many body systems affected, so clinical diagnosis of distinct syndromes important.

the scope of this book, it is a common cause of vaginal discharge and should be sought; detailed methods for its isolation and identification will be found elsewhere (4).

1.3 Pathogens associated with specific clinical conditions

To ensure efficient use of laboratory time and resources it is important to investigate specimens only for the appropriate pathogen associated with a particular condition. Table 2 shows the most commonly encountered clinical problems which require examination of an HVS or other specimen from the genital tract and the pathogens likely to cause each of those conditions.

2 Collection and transport of specimens

The type of specimen required varies with the presenting complaint. Unfortunately, a specimen commonly received in many laboratories is a low vaginal swab, which yields information about the perineal flora only. A cervical swab, preferably collected with the help of a speculum to avoid perineal contamination, is desirable. Triple swabs are required for the isolation of *Neisseria gonorrhoeae*, with specimens taken from the cervix, urethra, and rectum, and a separate swab for the identification of *Chlamydia trachomatis*, which should be placed in chlamydia transport medium immediately and held at 4 °C; if not cultured within 24 hours the swab should be frozen at −70 °C. Culture is now usually reserved for medico legal cases and a separate swab EIA/PCR should be placed in the appropriate transport medium and stored according to the manufacturer's instructions. It is unrealistic to expect to diagnose a microbial cause of pelvic inflammatory disease (PID) from an HVS alone. PID caused by *N. gonorrhoeae* requires an endocervical swab, while chlamydial PCR, serology, or culture may implicate *C. trachomatis*. A mixture of aerobes or anaerobes from the vagina, possibly after a primary infection with *N. gonorrhoeae*, is responsible for some cases of PID. Fluid from the pouch of Douglas is a more relevant specimen for the investigation of PID than an HVS, but the latter specimen is more likely to be sent to the laboratory (9). Urethral swabs from males should be obtained by inserting a cotton wool-tipped wire swab 4 cm into the urethra, rotating, and gently withdrawing. The swab should be placed in Stuart's or Amies' transport media (both suitable) and examined in the laboratory that day, although heavily inoculated swabs held in cool conditions may retain culture viability for several days. It is important to ensure that the swabs or transport media used are not toxic to *N. gonorrhoeae*; the addition of activated charcoal can remove toxic substances. A convenient medium and pre-sterilized swab kit (Transwab MW171) is available from Medical Wire and Equipment Ltd.

Table 2 Pathogens sought in genital specimens grouped by clinical diagnosis

Group	Clinical diagnosis		Pathogens sought	Suggested media[a]
I	Vaginal discharge	age 15–50	Neisseria gonorrhoeae	VCNT
			Trichomonas vaginalis	SAB
			Chlamydia trachomatis	
	Urethral discharge	>50, include	Streptococcus pyogenes and S. agalactiae	CHLT
			N. gonorrhoeae	
			C. trachomatis	
			S. pyogenes and Staphylococcus aureus	
II	Post-partum/gynaecological		S. pyogenes and Staphylococcus aureus	BA
	surgery		S. agalactiae	NEO
	Septic abortion		N. gonorrhoeae	VCAT
	Infected Bartholin's gland		'Coliforms'	MAN
			Clostridium perfringens	
			Mycoplasma hominis	
			Prevotella spp.	
			Anaerobic streptococci	
III	Acute cervicitis (non-peurperal)		All the above plus:	BA
	Vulvovaginitis		Chlamydia trachomatis	NEO
	Pelvic inflammatory disease		(Ureaplasma urealyticum)	VCAT
	Salpingitis		M. hominis	MAC
	Urethritis		M. genitalium	CHLT
	Discharge associated with IUCD		Actinomyces spp.	

Organism/media in brackets are given a low priority by many laboratories.
Vaginal specimens give a poor yield of N. gonorrhoeae, culture for this organism optional (G.P. specimens may only be HVS).

[a] SAB: Sabouraud's agar for C. albicans.
VCNT: vancomycin, colistin, nystatin, trimethoprim added to chocolate agar incubated in 5% CO_2 for N. gonorrhoeae, some laboratories use amphotericin instead of nystatin. As some strains of N. gonorrhoeae are sensitive to vancomycin, some laboratories may wish to include a chocolate agar plate *without* antibiotics in addition to VCNT, particularly in culture-negative suspected cases or Gram film positive, culture-negative cases.
BA: blood agar incubated in 5% CO_2.
NEO: neomycin blood agar for anaerobic bacteria.
MAC: MacConkey's agar for coliforms.
CHLT: transport medium for Chlam. trachomatis prior to culture or immunofluorescence.

3 Assessment of specimens in the laboratory

The clinical details, age of the patient, and ward or clinic from which the specimen was sent will determine the way in which it is examined. The scheme in Table 2 correlates the clinical details with presumed pathogens, and the specimen will then be examined in one of three ways. In group one, *Trichomonas vaginalis*, *Candida* spp., *N. gonorrhoeae*, *Chlamydia trachomatis*. The second group includes the aerobic and anaerobic bacteria listed, while all the above pathogens are sought in group three as well as, if possible, *M. hominis*, *Ureaplasma* spp., and *Actinomyces* spp. (rarely). The paucity of clinical details on some forms can cause problems in allocating specimens to one of these groups. One approach is simply to return the form and specimen and ask for relevant clinical details. The problem here is the possible delay in isolating an important pathogen, and microbiology departments should come to an understanding with the departments they serve about the need for full information, including clinical details, recent antibiotic therapy, and the age of the patient.

3.1 Microscopy

3.1.1 Gram films and wet preparations

Examination of a wet preparation of the swab for *Trichomonas vaginalis* should be performed on all specimens, along with a Gram stain. Examination of a wet preparation is often more useful than a Gram stain. The relative numbers of epithelial cells and pus cells provide helpful information. Infection with trichomonas is usually associated with an increased number of pus cells, the usual finding being approximately one pus cell per epithelial cell. In bacterial vaginosis (BV), previously known as non-specific vaginitis (NSV), and candidiasis there are usually relatively few pus cells, such that a large number of pus cells should lead to suspicion of a second pathogen.

Endocervical secretions should always be Gram stained. The cervical discharge usually contains some pus cells, so that large numbers of pus cells are required to diagnose cervicitis. Gram staining for *N. gonorrhoeae* produces many false negative results, and care must be taken in early infections to distinguish pathogenic intracellular Gram-negative diplococci from extracellular Gram-negative diplococci which may be non-pathogenic *Neisseria* spp. or *Acinetobacter* spp., which can colonize the normal female genital tract. The Gram stain will show the presence of pus cells and may also, in BV, show the characteristic clue cells, which are epithelial cells studded with 'Gram-variable' diphtheroid-like organisms. The presence of these clue cells, a mixed microbial flora and an absence of lactobacilli together with appropriate clinical details will indicate the possibility of BV. *C. albicans* should be looked for on microscopy, where both spores and mycelia stain Gram-positive. Examination of Gram stained smears of exudate can reveal the characteristic Gram-negative diplococci of *N. gonorrhoeae*, often intracellular in early infections, but frequently predominantly extracellular in the later stages. This method is cheap and rapid, and should be carried out in the clinic before the patient leaves. Unfortunately whilst the procedure will detect over 90% of male infections, only 60% of female infections are detected (10). The test can be made more specific and easier to read if an anti-gonococcal fluorescein-conjugated stain is applied. Unfortunately, most commercial reagents lack adequate specificity and fail to penetrate mucus. Autofluorescence of polymorphonuclear cell granules leads to false positive results, thus rendering this test unsuitable for routine use. Modern monoclonal antibodies have improved specificity but results are still little better than the ordinary Gram film examination.

3.1.2 Dark-ground illumination microscope

As it is not possible to culture *Treponema pallidum* on artificial media, direct microscopy of material from primary lesions and serological tests are the main diagnostic methods used.

Lymph, collected carefully from a suspected primary chancre or a secondary lesion, should be examined by dark-ground microscopy for the presence of spirochaetes. It is difficult to distinguish between *T. pallidum* and the various non-pathogenic commensal spirochaetes commonly found in moist areas of the body. The syphilis spirochaete is non-refractile, white, and it has between 6 and 20 waves of 1 mm pitch. It is best recognized by the experienced observer, so every opportunity should be taken to 'learn' the appearance of this organism by first-hand observation. Syphilis spirochaetes may also be demonstrated after fixation of smears using a modified absorbed fluorescent treponemal antigen test (FTA), and previously in tissues by silver staining. PCR offers a more specific and sensitive test for tissue specimens (11).

3.1.3 Fluorescence microscope

Fluorescent labelled antibodies to chlamydia permit the organisms to be directly detected in smears from mucosal surfaces. This technique is particularly appropriate for the examination of small numbers of specimens, and where distance makes transporting a specimen for culture difficult. It also allows for rapid diagnosis, which may be particularly useful in the case of ophthalmic infections, as the procedure takes only 30 minutes per specimen. Unfortunately, each specimen will require prolonged and careful microscopic examination, which will curtail the number of specimens that can be examined on any day. The test relies upon the specific staining, with fluorescein labelled monoclonal antibodies, of carefully made smears of genital or ocular mucosal surfaces. Results obtained compare favourably with culture (12–14). Indeed, because of its good results and its technical simplicity, it is now replacing culture techniques in most laboratories. The specimens must be taken very precisely and must contain cells which are carefully transferred by rolling the swab onto a slide. The antibodies are either directed against the elementary bodies and are predominantly species-specific (Microtrak, Genetic Systems Corporation, Syva UK; Chlamydiaset, Orion Diagnostica, Seward Laboratories) or are genus-specific (Imagen, Boots Celltech) and are directed against the lipopolysaccharide of earlier stages of the life cycle. Clearly, the species-specific reagents will tend only to detect genital chlamydia whereas the genus-specific reagent will also react with *C. psittaci* strains. A method for using these kits is given in Protocol 1.

Protocol 1

Immunofluorescent detection of *Chlamydia trachomatis* antigen

Equipment and reagents

- Commercial detection kit
- Specimen swab
- Fluorescent microscope

Method

1 Reconstitute the FITC-conjugated antibody[a] according to the manufacturer's instructions and date the bottle.[b]

2 Roll the specimen swab firmly across the well of the slide provided in the kit, remove as much material as possible from the swab.

3 Flood the well with 500 μl acetone and allow to evaporate.

4 Apply 30 μl of antibody conjugate to the well to cover the specimen (20 μl may be adequate). Do not dilute the reagent.

5 Incubate for 15 min at room temperature in a moist box (a plastic sandwich box with wet blotting paper is ideal).

6 Remove the excess antibody conjugate with a Pasteur pipette, gently rinse in distilled water for 10–20 sec.

7 Drain the slide using blotting paper to remove excess water from outside the area of the specimen and allow to air dry.

8 Add a drop of mounting fluid followed by a coverslip and examine using incident light and ×40 objective. Look for the bright green pin-point fluorescent elementary bodies against the dull red fluorescence of the cells. Specimens with no cells cannot be evaluated. Positive specimens should have >5 bodies.

[a] Commercial kits such as Microtrak or Imagen should be used.

[b] Store for a maximum of three months at 4 °C and use at room temperature.

3.2 Detection of antigen in specimens by enzyme immunoassay

Enzyme immunoassay of *C. trachomatis* antigen using EIA is available as a number of commercial kits, Chlamydiazyme (Abbott Laboratories), IDEIA (Boots Celltech Diagnostics Ltd.), and Microtrak EIA (Behring) being widely used.. These tests produce rapid results and are not susceptible to loss of viability of the specimen in transit; they are usually less sensitive than culture and vary in their individual performance (15). There is a wide range of limits of detection of *C. trachomatis* for different methodologies of which the user should be made aware (Figure 1). EIA assays require a degree of mechanization and are most suited to the larger

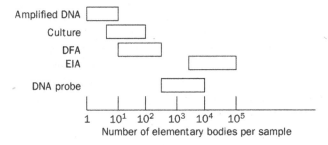

Figure 1 Detection limits of different methods for detection of *C. trachomatis* (modified from ref. 15).

laboratory which would find the immunofluorescence technique too demanding for the numbers of specimens examined.

There is interest in using urine for EIA, in which case it must be centrifuged and the sediment used. They are less sensitive than DNA amplification techniques (15). Recently a number of 'near to patient' tests based on EIA methods in various formats have been introduced. Although easy to perform they are qualitative and are less sensitive than laboratory-based EIAs (15).

4 Culture

The following sections describe the processing in the laboratory of each type of medium which is described in Table 2. Tests for the identification of suspected pathogens are included in each section.

4.1 Selective medium for the isolation of *N. gonorrhoeae*

N. gonorrhoeae is a fastidious bacterium, which is an obligate human pathogen that colonizes the anogenital tract. For successful isolation a highly nutritious medium is required with the addition of a cocktail of antibiotics to inhibit the normal flora and allow the pathogen to grow. Historically the agar base most commonly used was Columbia agar supplemented with horse blood or chocolatized blood to provide the iron source. However, in the last twenty years a specialized GC agar base which contains starch and peptones which can be supplemented either by blood or serum-free supplements, such as Vitox (Oxoid) or IsoVitaleX (BBL), has been used increasingly. The antibiotics of choice include vancomycin or lincomycin to inhibit Gram-positive organisms, colistin and trimethoprim to inhibit other Gram-negative organisms, and nystatin or amphotericin to inhibit yeasts. Lincomycin is sometimes preferred to vancomycin because strains of *N. gonorrhoeae* sensitive to vancomyin (*env* mutants) have been described. However, lincomycin is less inhibitory than vancomycin and overgrowth of normal flora on lincomycin containing media can occur, masking the gonococci. This is a particular problem for clinics and laboratories that receive large numbers of rectal samples. Combinations of these antibiotics, such as VCAT (LCAT) or VCNT, are available from commercial sources. Thayer–Martin Medium was the first of these media to be described but Modified New York City Medium is probably more often used, particularly in the UK. The use of any selective medium is a compromise and in an ideal situation both a non-selective and selective medium would be used. However, in most instances there are insufficient resources and the UK national guidelines recommend that if a single medium is to be used for the isolation of *N. gonorrhoeae* it should contain selective agents.

Specimens can be collected by either a disposable loop or a swab. If a loop is used the specimen should be inoculated directly onto the selective medium in the clinic, stored in a incubator, and then transported once or twice daily to the laboratory. If swabs are preferred then it is advisable to use a recognized transport medium such as Amies' that contains charcoal. Once the specimen has been taken the transport swabs should be stored in the fridge (+4 °C) until sent to the laboratory. Although transport medium is designed to maintain bacterial viability over time the highest recovery will be achieved if the swab reaches the laboratory within the same day or at the latest by the next morning. There is little evidence that either of these approaches is superior and therefore the choice between using a loop or a swab is dependent on the proximity of the clinic to the laboratory and preference of the microbiologist and clinician. Obviously if the specimens are to be collected at a site distant from the laboratory then transport swabs are advisable.

Once inoculated the culture plates should be incubated at 35–36 °C in a moist atmosphere of 5–10% CO_2 for a minimum of 48 hours before they are discarded as negative. In the UK incubation is usually in a CO_2 incubator but candle jars are still an adequate alternative where incubators are not available. A more expensive but useful alternative is the use of CO_2 pouches where one or two culture plates are placed in the plastic envelope which has its own CO_2 source. A number of commercially available systems (such as JEMBEC and Transgrow) combine selective culture medium with an individual supply of carbon dioxide (either by a citric acid/bicarbonate mixture or in a pre-gassed bottle) in a purpose-made container (16, 17). This immediately provides the necessary growth conditions, and if the system is incubated before transmission to the laboratory, very rapid results can be achieved. Survival in these systems is as good as other transport media.

The growth rate of colonies of *N. gonorrhoeae* is variable, dependent on the medium used, and is often retarded on selective media so primary isolation plates should be examined at 24 hours but if negative should be re-incubated for an additional 24 hours. The colonies are small (0.5–2 mm), shiny, and convex but the colour will vary on different media, grey on blood-containing media and cream on serum-free media. They may vary in size, and can become sticky as the culture ages. Suspect colonies should be screened for the presence of cytochrome oxidase, as follows:

(a) Prepare a 0.3–1% aqueous solution of tetramethyl-*p*-phenylene diamine hydrochloride in sterile water each day (reagent may be pre-weighed in plastic tubes and dissolved freshly each day).

(b) Soak a piece of filter paper in the reagent.

(c) If a strip of filter paper has been soaked it can be 'blotted' onto the colony. Alternatively, the colony can be rubbed onto the paper with a wooden stick or a platinum loop (Nichrome loops may give a false positive reaction).

(d) A deep purple colour appearing within 10 seconds indicates a positive result.

The suspect colony should also be Gram stained, whereupon the Gram-negative cocci, sometimes occurring as diplococci, which have their long axes parallel, will be seen. Isolates fulfilling these criteria, grown on selective media and isolated from a genital site are very likely to be *N. gonorrhoeae*, and a provisional report of 'presumptive *N. gonorrhoeae* isolated' may then be issued. In many parts of the world further identification is not performed because resources are not available and the presence of oxidase positive, Gram-negative cocci on specialized medium isolated from a genital site is highly predictive of *N. gonorrhoeae*. However, in the UK it is usual to confirm the identification as *N. gonorrhoeae* and to eliminate other species of *Neisseria* such as *N. meningitidis* and *N. lactamica*.

4.1.1 Identification of *N. gonorrhoeae*

There are two approaches to the confirmation of the identity of *N. gonorrhoeae*. There are tests that will identify *N. gonorrhoeae* and eliminate other *Neisseria* spp., using gonococcal-specific antibodies or the use of carbohydrate utilization test with or without the detection of preformed enzymes such as the aminopeptidases and β-galactosidase that will give the full speciation of the organism. The choice of approach is often decided by the workload, in that laboratories that handle large number of specimens for genitourinary medicine clinics and isolate gonococci regularly often use an immunological approach, at least in the first instance. Laboratories that rarely encounter *N. gonorrhoeae* often prefer to use kits which will give a full speciation. Presumptive *Neisseria* spp. that do not react in immunological tests should always be identified using full speciation. Any isolates from sexual or child abuse cases should be identified with a variety of tests, particularly as their primary isolation may have been on a non-selective medium and therefore commensal Neisseria need to be eliminated.

4.1.2 Identification by immunological methods

Identification by immunological means can be achieved using antibodies either linked to fluorescein (Syva Microtrak *Neisseria gonorrhoeae* Culture Confirmation Test, distributed by Launch Diagnostics in UK) (Protocol 2) or to staphylococcal protein A (Phadebact Monoclonal GC Test, distributed by Boule in UK) (Protocol 3). Both of these commercially available reagents contain a mixture of monoclonal antibodies raised to specific epitopes on the major outer membrane protein, Por. As both reagents contain several antibodies rather than a single antibody to a cross-reactive epitope, false negative reactions do occur, albeit relatively rarely. It is rather convenient that the mixtures in the two reagents do differ and false negatives with one reagent are often positive with the other reagent. The choice of reagent is largely personal preference although the co-agglutination seems more popular at this time.

Protocol 2

Identification of *N. gonorrhoeae* using Syva Microtrak reagent

In this reagent the antibodies have been attached to a fluorochrome, fluorescein, such that when the antibodies attach to specific gonococcal epitopes the organism fluoresces and appears bright yellow/green when viewed under UV light.

Equipment and reagents

- Fluorescence microscope
- Syva Microtrak reagent

Method

1. Select five colonies which have been presumptively identified as *N. gonorrhoeae* by oxidase test and Gram stain.
2. Place a 5 µl drop of water onto a slide well.
3. Touch each of the five colonies lightly and emulsify in the water. The smear should be very thin as thick smears may be difficult to interpret.
4. Allow the smear to air dry and gently fix by passing the slide, smear upwards, over a flame. (Do not overheat as this will lyse the bacteria.)
5. Place 30 µl of reagent on the slide well, ensuring that the entire surface of the smear is covered.
6. Incubate the slide for 15 min at 37 °C in a well humidified chamber.
7. Remove the excess reagent and wash for 5–10 sec in a stream of distilled or deionized water.
8. Gently shake off the excess water and thoroughly air dry the smears.
9. Examine under ×100 oil objective using a fluorescence microscope.

---

i. Identification of N. gonorrhoeae *using Phadebact Monoclonal GC test*

In this reagent the antibodies have been non-specifically absorbed onto staphylococci which are expressing protein A. When the supernatant of a dense boiled suspension of *Neisseria* spp. is mixed with the reagent, if the gonococcal-specific outer membrane protein, Por (either type IA or IB), is present, then the staphylococci will agglutinate (methylene blue is added to make the agglutination easily visible) (see Protocol 3). Two pooled monoclonal antibody reagents are provided, one detecting serogroup WI and the other WII/III (these correspond to Por IA and IB). The individual monoclonal antibody reagents can be used to designate a serovar, which combined with auxotyping, produces a system of strain characterization for research and medico legal purposes. Two sets of monoclonal antibodies are available for serotyping, a commercial set (Pharmacia) and a research set, which is in limited circulation.

Protocol 3

Identification of *N. gonorrhoeae* using the Phadebact Monoclonal GC test

Equipment and reagents

• Phadebact Monoclonal GC test kit

Method

1 Colonies should be presumptively identified as *N. gonorrhoeae* by oxidase and Gram stain (see Protocol 2).

2 Make a light suspension of the presumptively identified colonies in 0.5 ml normal saline.

3 Heat the suspension in a boiling water-bath for 5 min. (The suspension should be boiled immediately and NOT left to stand on the bench.)

4 Cool the suspension to room temperature.

5 Place one drop of each reagent (WI and WII/III) on the card provided in the kit.

6 Add one drop of the boiled suspension to each drop of reagent.

7 Mix the drops thoroughly but gently with a disposable loop or wooden stick, using a fresh one for each reagent.

8 Rock the slide gently and examine for agglutination, which should occur in one or other of these reagents within 1 min.

4.1.3 Identification by carbohydrate utilization

Traditionally the identity has been confirmed by detecting the acidification of glucose-containing media, but not those containing maltose, sucrose, or lactose. This is an oxidative and not a fermentative process. It is important that the basal medium is carbohydrate-free (if serum sugars are used, the serum should be checked for maltase activity). Cystine-tryptic digest semi-solid agar can be used, but the serum-free medium of Flynn and Waitkins is excellent (18). The basal medium is usually dispensed into small screw-capped bottles after supplementation with lactose, maltose, glucose, or sucrose, although drops of the medium can be dispensed into a sterile Petri dish when large numbers of isolates are to be tested and a more rapid result is required.

The inoculated plates or bottles are incubated in 5–10% CO_2 for 24 hours with the caps loosened and are then allowed to stand on the bench for 30 minutes to allow for any acidification due to dissolved CO_2 to dissipate. The disadvantage of this method is that it is slow, and requires a heavy, pure growth of gonococci. Further, some meningococci metabolize maltose slowly and may require at least two days for acidification of the conventional test system, and some gonococci can be slow to utilize glucose. Increased speed and possibly some increased sensitivity can be obtained by using lightly-buffered solutions of sugars and inoculating these with suspensions of putative gonococci (19). These will reveal pH changes within hours of inoculation but may still cause a delay of at least one day for obtaining a pure and sufficient growth of the culture.

Several commercial systems are available for the rapid detection of carbohydrate utilization, often in combination with aminopeptidases, in lightly-buffered media. Most kits consist of a plastic strip with microcapsules containing dehydrated reagents. Each capsule is inoculated with two or three drops of a heavy suspension of the organism in 0.85% (w/v) saline. The strip is sealed and the results read after two to four hours incubation at 37 °C. The reactions of commonly encountered neisseriae are listed in Table 3.

4.1.4 Identification by chromogenic detection of preformed enzymes

Detection of the aminopeptidases, γ-glutamyl and prolyl aminopeptidases together with β-galactosidase, using chromogenic substrates can enable identification to species level. This can be a useful alternative to the approaches above but should only be used on strains isolated from selective media, as certain non-pathogenic neisseriae give similar reactions to those given by *N. gonorrhoeae*. Reagents are available as commercial kits such as Gonochek II (EY Laboratories). In this system three chromogenic substrates are included in a single disposable plastic tube for ease of use.

(a) Remove, as a pair, red and translucent, stoppers from the tube.

(b) Rehydrate substrates with four drops of phosphate-buffered saline (PBS) pH 7.2.

(c) Inoculate several colonies of the test organism.

(d) Recap with both stoppers and incubate at 35 °C for 30 min.

(e) If the cell suspension is blue the organism is *N. lactamica* and if it is yellow the organism is *N. meningitidis*.

(f) If the colour is unchanged, both caps are removed, separated from each other, and the red cap returned to the tube. The tube is then inverted so that the bacterial suspension mixes with the substrate in the red cap and then the tube is returned to the upright position. If the liquid turns pink/red it is *N. gonorrhoeae*, if it remains unchanged or turns pale yellow the organism is *B. catarrhalis*.

Table 3 Characteristics of some human *Neisseria* spp. and *Branhamella catarrhalis*

Organism	Growth on		Acid production from				DNase	Butyrate esterase	γ-Glutamyl aminopeptidase	Propyl aminopeptidase
	Selective media	Nutrient agar at 35°C	Glucose	Maltose	Sucrose	Lactose				
N. gonorrhoeae	+	−	+	−	−	−	−	−	−	+
N. meningitidis	+	−	+	+	−	−	−	−	+	v
N. lactamica	+	+	+	+	−	+[b]	−	−	−	+
N. flavescens[a]	−	+	−	−	−	−	−	−	−	
N. cinerea	+	+	−	−	−	−	−	−	−	
B. catarrhalis	+	+	−	−	−	−	+	+	−	−

[a] Produces yellow pigment.
[b] Also gives positive β-galactosidase (ONPG) test.
V—Variable result.

The test appears to be as effective as traditional biochemical methods, but is more rapid and may well be increasingly used by laboratories. It should only be used on strains isolated from selective media, as certain non-pathogenic neisseriae give similar reactions to those given by *N. gonorrhoeae*.

4.2 Blood agar and blood agar with neomycin

The aerobic blood agar plate may reveal significant numbers *of Streptococcus pyogenes* and/or *Staphylococcus aureus*. Details of the characteristics and diagnostic tests applied to these organisms are found in Chapter 5, Section 4.1.4.

Listeria monocytogenes will grow on the aerobically incubated blood agar plate producing small, grey colonies with a narrow zone of β-haemolysis. Gram stained films of the colony reveal pleomorphic Gram-positive rods that on further testing are aesculin positive and catalase positive (lactobacilli are usually negative). If a six hour broth culture incubated at 25 °C is examined, the bacilli exhibit characteristic tumbling motility, whereas an identical culture incubated at 37 °C shows little or no motility.

Streptococcus agalactiae has overtaken *S. pyogenes* as the major streptococcal cause of neonatal death and *post-partum* sepsis. As it is present in the normal vaginal flora, assessment of growth from vaginal swabs is subjective; however, growth from gastric aspirates and deep ear swabs of 'septic' neonates may indicate a significant infection (20). The organism produces larger (compared to Lancefield group A) whitish/grey colonies surrounded by a narrower zone of β-haemolysis. Strains possess the Lancefield group B antigen; see Chapter 5, Section 4.1.4, for details of the method. Most laboratories will rely on the Lancefield grouping; however, if further identification is required, all group B strains will hydrolyze sodium hippurate (Appendix III) and give a positive CAMP test (as described by Christie, Atkins, and Munch-Petersen in 1944). The CAMP agent is an extracellular substance that enhances the lysis of red blood cells by staphylococcal β-lysin. Details may be found elsewhere (21).

The anaerobically incubated blood agar plate with neomycin will allow anaerobes such as *Clostridium perfringens*, *Bacteroides* spp., and anaerobic streptococci to be detected. Detailed methods will be found in Chapter 5, Section 3.3. Placing a 5 µg metronidazole disc on the second sweep of the plate will provide a zone of inhibition of anaerobic bacteria. Many laboratories may wish to add an anaerobically incubated blood agar plate without neomycin to their set of plates. *Gardnerella vaginalis* might be found growing on such a plate, but as its role in bacterial 'vaginosis' is unclear, not all laboratories will want to pursue it. Full details of its isolation and identification are given elsewhere (6, 7). It is a small, non-motile 'Gram-variable' bacillus often seen attached in large numbers to squamous epithelial cells. Good haemolysis is seen on human blood bilayer Tween agar which should be incubated in 5% CO_2; strains grow up to a 5 µg metronidazole disc, but not up to a 50 µg disc.

4.3 MacConkey's agar

This medium is selective for members of the Enterobacteriaceae and enterococci. The role of such bacteria in vaginal infections is doubtful, but if heavy pure growths are obtained, particularly from patients with retained products of conception, they should be reported as coliforms or enterococci and sensitivity tests performed and reported. Details of the identification of members of the Enterobacteriaceae are given in Chapter 6, Section 4.6. However, this should only be undertaken to 'match' a blood culture isolate.

4.4 Chlamydia transport medium

Culture is now largely used in reference centres for medico legal cases as it can no longer be regarded as the 'gold standard' for sensitivity. The difficulties of specimen transport and complexity of the method mean that very few laboratories now use the method. The method is described in detail (22).

5 Serological methods

5.1 Serological diagnosis of syphilis

This is the method of choice in later stages of the disease, but tests may not prove positive in early (primary) syphilis, when repeated examinations with appropriate tests should be continued until seroconversion occurs, or until an alternative diagnosis is reached. All patients with positive syphilis serology who have neurological signs or symptoms should undergo a CSF examination (23). In neonatal congenital syphilis a direct search for spirochaetes (in mucosal lesions or post-mortem specimens such as liver) and PCR can be helpful, as interpretation of serological data is difficult because maternal IgG will be present in the baby for two to three months. The diagnosis of congenital neurosyphilis benefits from the use of IgM immunoblotting and PCR assay (24). Serological tests use either cardiolipin antigens which detect 'reagin' antibodies or specific *Treponema pallidum* antigens. Selection of which test to perform will be dictated by clinical and laboratory factors (25). It is important to repeat any positive tests on a new serum sample to avoid clerical errors and to confirm the laboratory findings.

Protocol 4

VDRL test for reaginic antibodies in syphilis

Equipment and reagents

- Commercially available kit (e.g. from Oxoid Ltd. or Cambridge Biomedical Ltd.)
- Programmable automatic pipette (such as the EDP pipette, Rainin Instrument Co. Inc.)
- Rotary shaker

Method

1   Use this test in the commercially available kits format which involve the use of cards or a disposable WHO plate as described below.

2 Using a programmable automatic pipette, take up to 250 µl of the patient's serum. Deliver 100 µl into a well, then deliver the remaining 150 µl into a disposable plastic tube. Incubate at 58 °C for 20 min to provide the serum for the TPHA test which should be performed in parallel to the VDRL test. It is not practicable to do more than 30–40 tests at any one time, as the wells may begin to dry during shaking.

3 Include in each batch of tests a positive control prepared from a commercial positive control serum standard, diluted according to the manufacturer's recommendation. It is important that the standard is aliquoted and kept frozen until required and then freshly diluted for use each day.

4 Add 40 µl well-shaken carbon antigen (either from the kit or purchased separately).

5 Place WHO plate on a rotary shaker and shake for 8 min at 100 r.p.m.

6 Read the plate over a light box looking for flocculation as in the positive control.

7 All sera giving positive results to *any* syphilis test should be titrated, particularly if the TPHA test is positive and the VDRL negative, as prozone effects may give false negative results. It is usually sufficient to prepare doubling dilutions of the patient's serum up to 1 in 32.

5.1.1 Venereal disease reference laboratory (VDRL) and rapid plasma reagin (RPR) tests

Reaginic antibody tests rely for their activity on shared antigenicity of spirochaetes with the lipids in mitochondria. Originally colloidal suspensions of extracts from mitochondria-rich tissues such as heart muscle were used. These have now been superseded by chemically defined mixtures of lecithin and cholesterol (sometimes stabilized with choline), all detecting the same antibodies and known as lipoidal antigens. The VDRL test in its original format was a micro flocculation test carried out on a slide and is read with the aid of a low power microscope. A stabilized carbon-containing VDRL antigen and a very similar RPR test (in the USA) is now generally used as in this format, the test can be read by eye or automated, when results are read from the pattern of flocculated granules of carbon deposited on a ribbon of filter paper or in a plastic tray. The more recent RPR card test employs a choline-stabilized antigen which contains carbon. This test is performed on white plastic cards. The modifications allow it to be carried out on plasma as well as serum and to be read with the naked eye, so it has tended to replace the VDRL tests.

These tests have many advantages. They become positive early in the course of an infection and remain at substantial titres during the active stages, but fall on successful treatment or in old inactive 'burnt-out' syphilis. Thus they are very well suited to detect clinically active disease, and for this reason, and because they are cheap and simple to perform, are used extensively for screening purposes.

They may also be used effectively to monitor the efficacy of therapy in treated cases, because antibody levels reflect antigenic load in the body, and as this falls in the successfully treated case so the antibody titre declines.

Unfortunately, cross-reacting antibodies may also be produced in pregnancy, after immunization or after a variety of acute fevers, especially glandular fever. These are usually of low titre and tend to disappear after a few weeks or months. Sometimes, persistent antibodies appear at a high titre and are often associated with autoimmune disease or clotting defects. These are known as biological false positive (BFP) reactions. They can be distinguished from true positive reactions by performing any test which is specific for *Treponema pallidum* infection. Such tests for *T. pallidum* use the actual syphilis spirochaete as antigen. Sera with BFP are negative in *T. pallidum* tests that detect antibodies produced during both syphilis and any of the endemic non-venereal treponematoses such as yaws, bejel, and pinta. There is no certain way to distinguish between these last infections by serological means.

5.1.2 *Treponema pallidum* haemagglutination test (TPHA)

The original specific *T. pallidum* test was the *Treponema pallidum* immobilization (TPI) test. This relies upon the immobilization of live *T. pallidum* spirochaetes by the patient's serum in the presence of complement. The test is technically difficult and there is a risk of laboratory-acquired infection. It has been superseded by tests using dead whole or fractionated *T. pallidum* which can be stored for long periods, and are free from the risks of infection. They are also much cheaper, as they use far less of the expensive antigen per test. Unfortunately, they are not considered quite as reliable.

The TPHA test detects antibodies which will agglutinate a suspension of red blood cells which have been coated with sonicated *T. pallidum* spirochaetes. It was originally described by Rathlev in 1967 (26), and has now been developed as freeze-dried kits available from various manufacturers such as Mast Diagnostics Ltd. Bovine cells are used and the reaction takes place in a special buffer which contains ox red cell stroma and sonicated non-pathogenic (Reiter's) treponemes in order to avoid non-specific agglutination by antibodies often present in healthy persons, either to ox red cells or to commensal spirochaetes.

An alternative modification of the TPHA test has been developed in the UK by Sequeira and Eldridge (27). A method for this test based on a commercial kit is described in Protocol 5. This uses avian cells and so avoids the need to add mammalian red cell stroma. The Reiter treponeme sonicate is also omitted, apparently without loss of specificity. This test is known as the THA. Its properties are similar to those of the TPHA. Both variants of this test are easy to perform and to read. They tend to become positive rather later in the primary stage, or only in the secondary stage of the disease. Either variant of the test can be used as an ideal complement to the VDRL test for screening and diagnosis and will quickly reveal any BFP reactions. A further variant, the TPPA (*Treponema pallidum* particle agglutination) test, is now being used in which the antigen is attached to gelatin particles. Its performance is equivalent to TPHA type tests (28).

Protocol 5

Treponema haemagglutination (THA) test[a]

Equipment and reagents

- Standardized kit
- Automatic pipette

Method

1. Take up 190 μl of diluent into the automatic pipette, an air buffer, and then 10 μl of heat inactivated serum (Protocol 4). Dispense into the well of a disposable WHO tray.

2. Transfer 25 μl of 1 in 20 diluted serum to a well of a plastic microtitre plate with round-bottom wells using a new tip per sample.

3. Leave the diluted sera at room temperature for 20 min to allow absorption of cross-reacting antigens to occur and then add 75 μl well-mixed THA test cells, previously diluted 1 in 10 with THA diluent, to each well.

4. Mix by tapping the tray gently, cover, and leave undisturbed at room temperature for 60–90 min.

5. Read tray; negative wells have a tight button of sedimented red cells, the positive wells a well-defined granular ring.

6. Reconstitute the positive control serum according to the supplier's instructions, diluted 1 in 10 in saline and treat as in steps 1–5. The screening dilution for the sera is therefore 1 in 80 and 1 in 800 for the positive control.

7. Titrate any positive sera by preparing doubling dilutions of the 1 in 20 diluted serum from step 2 in a microtitre plate using 25 μl aliquots of THA diluent and 25 μl of diluted serum so that the final dilution of the serum is 1 in 1280. Dilute the positive control serum so that the manufacturer's titre can be reached.

8. Add 75 μl of THA test cells (diluted 1 in 10 in diluent) to each of the test and positive control dilution wells. Then add 75 μl of THA control cells to 25 μl of 1 in 10 diluted patient's serum to act as an agglutination control. Then test as steps 2–5. If agglutination is seen in the agglutination control, report the test as equivocal and perform an FTA-abs.

[a] Reagents for this test are only provided as a standardized kit consisting of absorbing diluent, lyophilized sensitized turkey cells, unsensitized control cells, and positive control serum. Do not mix reagents from kit to kit (Don Whitley Scientific Ltd., Shipley, West Yorkshire, UK).

5.1.3 Enzyme immunoassay (EIA) tests

Within the last ten years or so a number of commercial EIA tests have been developed. These tests were regarded as investigational tests in the USA but are increasingly being used as an alternative to the VDRL (RPR)/TPHA combination for screening, particularly in the UK (29). These tests in addition to having a high sensitivity and specificity are easily automated providing a further attraction for screening. The performance of different tests should be evaluated carefully, preferably as part of a major procurement programme as they can vary. It is also essential that all tests are controlled both by the manufacturer's internal QA standards and the laboratory participates in a recognized external QA scheme. The same test kit (manufacturer) should be used and preferably the same laboratory when monitoring response to therapy with tests such as VDRL carbon and RPR. A recently described immune capture EIA (ICE syphilis, Murex Diagnostics, Dartford, UK) which uses three recombinant antigens (TpN15, 17, and 47) has shown very promising performance in an evaluation against a native *T. pallidium* antigen EIA (30).

5.1.4 Fluorescent treponemal antibody test (FTA-abs)

The FTA-abs test may be useful when the results of other treponemal tests such as EIA and TPHA are discordant. This test employs fixed, whole *T. pallidum* spirochaetes on a slide. These are overlaid with the patient's serum, washed, and then treated with a fluorescein labelled anti-human antibody. The slide is subsequently examined by fluorescence microscopy, when positive sera will reveal fluorescent spirochaetes. Originally non-specific anti-treponemal antibody activity (which will otherwise produce spurious positive reactions) was diluted out by performing the test on serum diluted 1:200, but now antibodies are absorbed out by mixing the text serum with a 'sorbent' of heated Reiter treponeme culture filtrate or sonicate. This modification is known as the FTA-abs test. It becomes positive very early during the primary stage of the infection, and as with all the *T. pallidum* tests, once positive it remains so for very many years, if not for the patient's entire life. Details of the test are given in Protocol 6. A simple guide to the interpretation of syphilis serology is given in Table 4.

Table 4 Serological tests for syphilis and their interpretation

Test and result			Interpretation[a]
VDRL	TPHA	FTA	
+	−	−	Biological false positive.
+	−	+	Early syphilis.
+	+	+	Most stages of syphilis.
−	+	+	Syphilitic infection at some time.[b]
			Probably old and inactive or adequately treated.

[a] All positive tests should be repeated before establishing a clinical diagnosis.
[b] No test will differentiate between syphilis and the non-venereal treponematoses.

Protocol 6

Absorbed fluorescent treponemal antigen test (FTA-abs)

Equipment and reagents

- Antigen-coated slide
- Coverslip
- PTFE-coated slides (C. A. Hendley Ltd.)
- Serum
- FTA sorbent (Difco Bacto)
- PBS

- Fluorescent conjugate: Wellcome fluorescent anti-human globulin (sheep)
- Mounting fluid
- FTA antigen (Mast Diagnostics Ltd.)
- Methanol

A. Test

1 Dilute patient's inactivated serum and controls used 1 in 5 in FTA sorbent, i.e. 20 μl serum to 80 μl sorbent. The controls will be as follows.

   (a) + + + + reactive control.

   (b) + minimally-reactive control—serum (a) diluted in PBS.

   (c) Non-specific control (to check efficacy of absorption step).

   (d) Sorbent only.

   (e) PBS only.

2 Leave at room temperature for 10 min for absorption to occur.

3 Add 20 μl of diluted serum/controls to each spot on the antigen-coated slide.[a]

4 Incubate for 20 min at 37 °C in a moist chamber.

5 Rinse the slide with PBS using a wash bottle, diverting the jet from the spots and then immerse in PBS in a Coplin stain jar for 10 min, agitating from time to time.

6 Rinse in distilled water and allow to air dry (do not heat).

7 Add 20 μl of fluorescent conjugate (sheep anti-human globulin) and incubate for 30 min at 37 °C in a moist chamber. Do not refreeze conjugate or store for more than six months.

8 Repeat steps 5 and 6.

9 Mount the slide using Difco Bacto FA mounting fluid and a 70 × 20 mm coverslip.

10 Read as soon as possible (if not, store in dark) using non-fluorescent immersion oil and ×100 objective, preferably using incident light, an interference filter (DS500), and a blue barrier filter (LP515).

11 Controls (c)–(d) should not have any visible fluorescence. If the patient's serum exhibits fluorescence equal to the + control, report as positive, but if the fluorescence is less from the + control, report as negative.

B. Preparation of FTA-abs slides

1 Use slides with the antigen already deposited or prepare in the laboratory by soaking at least 20 PTFE-coated slides in 70% methanol, followed by polishing with lens tissue.

2 Reconstitute the FTA antigen. Draw up into a pipette at least 10 times to break up clumps of treponemes.

3 Dispense 10 μl of the antigen on to each test spot on the slide, air dry for 15 min.

4 Immediately fix in acetone for 10 min (no more than 60 slides/200 ml).

5 Allow acetone to evaporate and use slides immediately or pack in aluminium foil at −20 °C.

C. Titration of anti-human conjugates

1 Dilute 200 μl of reconstituted conjugate two-fold serially in PBS from neat to at least three dilutions beyond the stated titre.

2 Test each conjugate dilution against a ++++ positive, + positive, and PBS only control using the procedure in part A.

3 The working dilution is half the weakest dilution that gives strong fluorescence with the ++++ positive and weak fluorescence with the + positive. Treponemes in the PBS control area should not be stained by the 1 : 20 dilution of conjugate.

[a] Most slides have six spots, so one slide will hold all of the serum/controls for one patient.

In early (primary) infection serological screening tests may be negative so it is important that specific anti-treponemal IgM tests, usually an EIA, should be performed. FTA-abs tests are more difficult to perform than the TPHA and are tedious to read in more than small numbers. For these reasons the test is usually reserved for problem sera where the TPHA and VDRL give discordant results. The test can also be made specific for IgG and for IgM classes of anti-treponemal antibody by using immunoglobulin class-specific antisera. Unfortunately, excess IgG will tend to block any IgM in serum, so the tests must be carried out on fractionated sera if reliable results are to be obtained. There are indications that the presence of anti-treponemal IgM is associated with activity of the disease and that only IgG antibodies remain after cure, but this information is not needed in the assessment of adult syphilis. In untreated late infection specific IgM tests may be negative. However, serum fractionation is of great importance in the assessment of congenital syphilis in infants.

5.1.5 Syphilis serology and HIV infection

Although most HIV-infected individuals co-infected with *T. pallidum* respond normally in serological tests a number of variations have been described. They mainly relate to low absolute CD4 cell counts, with negative serological tests but a confirmed diagnosis of syphilis because of the presence of *T. pallidum* in material from lesions (24).

5.2 Serological diagnosis of chlamydial infections

In most cases of infection, either EIA (Section 3.2), direct immunofluorescence (Section 3.1.3), or PCR (Section 6) will be used; however, high levels of genus-specific antibodies are found in systemic chlamydial infections, especially in Lymphogranuloma Venereum (LGV), and psittacosis. These are detected by the complement fixation test. Only very low levels of antibodies are produced in response to mucosal infections by the oculo-genital strains. The test is performed using heated yolk sac (lipopolysaccharide) antigen and is conveniently carried out at the same time as other CFTs are being performed in the laboratory (Chapter 3, Section 3.4.2) by the method of Bradstreet and Taylor (31). It will be positive in patients who are suffering from systemic *Chlamydia trachomatis* infections (such as PID) caused by oculo-genital strains, and will also react in infections with *C. psittaci*, but it will not detect genital mucosal infections.

The micro-immunofluorescence test (32) is usually performed using pools of mixed antigen consisting of elementary bodies from the various serotypes of *C. trachomatis* (33). The egg-grown antigens are spotted on to holes in Teflon-coated glass slides, fixed, and then exposed to dilutions of patient's sera before staining with fluorescein-conjugated anti-human globulin and examining under a fluorescence microscope. Antibodies detected by this method can result from mucosal infections but will persist for long periods, making it difficult to distinguish between past and current infection (34). However, rising titres, and particularly high levels may be helpful in diagnosing systemic infection, especially if the sites concerned are inaccessible or if prior antibiotic treatment has rendered direct methods inappropriate. Detection of high levels of antibody in an infertile woman will suggest that her infertility may be due to previous chlamydial salpingitis. Specific IgM antibodies can be detected in neonatal chlamydial pneumonitis.

A number of tests for the detection of chlamydial antibodies by EIA have been described. They do however only detect genus-specific antibodies and are less sensitive than the MIF test (15).

6 Molecular methods

6.1 *Chlamydia trachomatis*

Because of the exquisite sensitivity combined with the considerable specificity the introduction of nucleic acid amplification techniques (NAAT) for the diagnosis of *C. trachomatis* infections has had a major impact on this diagnostic area.

The first commercially available NAAT was PCR based and developed by Roche Diagnostics (Amplicor) and became available in 1993. It has been extensively evaluated and has proved to be more sensitive than culture or serological diagnosis (Figure 1). NAAT can also be applied to first pass urine specimens as well as endocervical and urethral swabs making screening easy. The Ligase Chain Reaction (LCX, Abbott) and Strand Displacement Assay (BD ProbeTec ET, Becton Dickinson) have been widely used. LCX is no longer available. The principles and performance of these tests have been reviewed in detail elsewhere (35) and details of tests, which can also use automated platforms, will not be given here the reader being referred to the manufacturer's literature. The performance of the three test systems is largely similar as shown in a recent comparison and choice comes down to practicality and costs (36).

6.2 *Neisseria gonorrhoeae*

As with the diagnosis of *C. trachomatis* the sensitivity of NAAT compared to culture is considered superior (36). All three major NAAT systems include primers for the diagnosis of *N. gonorrhoeae* infection and give excellent performance, although not all laboratories can fund the increased cost and they are not commonly used in the UK.

6.3 *Treponema pallidum*

Although the first PCR for *T. pallidum* detection was described in 1991, they have not been widely used due to lack of sensitivity, inhibition, and contamination (24). PCR is valuable in congenital syphilis and could be useful in neuro syphilis and identifying new infections. A PCR based on the DNA polymerase I gene (*polA*) of *T. pallidum* has been described and when amplimer was detected with the ABI Prism Genetic Analyzer the detection limit was of the order of a single organism (37). This test may well be of utility in reference laboratories.

7 Antibiotic susceptibility testing

7.1 Antibiotic susceptibility testing of *N. gonorrhoeae*

In the treatment of gonorrhoea a single dose of antibiotic is often given at the patient's first visit to the clinic or the doctor and before the results of any susceptibility testing is known. It is, therefore, important that the levels of resistance in the population are known so that an antibiotic can be chosen that will give a high chance (>95%) of therapeutic success. This is most effectively achieved by surveillance programmes but can also be informed by sentinel studies at different geographical sites. A number of surveillance programmes exist, for example, Gonococcal Resistance to Antimicrobials Surveillance Programme (GRASP) in the UK and Gonococcal Isolate Surveillance Programme (GISP) in the USA. These programmes test a sample of gonococcal isolates each year, determine their susceptibility to a range of antimicrobial agents, and compare trends of resistance on an annual basis. Resistance is usually detected by determining the minimum inhibitory concentration and is performed in reference centres. If resistance to the antibiotic of choice is above 5% of isolates it is advisable to consider changing the first-line therapy.

It is also necessary, however, to detect resistance to the antimicrobial agent used for therapy and in most laboratories routine testing of all isolates of *N. gonorrhoeae* is performed. In particular it is advisable to test for high level resistance to penicillin and ciprofloxacin which are the agents most commonly used in the UK. The detection of penicillinase can be quickly and easily achieved using the chromogenic cephalosporin, Nitrocefin (Oxoid). The yellow reagent is spotted onto filter paper and then a small sweep of colonies is rubbed onto the filter paper using a disposable loop or wooden stick. If penicillinase is produced the colour turns from yellow to pink/red within a few seconds. There are alternative methods, such as iodometric or acidometric tests, but these are used infrequently for detecting penicillinase-producing *N. gonorrhoeae*.

Most laboratories will use inhibition around antibiotic-containing discs as the method of choice for detecting other types of resistance. Standard methodology has been described by the British Society of Antimicrobial Chemotherapy (BSAC) in the UK (40) and by the National Committee for Control of Laboratory Standards (NCCLS) in the USA. Care should be taken when performing disc testing as the breakpoints between sensitivity and resistance is dependent on the medium, disc content, and inoculum used. A simple alternative is to use an agar plate containing a single concentration of antibiotic which can be used as a breakpoint for resistance. For example: resistance to ciprofloxacin can be detected by growth on agar containing 0.5 mg ciprofloxacin (MIC ≥ 1.0 mg/litre).

7.2 Antibiotic susceptibility testing of other pathogens

General details of testing of other bacteria will be found in Chapter 7, Section 2.2.1. The testing of staphylococci and streptococci, anaerobic bacteria, and coliforms is detailed in Chapter 5, Sections 4.1.5, 3.4, and 5.1.6 respectively. Appropriate antibiotics to test against isolates of *Listeria monocytogenes* are benzylpenicillin, ampicillin, gentamicin, erythromycin, and tetracycline.

Acknowledgement

We are grateful to Dr Hugh Young, University of Edinburgh Medical School for helpful comments on the diagnosis of syphilis.

References

1. Hill, G. B., Eschenbach, D. A., and Holmes, K. K. (1984). *Scand. J. Urol. Nephrol.,* Suppl. **86**, 23.
2. Goidacre, M. J., Watt, B., Loudon, N., Milne, L. J. R., *et al.* (1979). *Br. Med. J.,* **1**, 1450.
3. Masfari, A. N., Duerden, B. I., and Kinghorn, G. R. (1986). *Genitourin. Med.,* **62**, 256.
4. Evans, E. G. V. and Richardson, M. D. (ed.) (1989). *Medical mycology: a practical approach.* IRL Press, Oxford.
5. Teberg, A. J., Yonelcura, M. L., Salminen, C., and Paylova, Z. (1987). *Pediatr. Infect. Dis. J.,* **6**, 817.
6. Taylor, E., Blackwell, A. L., Barlow, D., and Phillips, I. (1982). *Lancet,* **1**, 1376.

7. Ison, C. A., Dawson, S. G., Hilton, J., Csonka, G. W., *et al.* (1982). *J. Clin. Pathol.*, **35**, 550.

8. Platt, R., Lin, J. S. L., Warren, J. W., Rosner, B., *et al.* (1980). *Lancet*, **2**, 1217.

9. Hare, M. J. (1986). *Br. Med. J.*, **239**, 1225.

10. Barlow, D. and Phillips, I. (1978). *Lancet*, **1**, 761.

11. Burstain, J. M., Grimpel, E., Lukehart, S. A., Norgard, M. V., *et al.* (1991). *J. Clin. Microbiol.*, **29**, 62.

12. Tam, M. R., Stamm, W. E., Handsfield, H. H., Stephens, R., *et al.* (1984). *N. Engl. J. Med.*, **310**, 1146.

13. Thornas, B. J., Evans, R. T., Hawkins, D. A., and Taylor-Robinson, D. (1984). *J. Clin. Pathol.*, **37**, 812.

14. Alexander, I., Paul, I. D., and Caul, E. O. (1985). *Genitourin. Med.*, **61**, 252.

15. Black, C. M. (1997). *Clin. Microbiol. Rev.*, **10**, 160.

16. Martin, J. E. and Lester, A. (1971). *HMSHA Health Reports*, **86**, 30.

17. Martin, J. E., Arrnstrong, J. H., and Smith, P. B. (1974). *Appl. Microbiol.*, **27**, 802.

18. Flynn, J. and Waitkins, S. A. (1972). *J. Clin. Pathol.*, **25**, 525.

19. Young, H., Paterson, I. C., and McDonald, D. R. (1976). *Br. J. Vener. Dis.*, **52**, 172.

20. Ferrieri, P., Cleary, P. P., and Seeds, A. E. (1977). *J. Med. Microbiol.*, **10**, 103.

21. McFaddin, J. F. (1980). In *Biochemical tests for identification of medical bacteria*, p. 18. Williams and Wilkins, Baltimore.

22. Richmond, S. J., Bailey, J. M. G., and Mearns, G. (1985). In *Isolation and identification of microorganisms of medical and veterinary importance* (ed. C. H. Collins and J. M. Grange), SAB Technical Series, Vol. 21, p. 297. Society for Applied Bacteriology, Academic Press, London.

23. Clinical Effectiveness Group of Medical Society for the Study of Venereal Diseases. (2001). *UK National guideline for the management of late syphilis*. www.mssvd.org.uk

24. Larsen, S. A., Steiner, B. M., and Rudolph, A. H. (1995). *Clin. Microbiol. Rev.*, **8**, 1.

25. Michelow, I. C., Wendel, G. D., Norgard, M. V., Zeray, F., *et al.* (2002). *N. Engl. J. Med.*, **346**, 1792.

26. Rathlev, T. (1967). *Br. J. Vener. Dis.*, **43**, 181.

27. Sequeira, P. J. L. and Eldridge, A. E. (1973). *Br. J. Vener. Dis.*, **49**, 242.

28. Pope, V., Fears, M., Morrill, W. E., Castro, A., *et al.* (2000). *J. Clin. Microbiol.*, **38**, 2543.

29. Egglestone, S. I. and Turner, A. J. (2000). *Commun. Dis. Public Health*, **3**, 158.

30. Young, H., Moyes, A., Seagar, L., and McMillan, A. (1998). *J. Clin. Microbiol.*, **3**, 158.

31. Bradstreet, C. M. P. and Taylor, C. E. D. (1962). *Mon. Bull. Minist. Health Public Health Lab. Serv.*, **21**, 96.

32. Wang, S. P. and Grayston, J. T. (1971). In *Trachoma and related disorders, caused by Chlamydial agents* (ed. A. Nicholson), p. 217. Excerpta Medica, Amsterdam.

33. Treharne, J. D., Darougar, S., and Jones, B. R. (1977). *J. Clin. Pathol.*, **30**, 510.

34. Treharne, J. D., Dines, R. J., and Darougar, S. (1977). In *Non-Gonococcal urethritis and related infections* (ed. D. Hobson and K. K. Holmes), p. 249. Public Health Laboratory Service Monograph Series, 1. American Society for Microbiology, Washington DC.

35. Ostergaard, L. (1999). *APMIS*, Suppl. 1, **89**, 5.

36. Van Dyck, E., Ievan, M., Pattyn, S., van Damme, L., *et al.* (2001). *J. Clin. Microbiol.*, **39**, 1751.

37. Liu, H., Rodes, B., Chen, C-Y., and Steiner, B. (2001). *J. Clin. Microbiol.*, **39**, 1941.

38. Wilkinson, A. E., Tumer, G. C., and Ryeroft, J. A. (1972). In *Laboratory diagnosis of venereal disease* (ed. E. Wilkinson, C. E. D. Taylor, D. A. McSwiggan, G. C. Tumer, J. A. Ryeroft, and G. H. Lowe), p. 35. HMSO, London.

39. Jephcott, A. E. (1981). *Investigation of Gonococcal infection*. Association of Clinical Pathologists Broadsheet No. 100, British Medical Association, London.

40. Andrews, J. M. for the BSAC Working Party on Susceptibility testing. (2001). *J. Antimicrob. Chemother.*, Suppl. S1, **48**, 43.

Chapter 5

Bacteriology of superficial and deep tissue infection

Nicola Baker, Ann Bushell,[a] and
Peter M. Hawkey

Birmingham Laboratory, Health Protection Agency, Birmingham
Heartlands Hospital, Birmingham B9 5SS, UK.

1 Introduction

The range and variety of clinical samples seen and microbes grown from these infections is enormous. The approach will be to outline general methods, concentrating on the major pathogens, and then to examine specific techniques appropriate to different sites of infection, with cross-reference to other chapters.

To get the most useful results from these samples it is important to know the *site* (anatomical) and *nature* (primary/secondary, acute/chronic) of the infection. If the sample is of high priority (pus, tissue, and some fluids) then the laboratories must liaise with the clinicians, and expend maximum effort to obtain a microbiological diagnosis. If the sample is of lower priority (most 'wound swabs' fall into this category) then the laboratory may legitimately process the sample in a routine manner. The samples that deserve extra effort are not always immediately apparent, and it is part of the role of the clinical microbiologist to pick them out.

Finally, intelligent and informed interpretation of culture results and appropriate clinical liaison will make all the difference as far as the clinician (and patient) is concerned, between useful and useless laboratory reports.

1.1 Taking good samples

Pus or tissue is always preferable to a swab.

(a) *Pus.* This may be collected in a syringe, and then transferred into a sterile universal container. If the pus is very thick then it can be 'scooped' up or coaxed into a sterile container using a swab.

(b) *Swabs.* These must be well loaded, to saturation if possible. Sometimes duplicate swabs are useful, since one can be used for microscopy and the other for culture.

---

[a] During the preparation of this edition Dr Bushell died.

(c) *Non-discharging lesions* (e.g. cellulitis and early abscesses). These present a problem. Search very carefully for the entry wound and swab this if found. In cellulitis the characteristic clinical picture, together with the results of entry site cultures is often the most useful in selecting therapy. Although blood cultures and fine needle aspiration of the leading edge of lesions may be helpful, their yield is generally low (1).

(d) *Open lesions* (such as varicose, ischaemic, and diabetic ulcers, burns and pressure sores). Swabs taken from the surface of the lesion nearly always sample the surface flora. They yield mixed cultures of bacteria, many of which are surface colonizers of uncertain pathogenicity.

1.2 Transport

Pus, fluids, and tissue should be transported in a suitable sterile container. Swabs may be transported to the laboratory either dry or in transport medium (see Figure 1). The latter is preferable unless there is minimal delay in performing culture. Many types of transport medium are available commercially: they can be obtained in bijoux bottles into which a swab is broken off, or pre-packed in a plastic tube accompanied by a swab in a sterile pack. Swabs are available with a range of swab tips (cotton–wool, Dacron), shafts (wood, plastic), and transport media (Amies, Stuarts, and with or without charcoal).

The commercially prepared packs are the most convenient and widely used systems. It is up to the individual laboratory to determine which type of swab is most appropriate. Some of the plastic-shafted swabs can be very flexible and therefore difficult to use. Some transport media may show a tendency to 'pull out' of the tube when the swab is withdrawn in the laboratory.

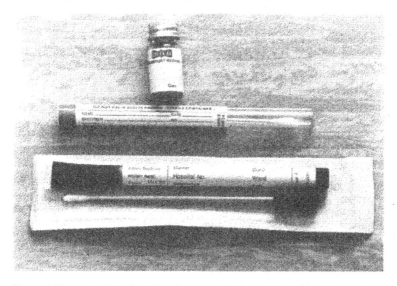

Figure 1 Two examples of swab and transport systems.

1.2.1 Transport medium for anaerobic bacteria

The common pathogenic anaerobes, such as *Clostridium perfringens* and the *Bacteroides fragilis* group are remarkably tolerant, and will survive well within pus, fluid, tissue, or swabs in good quality solid transport medium (2).

More exacting anaerobes, such as *Fusobacterium* spp., will also survive well in specimens, and providing they can be cultured within several hours, no special attention to transport is usually necessary. It should, however, be recommended that pus and fluids fill the container in which they are transported to minimize the exposure to air.

Fastidious anaerobes will not survive for long on a swab in ordinary transport medium. However, for routine swabs the use of a single transport system for the isolation of both aerobic and anaerobic organisms is most practical and cost-effective.

2 General methods

2.1 Pus

2.1.1 Macroscopic examination

The following characteristics should be noted:

(a) Colour—pyocyanin and other pigments, blood staining.

(b) Consistency—thin and watery or thick and purulent.

(c) Smell—many anaerobes have a foul odour.

(d) Presence of granules—actinomycosis.

(e) Fluorescence in long wave ultraviolet light—*Prevotella melaninogenica*, *Porphyromonas* spp. (usually only useful on pus from brain or lung abscess).

2.1.2 Microscopic examination

The commonest problem with making films is that the material tends to float or lift off the slide during staining. The following tips may help:

(a) Gently warm the slide first.

(b) Use a swab rather than a loop to apply the material.

(c) Keep the smear thin.

Once the material is on the slide, it should be allowed to dry, and heat fixed. A Gram stain must always be performed on pus. If no organisms are seen then a Ziehl–Neelsen (ZN) stain to detect mycobacteria should be considered. Mycobacteria may stain as weakly Gram-positive beaded bacilli. If clostridia are seen, then a spore stain (Appendix I) may be useful as spores may be more readily produced in pus than on culture.

The stain results should be telephoned to the clinician if:

(a) The pus is from a clinically important site (brain, lung, liver).

(b) The appearance of the organisms is diagnostic (staphylococci, streptococci, clostridia).

(c) Unusual organisms such as mycobacteria, actinomyces, or fungi are seen.

2.1.3 Direct methods for detecting bacteria

Methods for the direct detection of bacterial antigens have been described for a number of organisms, and are described in more detail in Chapter 2. However, the large range of possible pathogens in superficial or deep tissue infections makes these methods more difficult to apply than in meningitis, pneumonia, tonsillitis, or septicaemia.

In recent years the use of nucleic acid tests for the direct detection and identification of bacteria has shown increasing promise. Polymerase chain reaction (PCR) methods have been used to amplify the 16S ribosomal RNA gene. The gene sequences obtained can be used to identify bacterial pathogens using a large database. The approach has been shown to be useful in the diagnosis of a number of conditions including endophthalmitis, bacteraemia, and diabetic foot ulcers (3–5). Commercial kits for the identification of bacterial and fungal 16S rRNA gene sequences are available from PE Applied Biosystems. At the time of writing these kits have yet to be validated for routine clinical diagnostic use. However, they are likely to prove valuable in the future, particularly in the diagnosis of organisms that are difficult to culture.

2.1.4 Culture

A general description of the culture of pus is given below. See Section 3.2 and Protocol 1 for the full details of anaerobic culture which are necessary for the accurate diagnosis of anaerobic infections in samples from cerebral, lung, or liver abscesses. Methods for the culture of mycobacteria can be found in Chapter 3. Clinical information or microscopy of the pus may indicate whether any other special media are necessary.

(a) Using a sterile swab or loop to sample the specimen, inoculate the following media: blood agar (aerobic), blood agar (anaerobic, enriched if possible), selective blood agar (e.g. neomycin), MacConkey or CLED, enrichment broth (e.g. Robertson's cooked meat). Then follow the scheme outlined in Table 1.

(b) If organisms are seen on the Gram film, then 14 days incubation with terminal subculture of broth is needed before all the plates are discarded. If no organisms are seen, think again about unusual organisms such as mycobacteria, fungi, and actinomyces. Occasionally, bacteria seen on a Gram film fail to grow due to the presence of antimicrobial substances (usually antibiotics). The effect can be detected by applying a filter paper disc soaked in the pus to a lawn of *Staphylococcus aureus* and observing whether there is any inhibition of growth.

Table 1 Culture scheme for pus

Media	Atmosphere	Length of incubation (h)
1. Blood agar	Air or air + 5% CO_2	24
2. MacConkey or CLED agar	Air or air + 5% CO_2	24
3. Blood agar	Anaerobic	24
4. Enriched blood agar (with growth supplements for anaerobes—see Section 3.2)	Anaerobic	48
5. 'Selective' blood agar, e.g. neomycin blood agar plus metronidazole disc (Section 3.2)	Anaerobic	48
6. Anaerobic recovery broth, e.g. Robertson's cooked meat, Fastidious anaerobic broth (Lab M Ltd.)	Air or air + 5% CO_2	24

(c) If bacteria have grown on the culture plates, proceed to identify and carry out sensitivity testing, as described in the appropriate section according to the site of the infection. Even when there is good growth of bacteria on the 24 hour plates it is advisable to subculture the broth culture to ensure better recovery of anaerobes.

2.2 Swabs

Wound swabs are by far the commonest type of specimen received from soft tissue infections, and most laboratories receive large numbers every day. Because of this, and also because they are repeatable specimens and rarely come from life-threatening infections, culture methods are shorter and often less detailed than for samples of pus, fluid, or tissue.

2.2.1 Microscopic examination

Microscopy takes second place to culture unless more than one swab is received from the same site. Only a Gram stain is performed. Swabs are not suitable for examination for mycobacteria except in exceptional circumstances, since all the available material should be used for culture. In many hospital laboratories in the UK routine examination of films from swabs is not carried out.

2.2.2 Culture

Swabs should be cultured as outlined in Table 2. Any bacterial growth is dealt with as described in Sections 4–10 of this chapter, according to the site of infection.

Table 2 Culture scheme for routine clinical specimens (e.g. wound swabs)

Media	Atmosphere	Length of incubation (h)
1. Blood agar	Air or air + 5% CO_2	24
2. MacConkey or CLED agar	Air or air + 5% CO_2	24
3. Blood agar	Anaerobic	48
4. 'Selective' blood agar (e.g. neomycin) plus metronidazole disc plus (optional)	Anaerobic	48
5. Recovery broth (e.g. Robertson's cooked meat, BHI)	Aerobic	24 then subculture to media 1, 2, 3

2.3 Fluids

The general principles for dealing with a fluid sample are described here. The special processing methods needed for bile are covered in Section 5.4. Chapter 2 describes methods for cerebrospinal fluid, joint fluid, and peritoneal fluid.

2.3.1 Microscopic examination

(a) Provided there is sufficient volume, centrifuge the sample for 10 min at 1800 g.

(b) Remove all but 0.5 ml of the supernatant; resuspend the deposit in this and make a smear on a slide using a sterile loop or swab.

(c) Stain with Gram's stain. If no organisms are seen, consider a ZN stain if the clinical details warrant.

(d) Telephone a positive Gram stain result to the clinician.

2.3.2 Culture

The spun deposit is cultured in the same way as pus (Table 1). Bile fluid may need to be cultured for enteric pathogens; see Section 5.4.

2.4 Tissue

2.4.1 Microscopic examination

The tissue should be examined for the evidence of pus, and these areas sampled for microscopy, for which three methods are available:

(a) Press a freshly cut surface of the tissue firmly against a sterile slide. Stain the resulting imprint.

(b) Section—a histopathology section can be cut and stained.

(c) Ground smear—smear ground or crushed tissue on to a slide, and then stain.

2.4.2 Culture

Processing in containment level 3 facilities is recommended to protect the operator from the risk of aerosol infection.

Tissue which is likely to be contaminated, such as samples from superficial lesions or those taken *post mortem* must be washed in distilled water before being ground up for culture.

(a) Place a piece of tissue in a sterile container, add 5 ml of peptone water, and shake vigorously.

(b) With sterile forceps transfer the tissue to a fresh container and repeat the washing process twice.

(c) Keep the final peptone water washings for culture. The tissue is now ready for grinding.

Uncontaminated tissue can be ground up without washing.

(a) With a sterile scalpel blade cut the piece of tissue into 2–3 mm chunks in the lid of a sterile Petri dish.

(b) Then grind up the tissue with 1 ml peptone water.

Tissue (and washings) are cultured in the same way as pus (Table 1). Additional anaerobic techniques as described in Section 3.2 may be appropriate (for example for tissue from myonecrosis).

The micro-organisms found in tissue are usually present in smaller numbers than in pus and may be more 'unusual' and difficult to grow. For these reasons, the culture of tissue may need to be prolonged. Relevant information must be obtained from the clinician before culture is undertaken. The additional culture media necessary depends to a great extent on the source and nature of the tissue. This is discussed in more detail in Sections 4–10.

3 Anaerobic methods

3.1 Gas–liquid chromatography (GLC)

GLC is used to detect anaerobic bacteria in clinical material, and more commonly to identify them when cultured. The fermentation of carbohydrates by anaerobes results in the formation of volatile and non-volatile fatty acids (VFAs and NVFAs). These can be detected, after extraction, by GLC.

The relative types and amounts of fatty acids produced varies with both the genus and species of bacteria (Figure 2). The identification of bacteria based on these metabolic pathways is valid because they represent genetically conserved traits.

The extracted volatile components of the sample are carried along with a flow of specially prepared heated gas, through a long column of material that differentially slows down the flow of components based on their size and polarity. As the

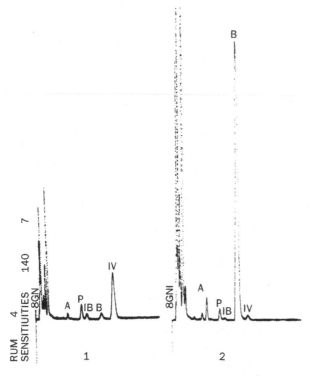

Figure 2 GLC trace using headspace analysis of two species of Gram-negative anaerobic bacteria. The bacteria were grown in FAB and the analysis was performed on a Perkin-Elmer Sigma 36/Sigma 15 machine with an HS6 headspace unit. The column was a 1/8″ × 6′ stainless steel column packed with 10% SP1000/1% H_3PO_4 on Chromosorb WHP 100/120 mesh. Trace 1 is *Bacteroides fragilis* and trace 2 is *Fusobacterium nucleatum*. Metabolic product abbreviations are as follows: IV, iso-valeric acid; B, butyric acid; IB, iso-butyric acid; P, propionic acid; A, acetic acid. (Courtesy of Dr P. G. R. Godwin, University of Leeds.)

components reach the end of the column they are detected by either a temperature change (thermal conductivity detector) or a change in ionization potential (hydrogen flame ionization detector), which are plotted on a chart recorder as a series of peaks. The peaks are identified by comparison with those obtained from known standards.

Gas chromatographs are available from a number of manufacturers (Pye-Unicam, Varian, Perkin-Elmer). The newest machines use microprocessor controls to stop and start the analysis, control the baseline, and to identify and quantify the peaks. Machines which undertake headspace gas analysis reduce the time spent on sample preparation.

Anaerobes are present in a clinical sample if the trace shows any VFA other than acetic acid. If only acetic acid is present then this could be due to facultative anaerobes such as *Escherichia coli* or *Staphylococcus aureus*. An NVFA trace may then be helpful: if more than lactic or succinic acid are detected then anaerobes are present. Enterobacteriaceae produce lactic and succinic acid, and so the detection of these two products alone is insufficient.

GLC is primarily used as a reference laboratory technique, and so a detailed description of the process is not indicated here. Further information may be found elsewhere (6, 7).

3.2 Culture of anaerobes

Clinical microbiology laboratories should be able to grow and presumptively identify the obligate anaerobes that are commonly associated with human infection. Obligate anaerobes do not use molecular oxygen and their growth is inhibited by it. The amount of oxygen they will tolerate varies from species to species, but most human pathogens (as opposed to commensals) are moderate anaerobes which tolerate 2–8% oxygen and exposure to air for a short time (8). Strict anaerobes, which are inhibited by more than 0.5% oxygen, are found amongst the indigenous flora but are rarely isolated as pathogens. Clinical laboratories must therefore direct their time to the culture of moderate anaerobes particularly the *Bacteroides fragilis* group and *Clostridium perfringens*. The key to successful anaerobic culture is the attainment of an atmosphere with no more than trace amounts of oxygen. The use of reducing agents such as thioglycollate, cysteine, and ferrous sulfide in media also enhances growth. Reducing agents have two effects: they lower the redox potential (Eh) and they remove oxygen from the medium.

3.2.1 Culture media

Three types of freshly prepared or pre-reduced media are necessary and should be used routinely for best results. Solid media should be incubated anaerobically, undisturbed for 48 hours. Liquid media can be subcultured after 24 hours incubation. A recommended culture media scheme is given in Protocol 1.

Protocol 1

Anaerobic culture scheme for specimens from serious infections, e.g. pus and tissue from brain, lung, and liver abscesses, myonecrosis and related infections

Equipment and reagents

- Enriched blood agar
- Selective blood agar
- Metronidazole disc
- Re-reduced cooked meat broth or fastidious anaerobic broth (FAB, Lab M Ltd.)

Method

1 Inoculate on to enriched blood agar. Incubate for 48 h and re-incubate for a further five days if there is no growth.

Protocol 1 continued

2 Inoculate on to selective blood agar+metronidazole disc. Incubate for 48 h and re-incubate for a further five days if there is no growth.

3 Inoculate in to re-reduced cooked meat broth or fastidious anaerobic broth. Incubate anaerobically for 48 h then subculture on to:
   (a) Blood agar. Incubate for 48 h aerobically.
   (b) Enriched blood agar. Incubate anaerobically for 48 h.
   (c) Selective blood agar. Incubate anaerobically for 48 h.

4 Re-incubate the broth for a further five days and subculture again if there is no growth.

5 Specimens from myonecrosis, gangrene, etc., also put up a Nagler plate for the identification of *Clostridia* spp. (see Protocol 4 for details).

(a) *Non-selective media.* A good quality blood agar, such as columbia agar base with 5–10% horse blood, supplemented with 5 mg/litre haemin and 1 mg/litre vitamin K, is recommended. Many other agar bases are suitable, for example fastidious anaerobic agar (Protocol 1).

(b) *Selective media.* This is necessary to avoid missing small numbers of anaerobes in mixed aerobic/anaerobic infections. The selective agent can be incorporated in blood agar or in an enriched blood agar. Selection is achieved by adding antibiotics which inhibit aerobes, especially Gram-negative bacilli. The most popular in the UK is neomycin, but gentamicin and nalidixic acid are acceptable. Kanamycin may not be sufficiently selective. Almost all obligate anaerobes are sensitive to metronidazole, and all aerobes are resistant, and so this property can be used to facilitate the detection of anaerobes in a mixed culture. Place a 5 mg metronidazole disc on the 'well' of the inoculum on either the selective or non-selective agar. The selective plate often gives the clearest results.

(c) *Liquid enrichment media.* Robertson's cooked meat broth and enriched thioglycollate broth are commonly used for enrichment culture. They may be supplemented with vitamin K and haemin and pre-reduced before use either by holding in an anaerobic atmosphere, or by steaming/heating in a boiling water-bath for 15 minutes to drive off oxygen. In practice few laboratories do this, and the broths may thus not support the growth of strict anaerobes. Fastidious anaerobe broth is an excellent recovery and enrichment broth (9). Broths should be routinely incubated for 24 hours, preferably in an anaerobic atmosphere with a loosened cap, and then subcultured aerobically and anaerobically.

3.2.2 Anaerobic incubation

(a) *Anaerobic jars.* These are made of plastic or metal with an air-tight clamped lid. The metal jars have two valved vents in their lid. The oxygen in the jar

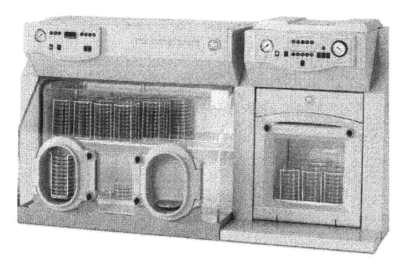

Figure 3 Anaerobic cabinet illustrating the airlock facility. (Model MG500, courtesy of Don Whiteley Scientific.)

may be removed by two methods. Evacuation systems are rarely used now. Gas generator systems (Gas Pak, Beckton-Dickinson; Gas Kit, Don Whitley; Gas Generating Kit, Oxoid Ltd.) are simple, quick, reliable, and ideal for small scale use. They consist of a transparent plastic jar, and work by the production of H_2 and CO_2 following the addition of water to sodium borohydride and sodium citrate. H_2 combines with O_2 in the presence of a catalyst to form water (see Protocol 2 for the method of use). CO_2 is necessary for the growth of most anaerobes.

(b) *Anaerobic cabinets.* For larger laboratories with many anaerobic cultures, stringent anaerobic conditions may be obtained using an anaerobic cabinet (Figure 3). These are air-tight, transparent walled incubator chambers fitted with gloved ports and an air-lock loading port for culture plates. Modern cabinets evacuate and refill with anaerobic gas (10% H_2, 5% CO_2, 85% N_2) automatically. They are designed for work to be done inside them, and allow for the inspection of anaerobic plates at any time without exposing them to the air. This is particularly useful when slow growing anaerobes such as *Prevotella* spp. are sought in pus specimens. Working inside the cabinet, however, requires a certain amount of practice and is unpleasant for long periods of time.

Protocol 2

Procedure for the use of a gas generator system

Equipment and reagents

- Gas generator system

Method

1 Renew the catalyst in the lid of the jar.

2 Load the jar with plates.

3 Open an indicator sachet (a paper strip impregnated with methylene blue); this turns colourless (white) when reduced, which takes 6 h. Place the strip so that it is visible from the outside.

4 Cut off the corner of the gas generator (a foil envelope) and add 10 ml of tap-water with a syringe.

5 Put the generator in the jar and clamp down the lid. Place the jar in the incubator.

6 Check after 30 min that the generator is working and the jar is air-tight, i.e. condensation on the inside of the jar and the lid feels slightly warm to touch.

7 Check the incubator strip at 6 h or before the jar is opened.

3.3 Identification of anaerobes

Only a small number of organisms or groups of organisms account for the majority of anaerobes isolated from clinically significant infections. These include; the *Bacteroides fragilis* group, the pigmented *Prevotella–Porphyromonas* group, *Fusobacterium* spp., *Peptostreptococcus* group, *Costridium perfringens*, and *Clostridium ramosum*.

In routine laboratories the extent of anaerobic identification will be limited based on the clinical relevance and level of capability. Presumptive identification based on a Gram stain and sensitivity to metronidazole is usually sufficient (10). This is particularly true for specimens which contain mixed anaerobic flora, such as those from wounds related to gastrointestinal or gynaecological surgery. Isolates from blood cultures and other normally sterile sites require further identification. In these situations it is advisable for laboratories without expertise to send isolates to reference laboratories.

It is not within the scope of this book to write a comprehensive guide to the identification of anaerobes and readers are referred elsewhere for further details (6, 7, 11).

A brief account follows of some of the methods that may be used.

The first step in identification is to ensure that the isolate is an obligate anaerobe. All isolates sensitive to a 5 μg disc can be assumed to be anaerobes, but the isolate should also be subcultured on to a blood agar plate and incubated in air + 5% CO_2 for 48 hours to confirm that it is not capable of aerobic growth.

3.3.1 Microscopic morphology

Perform Gram stains of both solid and liquid cultures of the isolates if possible. Note the Gram reaction, cell morphology, and presence/absence of spores.

Clostridia and peptostreptococci, especially in old cultures, over decolorize very easily and so appear to be Gram-negative. In the case of clostridia, cell shape and often the presence of spores makes misidentification unlikely. Cell morphology can be a helpful aid to identification at genus level. *Bacteroides* spp. are notably very pleomorphic, irregularly staining, parallel sided Gram-negative bacilli; *Fusobacterium* spp. have slightly swollen middles and tapering ends, but may also be pleomorphic. Actinomyces are branching Gram-positive bacilli.

Spores show as unstained areas on the Gram stain, but occasionally a spore stain may be helpful (Appendix I). The shape and position of the spores should be noted. *Clostridium perfringens* rarely forms spores in culture and this is a helpful 'negative' finding.

3.3.2 Colonial morphology

Note the size, pigmentation, shape, and edge of the colony, any swarming and haemolysis on blood agar.

Many anaerobes may be presumptively identified on the basis of their colonial and microscopic morphology:

(a) *Prevotella melaninogenica* and *Porphyromonas* spp.—black colonies of Gram-negative bacilli, fluoresce brick red in long wave UV light.

(b) *Bacteroides ureolyticus*—pitting of blood agar.

(c) *Clostridium perfringens*—typical double zone haemolysis, no spores.

(d) *Clostridium tetani*—fine swarming growth, drumstick bacilli (terminal spores).

3.3.3 Further identification tests

Laboratories should be able to identify those anaerobic bacteria common in human disease, particularly *Bacteroides fragilis* and *Clostridium perfringens*. A suggested scheme for the basic identification of some of the commoner anaerobic Gram-negative and Gram-positive rods is detailed in Protocol 3 and Figures 4 and 5.

Protocol 3

Methods for the identification of common anaerobic Gram-positive and Gram-negative rods

Equipment and reagents

- Petri dishes
- Coverslips
- Bacteroides bile aesculin agar (BBE)
- Thioglycollate broth
- Oxgall

- Blood agar plate
- Kanamycin and vancomycin discs
- Indole reagent: 1% *p*-dimethylaminocinnamaldehyde in 10% HCl
- Urease broth (Difco laboratories)

Protocol 3 continued

- H_2O_2
- Hitrate broth medium
- 1% HCl
- 0.2% sulfaniliamide
- 0.1% N-naphthylethylenediamine hydrochloride

Use a pure culture. Note the Gram stain and colonial morphology, and carry out the following tests as indicated, using Figures 4 and 5 to identify the organism.

A. Bile sensitivity

1 Anaerobes vary in their ability to grow in the presence of 20% bile.

2 Subculture isolates on to bacteroides bile aesculin agar (BBE), or into thioglycollate broth with and without the addition of 2% oxgall.

3 Incubate anaerobically for 48 h.

4 The *B. fragilis* group is bile tolerant and so will grow well in bile-containing media.

B. Susceptibility to antibiotics

1 Subculture isolates to an anaerobic blood agar plate.

2 Add kanamycin (1000 μg) and vancomycin (5 μg) discs to the plate.

3 Record sensitivities after 48 h incubation.

C. Spot indole

1 Soak a filter paper in the bottom of a Petri dish with indole reagent (1% *p*-dimethylaminocinnamaldehyde in 10% HCl).

2 Using a stick or loop rub a portion of the colony on the filter paper.

3 Rapid development of a blue colour indicates a positive test, whilst a pink colour is negative.

D. Urease test

1 Incoulate a urease broth with a heavy incoulum of the isolate.

2 Incubate aerobically for up to 4 h.

3 A positive result is indicated by the development of a bright pink/red colour.

4 A disc test is also available.

E. Catalase

1 Place a drop of 3% H_2O_2 on a glass slide.

2 Touch a colony of the isolate with the edge of a glass slide.

3 Lower the coverslip on to the slide with the colony side down.

4 Observe for the evolution of bubbles which indicates a positive test.

Protocol 3 continued

F. Nitrate reduction

1 Inoculate a nitrate broth medium and incubate overnight.

2 Acidify with a few drops of 1% HCl, and add 0.5 ml each of 0.2% sulfaniliamide and 0.1% N-naphthylethylenediamine hydrochloride.

3 A pink colour denotes nitratase activity, but some organisms further reduce nitrite. If no colour is produced add a small amount of zinc dust.

4 Any nitrate present will be reduced to nitrite, producing a pink colour, i.e. a pink colour here indicates a negative test with no nitratase activity, and no colour indicates that the nitrates have been completely reduced.

5 A disc test is also available.

Km = Kanamycin, Vm = Vancomycin
S = susceptible (zone > 10 mm), R = resistant (zone < 10 mm)

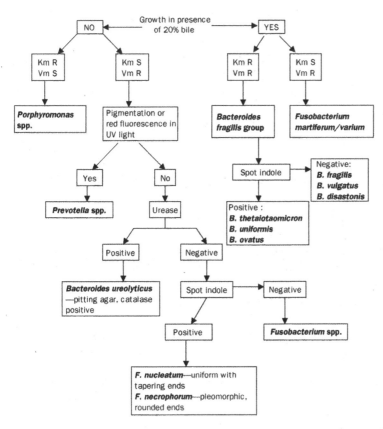

Figure 4 Simplified scheme for the identification of anaerobic Gram-negative bacilli (adapted from ref. 12).

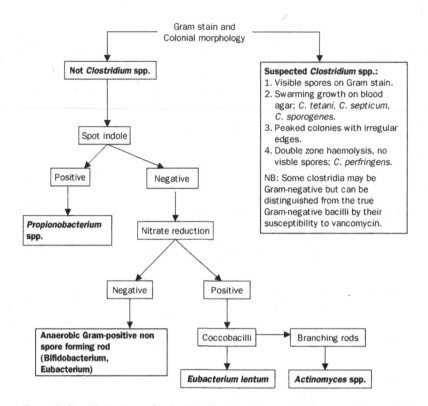

Figure 5 Simplified scheme for the identification of anaerobic Gram-positive bacilli (adapted from ref. 12).

Clostridia should be speciated as much as possible in order to distinguish those which are pathogenic in wounds, i.e. *Clostridium perfringens*, *C. tetani*, *C. noyvi A*, *C. septicum*, *C. histolyticum*, *C. bifermentans*, *C. ramosum*, from those that are not. A scheme for the identification of *Clostridium* spp. is shown in Protocol 4 and Table 3. In practice most laboratories identify isolates using commercial kits as described in Section 3.3.4. *Clostridium botulinum* is rarely encountered as a wound pathogen and is not discussed further here. *C. tetani* has such characteristic fine swarming growth and drumstick appearance on Gram stain, that it is rarely misidentified. The diagnosis of tetanus, however is clinical and should not rely on isolation of the organism.

The reverse CAMP test may be used in some laboratories as an alternative to the Nagler test for the identification of *C. perfringens*. Details on how to perform the test are given in more detail elsewhere (14).

An agar plate system has been developed by the CDC Anaerobic Laboratory for the identification of anaerobic bacteria. The system uses three quadrant plates—Presumpto plates I, II, and III—each containing various different substrates incorporated into Lombard–Dowell agar. The method is reviewed in more detail elsewhere (13).

Table 3 Identification of clostridia (adapted from refs 14 and 15)

Organism	Sugar fermentation				Gelatinase	Urease	Indole	Nagler	Lipase	Spores
	Glucose	Maltose	Lactose	Sucrose						
C. perfringens[a]	+	+	+	+	+	−	−	+	−	Rare, terminal
C. septicum	+	+	+	−	+	−	−	−	−	Oval, subterminal
C. noyvii (A)	+	+	−	−	+	−	−	+	+	Oval, subterminal
C. bifetmetans	+	+	−	−	+	−	+	+	−	Variable
C. sordellii	+	+	−	−	+	+	+	+	−	Variable
C. sporogenes	+	+	−	−	+	−	−	−	+	Oval, subterminal
C. histolyticum[b]	−	−	−	−	+	+	−	−	−	Oval, subterminal
C. tetani	−	−	−	−	+	−	−	−	−	Round, terminal
C. ramosum[a]	+	+	+	+	−	−	−	−	−	Rare, terminal
C. tertium[b]	+	+	+	+	−	−	−	−	−	Oval, terminal

[a] Non-motile.

[b] Aerotolerant—capable of aerobic growth.

+ positive, − negative.

Protocol 4

Identification scheme for clostridia isolated from clinical material

Equipment and reagents

- See Protocol 3
- Egg yolk agar plate
- Antitoxin
- 10% sugar solution (glucose, maltose, lactose, and sucrose)
- Blood agar plates
- Gelatin disc containing carbon black particles

A. Nagler test

1 Egg yolk agar is used to detect alphatoxin by neutralization with specific antitoxin.

2 Spread a loopful of antitoxin over one-half of an egg yolk agar plate and allow it to dry for 15 min.

3 Streak the isolate across the plate from the non-antitoxin side. Streak a positive control (*C. perfringens*) on each plate.

4 Incubate for 24 h.

5 Alphatoxin-producing organisms produce a diffuse opaque halo in the medium surrounding the colonies on the untreated half of the plate. On the half treated with antitoxin there is no halo (Figure 6).

B. Lipase production

1 Use an egg yolk agar plate as described above.

2 Incubate for 48 h.

3 Lipase-producing organisms produce a restricted opacity immediately beneath the colonies, and a pearly oil-slick layer on top of the colonies. This opacity is not affected by antitoxin.

C. Sugar fermentation

1 Pipette 1 ml of a 10% sugar solution (glucose, maltose, lactose, and sucrose) on to the surface of separate blood agar plates. Rock to spread over the surface.

2 Tip off the excess and dry in an incubator.

3 Spot the isolates on each plate, using a control (*C. perfringens*) for each plate.

4 Incubate anaerobically for 48 h.

5 Remove plugs of agar containing each colony, and add two or three drops of bromophenol purple. If the sugar has been fermented, the acid produced changes the indicator from purple to yellow.

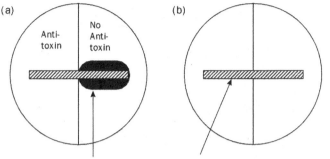

Diffuse halo = Lethinase C production   Lipase opacity__no diffusion into medium

Figure 6 Reactions seen on egg yolk agar. (a) α-toxin producing organism. (b) Non α-toxin producing organism which does however produce lipase.

Protocol 4 continued

D. Urease test

1 See Protocol 3.

E. Spot indole

1 See Protocol 3.

F. Gelatin liquefaction

1 Add a gelatin disc containing carbon black particles to a broth culture of the isolate.

2 Incubate for 48 h.

3 A positive result is indicated by the release of carbon particles into the medium.

3.3.4 Commercial identification kits

Several pre-packaged identification kits are available (Figure 7), and widely used in clinical laboratories.

(a) *Microtube systems* (API 20A, bioMerieux, France; Minitek, Beckton-Dickinson, UK). These kits rely on the metabolic breakdown of substances and production of specific end-points during bacterial growth. The organism is added to test wells and incubated anaerobically for 24–48 hours. The tests are read according to colour changes after the addition of required reagents. The results are scored numerically, and the final numerical profile obtained corresponds to the species identification.

(b) *Preformed enzymes* (RapID ANA II, Innovative Diagnostic Systems Inc., Atlanta; Rapid ID 32A, bioMerieux, France). These are rapid identification systems that do not require growth, but instead rely on substrate breakdown by preformed enzymes. The results are read after only four hours, to generate a numerical profile as described above.

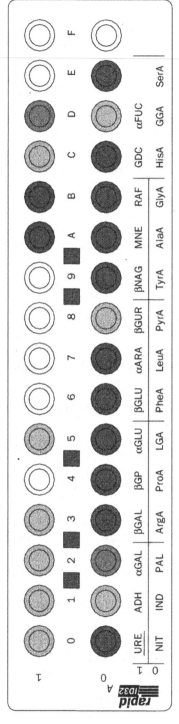

Figure 7 Disposable rapid biochemical identification strip for anaerobic bacteria (Rapid ID 32A system, courtesy of bioMerieux SA).

Despite their widespread use and general acceptability these identification kits do have drawbacks. Many of the commonly encountered anaerobes of the *Bacteroides* spp. are correctly identified by these systems, but their overall accuracy is no more than 60–70% (10, 16). Since they rely on a colour change, reading the tests is often subjective.

The kits must be supplemented with additional tests for accurate identification of many groups of anaerobes. It is still necessary to interpret correctly Gram stains, microscopic and colonial morphology. The enzyme kits should be supplemented with egg yolk agar reactions for the clostridia (Figure 6). The misidentification of organisms is possible, and so alternative methods or a reference laboratory should always confirm the identification of rare species.

3.4 Anaerobic sensitivity testing

The antimicrobial susceptibility pattern of clinically significant anaerobes has become increasingly unpredictable in recent years (17). Methodology is outlined in Chapter 7. Testing of the following antibiotics is suggested for all species: metronidazole (5 μg); penicillin (1 unit); Augmentin (20 + 10 μg); erythromycin (10 μg).

Additional antibiotics to test may include: clindamycin (10 μg); cefotaxime (10 μg); Piperacillin–Tazobactam (30 μg); imipenem (30 μg). The newer quinolones (e.g. moxifloxacin) are also likely to prove useful in the treatment of anaerobic infections. Report antibiotics according to local policy.

4 Skin and soft tissue infections
4.1 Pyoderma and cellulitis

These include primary skin infections such as boils, furunculosis, impetigo, cellulitis, erysipelas, infected sebaceous cysts, soft tissue abscesses, and erysipeloid.

4.1.1 Types of samples

Samples may be pus/pus swabs, with the occasional biopsy, curretage, or needle aspirates.

4.1.2 Expected organisms

(a) Common: *Staphylococcus aureus*, typically associated with pustular lesions but also with cellulitis. Group A β-haemolytic streptococci, typically associated with cellulitis.

(b) Less common: *Haemophilus influenzae* (facial cellulitis in children); other β-haemolytic streptococci, usually group G, occasionally groups F, B, C, but rarely D; anaerobic cocci (infected sebaceous cysts), *Bacteroides* spp., *Clostridium* spp. (anaerobic cellulitis); *Candida albicans* (paronychia, mucocutaneous candidiasis).

(c) Uncommon: *Erysipelothrix rhusiopathiae* (erysipeloid); *Corynebacterium minutissimum* (erythrasma); *Corynebacterium diphtheriae* (cutaneous diphtheria); *Bacillus anthracis* (anthrax); *Mycobacterium marinum, ulcerans,* and *kansasii; Pseudomonas mallei* (melioidosis); *P. aeruginosa* (folliculitis); *Sporothrix schenkii* (sporotrichosis); dermatiaceous fungi of mycetoma; *Nocardia* spp.; *Lymphogranuloma venereum* (inguinal lymphadenitis with discharging sinuses).

4.1.3 Special processing

Additional processing to that described in Sections 2.1 and 2.2 is necessary only for the uncommon causes. The laboratory needs to be alerted by the clinical details (e.g. foreign travel, occupation).

The following points may be helpful.

(a)	Cellulitis in a child	Put up a chocolate agar plate for *Haemophilus influenzae.*
(b)	Cellulitis in butcher's or meat/fish handlers	Check all β-haemolytic colonies, they may be *Erysipelothrix rhusiopathiae* which is catalase negative, H$_2$S positive.
(c)	Chronic infections and infections in immunosuppressed patients	Consider a ZN film if Gram film negative and culture for mycobacteria and nocardia (Chapter 3).
(d)	Foreign travel	Consider exotic fungi (e.g. *Sporothrix schenkii*), protozoal infections (e.g. leishmaniasis), and *Corynebacterium diphtheriae.*

Culture and identification methods for the more exotic organisms can be obtained from major texts (11, 14, 18).

4.1.4 Identification methods

The identification of the common pathogens *Staphyloccocus aureus* and the β-haemolytic streptococci is described here. For *Haemophilus* spp. identification see Chapter 3; and for anaerobes see Section 3.3.

i. Staphylococcus aureus

(a) *Pus:* often has little odour and is thick and creamy. The Gram stain shows many polymorphonuclear leukocytes with Gram-positive cocci which are

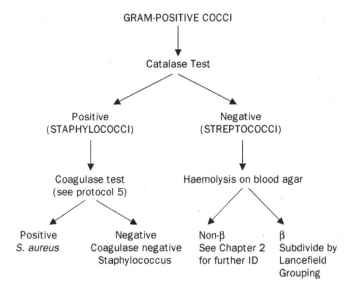

Figure 8 Simple scheme for the identification of Gram-positive cocci in clinical specimens.

intracellular and/or extracellular, and tend to form clumps or pairs. Dead bacteria stain Gram-negative.

(b) *Culture*: at 18–24 hours good growth is visible on the blood agar and the CLED or MacConkey plates. The best growth is seen on the aerobic blood plates where the colonies are 1–2 mm in diameter, opaque or creamy white, with a smooth edge. The classical golden colour may take 48 hours to become apparent, a narrow zone of α-haemolysis is fairly common. On CLED agar the colonies are often bright yellow/green; on MacConkey agar, deep opaque pink. A few strains are CO_2 or nutritionally dependent, and the colonies correspondingly small on ordinary media, especially if not incubated in CO_2.

(c) *Identification*: the simplified scheme shown in Figure 8 outlines the steps in the identification of *S. aureus*. Perform Gram stains (refer to Appendix I) and catalase test (described in Protocol 3).

The most simple and reliable method for identifying *S. aureus* is the presence of coagulase. This distinguishes *S. aureus* from the majority of coagulase negative staphylococci and micrococci. The enzyme coagulase converts fibrinogen to fibrin, so causing the organism to coagulate in small quantities of plasma. The slide coagulase test (Figure 9) detects cell bound coagulase (or clumping factor). Some strains of the human coagulase negative *S. lugdenensis* and *S. schleiferi* also produce clumping factor, and so may be positive with the slide coagulase test. 5–10% of strains of *S. aureus* are slide coagulase negative, and yet produce free coagulase,

143

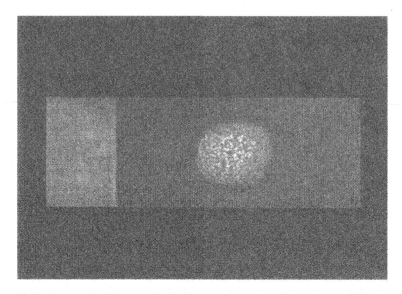

Figure 9 A positive slide coagulase test.

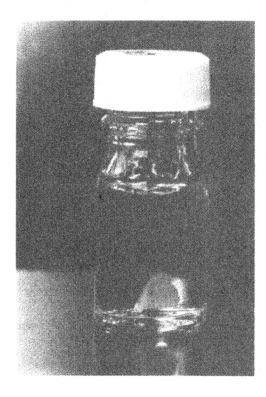

Figure 10 A positive tube coagulase test; the plasma clot can be seen at the bottom of the tube.

which can be detected using the tube coagulase test (Figure 10). In the laboratory, all staphylococci which are slide coagulase negative should have a tube coagulase test carried out. These tests are described in Protocol 5.

Protocol 5

Methods for the detection of staphylococcal coagulase

Equipment and reagents

- Slide
- Small test-tube
- Rabbit plasma
- Saline
- Broth

A. Slide coagulase

This test should not be performed on colonies from high salt content media as false positive results may be obtained.

1 Emulsify several colonies in a drop of water on slide to make a heavy suspension. A second suspension should be prepared alongside to act as a control for auto-agglutination.

2 Stir in a loopful of undiluted rabbit plasma.

3 Rock the slide gently for 5 sec. Agglutination within 5 sec indicates a positive result (see Figure 8).

B. Tube coagulase

1 Add 40 μl of rabbit plasma to 360 μl of normal saline in a small test-tube.

2 Either add 40 μl of an overnight broth culture, or emulsify several colonies straight into the diluted plasma and add a drop of nutrient broth.

3 Set up controls with each batch of tests: coagulase positive (e.g. NCTC 6571), coagulase negative (e.g. NCTC 7944), uninoculated plasma.

4 Incubate at 37 °C and examine at 1, 3, and 6 h and after overnight incubation. Clotting of the plasma into a gel (see Figure 9 for appearance) represents a positive result.

Several commercial agglutination test kits are available which are designed to differentiate *S. aureus* from coagulase negative staphylococci. Many of these kits (Staphaurex, Murex; Slidex Staph, bioMerieux-Vitek; Staphylatex, MicroScan), use coated latex particles and/or sensitized sheep erythrocytes to identify *S. aureus* by the simultaneous detection of clumping factor and staphylococcal protein A. Colonies of staphylococci are emulsified in a drop of test reagent. A positive test results in rapid agglutination.

These kits are reliable, quick and easy to use, and comparable to the slide coagulase test. However, there have been reports of false negative results among methicillin-resistant strains of *S. aureus* (19). Newer products (Slidex Staph Plus, bioMerieux; Staphaurex Plus, Murex Diagnostics Ltd.), utilize latex particles coated with human fibrinogen, and monoclonal antibodies for the simultaneous detection of clumping factor, protein A, and group-specific antigens on the *S. aureus* cell surface. Evaluation of these kits has shown sensitivities and specificities comparable to the tube coagulase test (20). As with the slide coagulase test false positive results may occur with *S. lugdenensis* and *S. schleiferi*, due to the presence of clumping factor. *S. haemolyticus* may also produce false positive results.

If there is any doubt about diagnosis, further identification tests may be performed. *S. aureus* produces both DNase and a thermostable endonuclease (TNase). Whilst not infallible, detection of these will aid identification and differentiation from the coagulase negative staphylococci. The methods used are described in Protocol 6. The TNase test may be used directly on blood culture broth. In this situation 2 ml of the blood culture broth is boiled and the supernatant added to the test wells as described in Protocol 6. Although able to give rapid information as to the potential significance of blood culture isolates, false negative results may occur, particularly when using the newer ventless blood culture bottles (21).

If there is still any doubt about the identification of isolates, then an API Staph (bioMerieux) may be performed.

Protocol 6

Methods used for the detection of DNase and thermostable deoxyribonuclease (TNase)

Equipment and reagents

- DNase agar (Oxoid Ltd.)
- 10% HCl
- Brain heart infusion (BHI) broth
- TDA medium (Appendix II)

A. DNase test

1 Spot inoculate the organism to be tested on to DNase agar. Use a positive (*Staphylococcus aureus*) and negative (*Escherichia coli*) control.

2 Incubate overnight.

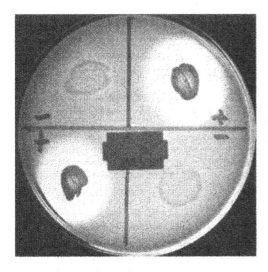

Figure 11 Agar plate DNase test. Unaltered DNA has been precipitated with 10% (v/v) HCl and clear zones where DNA has been denatured are seen around the inocula labelled as positive, which are *Staphylococcus aureus*. The DNase negative isolates are *S. epidermidis*.

Protocol 6 continued

3   Flood the plate with 10% HCl. This causes precipitation of nucleic acid which makes the medium cloudy. Where the medium has been hydrolysed by DNase, there is no precipitation (Figure 11).

B. Rapid TNase test

1   Inoculate several colonies into 1 ml of brain heart infusion (BHI) broth, and incubate for 2 h at 37 °C.

2   Boil in a water-bath for 15 min.

3   Punch a well in TDA medium—the large end of a sterile pastette works well. Fill the wells with cooled broth suspension.

4   Incubate the plate at 37 °C, and inspect after 1 h and 2 h.

5   A positive result is indicated by a pink halo around the well. The pink halo is evidence of DNA breakdown since toluidine blue dye is blue when complexed with intact DNA, but pink when complexed with nucleotides. A small clear zone around a well is not a positive test, since some coagulase negative staphylococci can destroy the dye without denaturing DNA.

ii. β-haemolytic streptococci

Lancefield groups A (*Streptococcus pyogenes*) and G are the commonest pathogens in soft tissue infections, although groups F, B, and C may also be found. These streptococci do not invariably show β-haemolysis, so non-haemolytic or α-haemolytic streptococci which appear to be playing a major part in infection should be grouped and biochemically identified.

(a) *Pus*: usually thin and watery, if present at all, although infections caused by group F streptococci (*S. milleri*) can result in the formation of large amounts of thick pus. The Gram stain shows Gram-positive cocci in short or long chains.

(b) *Culture*: β-haemolysis is seen as a complete clearing of the blood agar medium around the colonies, enhanced after anaerobic incubation. α-haemolysis is seen as a zone of greenish discoloration. Colonies of groups A, B, C, and G are whitish/grey and about 1 mm in diameter; group F colonies may be pin-point in size. Zones of β-haemolysis are largest around group C and G streptococci. Group B streptococci show a narrow zone of haemolysis and the colonies themselves are large, with a characteristic pink tinge.

(c) *Identification*: streptococci are identified in the laboratory primarily by the simple tests shown in Figure 7 and their haemolytic action on blood agar (α, β, γ, α', or non-haemolysis). α'-haemolysis consists of an inner zone of partial haemolysis surrounded by an outer zone of complete haemolysis which macroscopically resembles β-haemolysis.

β-haemolytic streptococci are further identified by the specific action of cell wall carbohydrate antigens, first characterized by Rebecca Lancefield. Eighteen distinct antigenic groups are recognized: groups A–H and K–T. Some groups contain largely one species as defined by their biochemical reactions, e.g. group A, *S. pyogenes*; group B, *S. agalactiae*. Others groups contain a number of species, e.g. group C, *S. equisimilis*, *S. dysgalactiae*, *S. equii*. The β-haemolytic streptococci are usually identified only to Lancefield group level, and not given species names in most laboratories.

The β-haemolytic streptococci which are pathogenic in man are groups A, B, C, D, F, G, and R (acquired from contact with pigs), but rarely any other group. Methods for grouping therefore only need to detect these antigens. Some commercial grouping methods exclude groups D (*Enterococcus* spp.) and F: D because these species can usually be recognized by their ability to grow on MacConkey's agar and a positive aesculin test, and F because these are uncommon outside certain specific clinical situations.

All grouping methods use specific antibodies to detect group antigens, and the immunological recognition is visualized by precipitation or agglutination. The original Lancefield hot acid technique is now rarely used as a grouping method. Most laboratories in the UK use commercially produced grouping kits in which grouping is performed by a slide agglutination test. In these kits the specific antibodies are conjugated to either latex particles or specially prepared protein A-rich staphylococcal cells. These carrier particles are so large that agglutination can be seen with the naked eye.

A number of kits are available which can be used on small numbers of colonies from solid media. Some may also be used with extraction to detect β-haemolytic streptococci directly from swabs (22). The time taken for the test varies from 1 min to 1 h depending on whether the method includes antigen extraction. Some of

Table 4 Examples of streptococcal grouping kits

Name	Principle	Groups detected	Manufacturer
Streptex	Latex agglutination	ABCDFG	Murex Diagnostics
Phadebact	Co-agglutination	ABCG	Boule Diagnostics
Prolex streptococcal grouping kit	Latex agglutination	ABCDFG	Pro-Lab Diagnostics
Oxoid streptococcal grouping kit	Latex agglutination	ABCDFG	Oxoid Ltd.

the kits available are listed in Table 4. The performance and costs are varied, and choice is a matter for individual decision.

Cross-reactions can occur with the grouping sera, most notably with groups D and G, leading to misidentification. For this reason group D streptococci which have been isolated from a clinically significant site should be further identified using an aesculin test and biochemical reactions (e.g. API system). Pneumococci can on occasions agglutinate with group C antibodies. The distinctive colonial morphology of *S. pneumoniae* should prevent confusion but if there is any doubt then identification of the presumed pneumococcus with optochin and bile solubility tests should be undertaken.

The streptococci in group A and a few other groups can be further classified into serological types on the basis of their protein antigens, M and T. Typing of the haemolytic strains, particularly group A, is necessary for epidemiological purposes and is carried out in reference laboratories. Classification of the M protein using precipitin tests has now largely been replaced by a gene typing system based on sequence analysis of the *emm* gene which encodes the surface M protein (23).

4.1.5 Sensitivity testing, interpreting, and reporting

Most patients with pyoderma or cellulitis in the UK are treated empirically with penicillin and/or flucloxacillin or with erythromycin if allergic to penicillin. The intravenous route should be used in serious infections. Topical antibiotics are not recommended.

Direct disc sensitivity testing with appropriate antibiotics is useful if a recognized pathogen is seen on the Gram stain; otherwise the microbiologist should wait for the cultures. Suggested antibiotics to test and report for the common pathogens follow. Any antibiotics that the patient is taking should always be reported (together with comment on appropriateness).

(a) *Staphylococcus aureus*

First-line antibiotics
  i. *Test*: penicillin, erythromycin, trimethoprim, fusidic acid, gentamicin, vancomycin, and methicillin or oxacillin at 30 °C.
  ii. *Report*: all on local antibiotic policy. Consider not reporting fusidic acid or gentamicin, unless the organism is resistant.

149

Second-line antibiotics: These are tested if the organism is methicillin resistant or if there is clinical reason for doing so.

  i. *Test*: tetracycline, rifampicin, clindamycin, ciprofloxacin, mupirocin.

  ii. *Consider*: teicoplanin, tobramycin, amikacin.

Note that >90% of all *S. aureus* isolates are now penicillinase producing, regardless of their origin. Telephone the clinician, and inform the infection control doctor or nurse if a methicillin-resistant *S. aureus* (MRSA) is isolated.

Several rapid methods are available for the detection of MRSA. These are discussed in more detail in Chapter 7 and have been reviewed elsewhere (24).

(b) β-haemolytic streptococci

  i. *Test*: penicillin, erythromycin, tetracycline, clindamycin, cephalosporins (e.g. cephradine, cefuroxime).
Enterococci should be tested for ampicillin, vancomycin, teicoplanin, and high level gentamicin sensitivity.

  ii. *Report*: all on local policy.

Penicillin is preferred to ampicillin except in enterococcal infections. Streptococci of groups A, B, C, and G are almost universally susceptible to penicillin.

4.2 Wound infections

Wound infections follow surgery or trauma that disrupts the skin or mucosal surface (e.g. road traffic accidents and bites). Post-operative wound infections commonly follow gastrointestinal surgery and some gynaecological surgery. These are discussed further in Sections 5 and 6 respectively.

4.2.1 Expected organisms

The type of infecting organism depends on the site and nature of the surgery or trauma. Wound infections following colorectal surgery often contain bacteria from the large bowel (*E. coli*, *Bacteroides* spp., etc.). Wound infections following bites will contain mouth organisms from the biting animal.

Wound infections are often caused by organisms resident on the skin surface which has been breached. The main culprit here is *S. aureus*, and this is the only constituent of the normal skin flora that is worth looking for routinely.

(a) Common: *S. aureus*; β-haemolytic streptococci; *E. coli*; *Bacteroides fragilis* group; *Proteus* spp.; other Enterobacteriaceae; *Cl. perfringens*; anaerobic cocci.

(b) Less common: micro-aerophilic streptococci; *Pasteurella multocida* (animal bites); other clostridia, other bacteroides; *Fusobacterium* spp.; *Pseudomonas* spp.; *Salmonella* spp.; *Capnocytophaga* spp.

(c) Rare: vibrios (infected marine wounds); *Cl. tetani*; fungi.

4.2.2 Special processing methods

None are necessary for the common pathogens. Inoculation of TCBS (thiosulfate/citrate/bile/sucrose) agar will aid in the recognition of marine vibrios.

4.2.3 Identification and sensitivity testing

(a) Do not identify or carry out sensitivity testing further than necessary for the normal skin commensals (e.g. coagulase negative staphylococci, micrococci, diphtheroids, propionobacteria).

(b) Identify and carry out sensitivity tests on *S. aureus* and β-haemolytic streptococci: Sections 4.1.4 and 4.1.5.

(c) Identify and carry out sensitivity tests on anaerobes: Sections 3.3 and 3.4.

(d) Look for *Pasteurella multocida* in swabs from infected animal bites. Direct microscopy of material from the swab is rarely helpful.
Identification: smooth greyish colonies on blood agar, poor growth at 18–24 h, colonies reaching 2 mm at 48 h. No growth on MacConkey or CLED agar. Gram stain of colonies reveals Gram-negative coco-bacilli They are oxidase positive and penicillin sensitive. Complete identification is by API 20E (bioMerieux) or suitable sugar fermentation, urea and indole tests (11).
Sensitivity testing and reporting: test and report, penicillin, ciprofloxacin, tetracycline, and cephalosporins.

(e) Animal bites may also yield *Capnocytophaga* spp. particularly in patients with DIC/ septicaemia and splenectomy/alcoholism.
Identification: colonies only visible after 48–72 h incubation on blood in CO_2, greyish/purple on the plate, but distinctly yellow when removed on a loop. Older colonies have flat, spreading finger-like edges on account of the cells exhibiting gliding motility. *C. canimorsus* and *C. cynodegmi* are both oxidase/catalase positive (25), whereas the former DF1 group (now separated into three species, *C. ochracea* being the most frequently encountered) are negative for both tests.
   Microscopy shows slender or filamentous Gram-negative rods with tapered ends. *C. ochracea*, and the very closely related species *C. sputigena/C. gingivalis* may be isolated from oral associated soft tissue sepsis but is more common as a cause of septicemia in neutropenic patients (26).
Sensitivity testing and reporting: test and report penicillin, amoxicillin-clavulinate, cephalosporins (some strains produce ESBLs), tetracycline, quinolones, and imipenem.

4.2.4 Interpretation and reporting

The presence of a normal commensal skin flora (apart from *S. aureus*) is common, and although it may be recorded on the report, is rarely significant.
   The main problem with reporting wound swab cultures is that, apart from the major pathogens such as β-haemolytic streptococci, *S. aureus*, and *Bacteroides* spp., it can be difficult to judge the pathogenic nature of the organisms isolated. This difficulty applies particularly to coliforms, *Proteus* spp., and *Pseudomonas* spp., which are often only colonizing the wound. There are occasions when these infections need to be treated, such as when deeper foreign material is present, or in certain clinical conditions such as immunocompromised patients or diabetes

mellitus. They may also be deemed to be significant if isolated in pure growth from a wound.

These problems with interpretation are often left for clinicians to resolve. However, discussion with the clinical microbiologist often ensures appropriate therapy is used. The practical approach in the laboratory is to identify and carry out sensitivity testing on all isolates except the skin commensals and those thought to be colonizing the wound, as described in Sections 4.2.3 and 5.1.4.

If there is a collection of pus in a wound then surgical drainage is the most important step. Antibiotics alone will be ineffective.

The presence of pathogens in the absence of clinical signs may not require antibiotic therapy (with the possible exception of group A β-haemolytic streptococci). This is particularly relevant for the pathogenic clostridia such as *Clostridium perfringens*, which are commonly isolated from wounds as a consequence of faecal contamination.

4.3 Gangrene, myositis, and fasciitis

Extensive serious infections include, clostridial myonecrosis (gas gangrene), necrotizing fasciitis, and synergistic necrotizing cellulitis.

Localized infections include pyomyositis (most commonly due to S. *aureus*), infected vascular gangrene (in patients with peripheral vascular insufficiency, usually a low grade infection), and psoas muscle abscess (S. *aureus* and *Mycobacterium tuberculosis*).

4.3.1 Expected organisms

(a) Anaerobes. Pathogenic clostridia: *C. perfringens*, *C. ramosom*, *C. septicum*, *C. noyvii A*. Anaerobic cocci. *Bacteroides* spp., *Fusobacterium* spp.

(b) Aerobes. Group A β-haemolytic streptococci. Microaerophilic streptococci. *Staphylococcus aureus*. Rarely coliforms and other Gram-negative bacilli (usually in patients with diabetes mellitus).

Necrotizing fasciitis and synergistic necrotizing cellulitis frequently yield mixed cultures of anaerobic and facultatively anaerobic bacteria.

4.3.2 Special processing

Process swabs, pus, and tissue as described in Sections 2.2, 2.3, and 2.4, respectively. Pay particular attention to anaerobic culture (Section 3.2).

4.3.3 Identification and sensitivity testing

(a) Identify and carry out sensitivity testing on all anaerobic isolates: Sections 3.3 and 3.4.

(b) Identify and carry out sensitivity testing on all S. *aureus* and β-haemolytic streptococci: Sections 4.1.4 and 4.1.5.

(c) Identify and carry out sensitivity testing on other organisms if warranted by the clinical picture, and particularly in diabetic patients.

4.3.4 Interpretation and reporting

Since the pathogens involved are well defined and often isolated from normally sterile sites, there is rarely any difficulty in interpreting culture results. Coliform organisms are so rarely involved that unless they are isolated from pus or tissue, or seen in pure growth, they are assumed to be secondary invaders or colonizers. Blood cultures may be a useful adjunct to diagnosis in the severe infections of this group.

4.4 Burns, varicose ulcers, ischaemic ulcers, pressure sores

These lesions are universally colonized with various potentially pathogenic bacteria. This makes interpretation of culture results nearly impossible. The best practical approach is to identify and carry out sensitivity tests as suggested for wound infections. The clinician, sometimes with advice from the clinical microbiologist, decides on clinical grounds when to use systemic antibiotic therapy instead of cleansing and antiseptics. Cellulitis would be a deciding factor, as would accompanying bacteraemia or proposed skin grafting.

4.5 Sinusitis

Chronic sinusitis are associated with the drainage of underlying deep-seated infection. The commonest of these is chronic osteomyelitis, and the processing of such samples is described in Section 7.2. Other conditions in which sinuses are found are all uncommon in the UK and include lymphogranuloma venereum, actinomycosis, Nocardia infections, tuberculosis, and atypical mycobacterial infection.

Basic laboratory methods for culture and identification of actinomycetes follow, see also Section 6.3. For detailed accounts, see the reference texts (6, 7, 11).

4.5.1 Actinomycosis

Lesions consist of purulent foci surrounded by dense fibrous tissue, forming a hard granulomatous mass which frequently discharges to the skin surface in multiple sinuses. The most common sites of infection are the jaw (cervico-facial), the ileocaecal region, the lungs, and the pelvis (often in association with intrauterine contraceptive devices). Cerebral abscesses may result from extension of cervico-facial disease. Haematogenous spread can lead to infection in the kidneys, brain, spleen, musculoskeletal system, or soft tissues.

4.5.2 Types of samples

Pus or biopsy tissue are preferred, but often all that can be obtained is the dressing from the discharging lesion. Swabs should not be processed unless no other sample can be obtained.

4.5.3 Microscopic examination

(a) Place pus, fluid, IUD, or dressings in a Petri dish and examine for sulfur granules with a plate microscope ($\times 7$ to $\times 15$ magnification). Sulfur granules are

153

macro-colonies of actinomycete bacteria. They are yellowish white, 0.2–2 mm in diameter, and irregular in shape.

(b) Crush a granule together with a drop of water between two microscope slides. Remove one slide, heat-fix the preparation, and stain with Gram's stain. The typical and diagnostic appearance is a central mass of Gram-positive branching and non-branching filaments surrounded by Gram-negative club-shaped forms.

4.5.4 Culture

(a) Culture pus, fluid, or tissue on blood agar in air +5% CO_2, anaerobically and in broth medium as described in Section 2.

(b) To culture a dressing for actinomyces, pick the most contaminated part (complete with granules if seen) and place it in either fastidious anaerobe broth (Lab M), pre-reduced cooked meat broth, or thioglycollate broth.

(c) Incubate, preferably anaerobically with the cap loosened, for 48 h, then centrifuge the broth and culture the deposit as above.

(d) Incubate culture plates initially for 48 h. If they are sterile re-incubate for five to seven days and re-examine. If still sterile then re-incubate for a further two weeks before discarding.

(e) *Actinomyces israelii* grows on the anaerobic plates only. Smooth strains grow after two to three days and are unremarkable 1–2 mm white, opaque, smooth colonies. The more typical rough strains usually take five to seven days to grow and appear as 1 mm raised, irregular, white, opaque colonies which look like very rough molar teeth.

4.5.5 Identification

Typical sulfur granules in clinical material are diagnostic. If absent, definitive identification of actinomyces is more difficult. Gram's stain of colonies shows Gram-positive bacilli, sometimes filamentous and sparsely branching. Formal identification and differentiation from the other anaerobic Gram-positive non-spore forming bacilli may be accomplished by gas–liquid chromatography and biochemical tests (6, 7, 11).

4.6 Fistulae

Swabs from fistulae yield the indigenous flora of the underlying viscus as well as skin flora. The interpretation of the bacteriology of such swabs is impossible and has little clinical relevance, since treatment of the bacteria will not 'cure' the fistula. The underlying cause must be sought.

4.7 Vesicles and bullae

Bacterial infections include the neonatal scalded skin syndrome and toxic epidermal necrolysis (*S. aureus*); cellulitis with bullae (β-haemolytic streptococci);

gangrene with bullae (*Pseudomonas aeruginosa* and *Clostridium* spp.). Viral infections include chickenpox and shingles (*Varicella zoster*); cold sores and genital herpes (*Herpes simplex*) and orf.

4.7.1 Type of sample

These may be vesicle or bulla fluid or swabs or swabs from the base of the vesicle or blister.

4.7.2 Expected organisms

(a) Common: *Varicella zoster*, *Herpes simplex*.

(b) Less common: group A β-haemolytic streptococci, *Clostridium* spp., *S. aureus*, orf virus.

(c) Rare: *Pseudomonas aeruginosa*.

4.7.3 Special processing methods

Process for bacterial pathogens as for wound swabs (Section 2.2). The viral infections are often diagnosed clinically, but the diagnosis may be confirmed by electron microscopy or by viral culture. Fluid is required for electron microscopy. For culture swabs should be taken from the base of the lesion (i.e. containing epithelial cells) and placed in viral transport medium.

4.7.4 Identification and sensitivity testing

Identify and carry out sensitivity tests on group A β-haemolytic streptococci and *S. aureus* (Section 4.1). If the clinical information is suggestive, such as presence of gangrene or immunosuppression then identify and carry out sensitivity tests on *Clostridium* spp. (Sections 3.3 and 3.4), and *Pseudomonas* spp. (Sections 5.1.3 and 5.1.4).

4.7.5 Interpretation and reporting

This is usually straightforward, since the clinical picture often suggests the aetiology. Sometimes coliforms, *Pseudomonas*, or *Proteus* are isolated from such lesions. This nearly always represents colonization of the wet surface of a broken vesicle or bulla. Rarely *Pseudomonas aeruginosa* is found as a primary pathogen in immunosuppressed patients—a type of ecthyma gangrenosum.

4.8 Suppurative lymphadenitis

Commonly, the infection is an uncomplicated acute pyogenic infection. Rare conditions include tuberculosis, tularaemia, plague, meliodosis, sporotrichosis, and glanders. Needle aspirates or lymph node biopsies are the most useful specimens.

4.8.1 Expected organisms

(a) Common: *S. aureus*; group A β-haemolytic streptococci.

(b) Less common: *Mycobacterium tuberculosis*, *M. bovis*, *M. avium-intracellulare* complex.

(c) Rare: *Francisella tularensis* (tuleraemia), *Yersinia pestis* (plague), *Pseudomonas mallei* (glanders), *Pseudomonas pseudomallei* (melioidosis), *Coccidioides* spp., *Sporothrix schenkii* (sporotrichosis), *Bartonella henselae* (cat scratch disease).

4.8.2 Special processing

The aspirate or tissue should be processed as described in Section 2.4. For mycobacteria see Chapter 3, for fungal pathogens see Evans and Richardson (27). Some of these organisms, e.g. *Mycobacterium tuberculosis*, *Yersinia pestis*, *Francisella tularenesis*, are in ACDP (UK Advisory Committee on Dangerous Pathogens) Hazard Group 3, and so consideration must be made to ensure specimens are processed at a suitable containment level. *Yersinis pestis* and *Pseudomonas pseudomallei* will grow on 'ordinary' media. Others are fastidious and need additional media, e.g. *Francisella tularensis*, Dorsets egg medium; *Pseudomonas mallei*, 4% glycerol blood agar.

4.8.3 Identification and sensitivity testing

Identification and sensitivity tests should be performed on *S. aureus* and β-haemolytic streptococci (Sections 4.1.4 and 4.1.5). Provided the tissue or aspirate has not been contaminated by the laboratory, any growth must be regarded as significant and must be fully identified with sensitivity tests. The rare organisms which need special media will not normally be seen on routine culture. Those that grow on routine culture will appear as small, unusual-looking Gram-negative bacilli. Laboratories with no experience of these organisms may wish to refer suspect colonies or even the original specimens to reference centres. *Bartonella henselae* infection can be diagnosed either serologically or by PCR.

4.9 Chronic ulcers

The following clinical conditions are found: atypical mycobacterial infections, for example swimming-pool granuloma, fish-tank granuloma (*M. marinum*); Buruli ulcer (*M. uicerans*); sporotrichosis (*Sporothrix schenkii*); glanders (*Pseudomonas mallei*); anthrax (*Bacillus anthracis*); leishmaniasis and paracoccidioidomycosis (muco-cutaneous ulceration). There are also chronic ulcers associated with the sexually transmitted diseases, syphilis, yaws, chancroid, and lymphogranuloma venereum. Samples from these ulcers should be either aspiration or biopsy samples.

Reference should be made to Chapter 3 for mycobacteria; to mycology textbooks for the fungi (27) and to Chapter 4 for the sexually transmitted infections; and to major texts for the remainder. If leishmaniasis is suspected, the aspirate or biopsy should be stained for Leishman–Donovan bodies; see other texts (11, 14, 28).

5 Infection associated with the gastrointestinal tract

5.1 Intra-abdominal abscess

Subphrenic abscesses, pelvic abscesses, appendix abscesses, diverticular abscesses, Crohns disease abscesses, and para-colic abscesses may be encountered.

5.1.1 Expected organisms

Bacteria from the bowel most commonly occur, for example *Escherichia coli*, *Proteus* spp., other Enterobacteriaceae, enterococci, and other streptococci, *Bacteroides* spp., anaerobic cocci, and other anaerobes. Infections are commonly polymicrobial.

Staphylococcus aureus infections are less common and probably follow a bacteraemia.

5.1.2 Processing methods

(a) Process pus and swabs as described in Sections 2.1 and 2.2. Gram stains usually confirm mixed infection but many unexpectedly reveal a pure staphylococcal infection.

(b) Gas chromatography is rarely useful since the presence of anaerobes is almost universal.

5.1.3 Identification methods

(a) Identify enterococci using the bile aesculin test, or other biochemical tests. Their presence may often be inferred from sensitivity testing of β-haemolytic streptococci (enterococci are penicillin and cephalosporin resistant).

(b) Identify *S. aureus* as described in Section 4.1.4.

(c) Identify the anaerobes as described in Section 3.3.

(d) Identify the aerobic Gram-negative bacilli as outlined in the scheme shown in Figure 12. Full species identification of all the Gram-negative bacilli may be appropriate in certain clinical situations, but is not routine. Oxidase negative, lactose fermenting bacilli can be identified using a number of commercial kits, e.g. API 20E (bioMerieux, France). Oxidase positive or non-lactose fermenting bacilli can be more easily identified using kits such as the API 20NE (bioMerieux).

5.1.4 Sensitivity testing and reporting

(a) Test and report *S. aureus* as described in Section 4.1.5, and anaerobes as described in Section 3.4.

(b) Test and report sensitivity of enterococci to ampicillin, vancomycin, and teicoplanin, together with high level gentamicin. Test other streptococci to penicillin and cephalosporins.

157

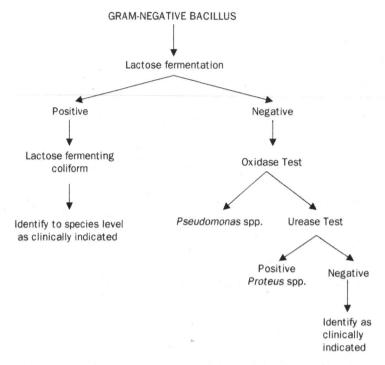

GRAM-NEGATIVE BACILLUS

Lactose fermentation

Positive

Negative

Lactose fermenting
coliform

Oxidase Test

Identify to species level
as clinically indicated

Pseudomonas spp.   Urease Test

Positive
Proteus spp.   Negative

Identify as
clinically
indicated

Figure 12 Simple scheme for the identification of Gram-negative bacilli in clinical specimens.

(c) Test and report sensitivity of aerobic Gram-negative bacilli, other than *Pseudomonas* spp., to ampicillin, cefuroxime, trimethoprim, gentamicin, ciprofloxacin, and ceftazidime. Second-line antibiotics (piperacillin, piperacillin–tazobactam, imipenem, meropenem) should be tested if the organism is resistant to more than three of the antibiotics. Consider testing amikacin, tobramycin, and aztreonam.

(d) *Pseudomonas* spp. should be tested against gentamicin, tobramycin, ceftazidime, piperacillin, piperacillin–tazobactam, imipenem/meropenem, and ciprofloxacin. Second-line antibiotics are amikacin and aztreonam.

(e) Report all antibiotics on local antibiotic policy.

Antibiotics alone without surgical drainage of the abscess will not be effective.

5.2 Peritonitis

Primary peritonitis (spontaneous bacterial peritonitis) occurs when there is no evident focus of infection. The condition may occur following a bacteraemia, but is increasingly recognized in patients with cirrhosis and in children with nephrotic syndrome, in which ascites accumulate.

Secondary peritonitis follows rupture or surgical opening of an abdominal viscus, trauma, or preceding intra-abdominal infection (liver abscess, salpingitis, etc.).

5.2.1 Types of samples

Usually a swab of free peritoneal fluid is received. Occasionally, especially in primary peritonitis, peritoneal fluid itself is sent, and this is very often more helpful.

5.2.2 Expected organisms

(a) Primary peritonitis: In the past the commonest causes described were *Streptococcus pneumoniae* and group A β-haemolytic streptococci. In recent years the relative frequency of other organisms has increased, particularly the Gram-negative bacilli and enterococci. *S. aureus* and anaerobes are rare causes.

(b) Secondary peritonitis: The infecting organisms are often related to the underlying cause. *E. coli*, other Enterobacteriaceae, and anaerobes are the most commonly encountered isolates. If the underlying problem is associated with the genital tract (e.g. salpingitis), then *Neisseria gonorrhoeae* and *Chlamydia trachomatis* may also be seen.

Tuberculous peritonitis may be primary or secondary, due to spread from an adjacent tuberculous focus. Although rare the condition needs to be considered because of difficulty in making the diagnosis.

5.2.3 Processing methods

(a) In primary peritonitis perform an urgent Gram stain. If negative or if there is any doubt about the organisms seen, direct testing for pneumococcal or group A β-haemolytic streptococcal antigens may be performed using latex agglutination tests.

(b) Process fluid as described in Section 2.3.

(c) Culture on additional media if *N. gonorrhoeae* or *Chlamydia* are suspected. See Chapter 4.

5.2.4 Identification methods, sensitivity testing, and reporting

For *S. pneumoniae*, *N. gonorrhoeae*, and *C. trachomatis* see Chapters 3 and 4. For group A β-haemolytic streptococci, see Sections 4.1.4 and 4.1.5. For aerobic Gram-negative bacilli see Sections 5.1.3 and 5.1.4. For anaerobes see Sections 3.3 and 3.4.

5.2.5 Interpretation

The precise value of peritoneal swabs in many cases of secondary peritonitis is difficult to assess. They are often taken routinely in acute appendicitis. The bacteriology never influences antibiotic therapy, which is given empirically on clinical indications for short periods, sometimes ending at about the time the full bacteriology results are available.

5.3 Wound infections

5.3.1 Samples and expected organisms

Almost invariably 'wound swabs' with the occasional sample of pus will be sent to the laboratory. The organisms found in wound infections relate either to the skin or to the site of the surgery (gastrointestinal tract, genital tract). Of the skin organisms, S. *aureus* is the major pathogen; see Section 4.1. The organisms from the gastrointestinal tract vary; from oesophagus and stomach they tend to be of mouth and upper respiratory tract type; from the duodenum, mainly streptococcal with a few coliforms and anaerobes; from the ileum, there are more coliforms and anaerobes; from the large bowel, coliforms and anaerobes predominate. Large numbers of coliforms may be found in the stomach and duodenum if the gastric acidity is reduced (usually by H_2 antagonists or proton pump inhibitors). Following gynaecological surgery, anaerobes, group B, and other streptococci as well as coliforms are commonly found in wound infections.

5.3.2 Processing and identification methods and sensitivity testing

(a) Process as for pus and swabs in Sections 2.1 and 2.2. No special techniques are necessary.

(b) Identify and carry out sensitivity tests on S. *aureus* and β-haemolytic streptococci as described in Sections 4.1.4 and 4.1.5.

(c) Identify and carry out sensitivity tests on anaerobes as described in Sections 3.3 and 3.4, and on aerobic Gram-negative bacilli and enterococci as described in Sections 5.1.3 and 5.1.4.

5.3.3 Reporting and interpretation

This can be extremely difficult. The decision as to whether to treat a 'wound infection' depends more on the clinical picture than on the organisms isolated, with the exception of β-haemolytic streptococci. Unless the laboratory wishes to have a dialogue with the clinician over every wound swab, it is more practical on culture to identify organisms as far as seems appropriate and perform selected sensitivity tests.

5.4 Biliary infections

These include acute cholangitis, acute cholecystitis, empyema of gall bladder, and infection associated with external biliary drainage (T-tubes).

5.4.1 Type of sample

Bile collected from a drainage bag is unacceptable; the sample must be from the T-tube catheter itself. Operative specimens of pus, swabs, and bile are often received. Blood cultures may be the only sample that can be sent in acute cholangitis and they are often positive.

5.4.2 Expected organisms

Typically gastrointestinal tract organisms, and often a mixed flora, are isolated. The bacteria most commonly encountered are: *E. coli*, *Proteus* spp., other Enterobacteriaceae, *B. fragilis*, *C. perfringens*, anaerobic cocci, other anaerobes, and streptococci usually enterococci.

In addition, *Pseudomonas aeruginosa* is frequently associated with biliary T-tube drainage, although it is often only colonizing. *Salmonella* spp., including *S. typhi*, may be isolated from biliary carriers.

5.4.3 Processing methods

(a) Process pus and swabs as described in Sections 2.1 and 2.2.

(b) Bile fluid should be centrifuged at 1800 g for 10 min. Make a Gram stain of the deposit and culture as described in Section 2.1.

(c) Set up additional media for enteric pathogens, such as DCLS, DCA, or XLD and selenite broth (see Chapter 6), if the clinical details are appropriate.

(d) Gas chromatography can be carried out directly on bile, and of course pus, but is rarely used in clinical laboratories.

5.4.4 Identification methods and sensitivity testing

The methods described in Sections 5.1.3 and 5.1.4 are appropriate. Gram-negative bacilli which identify biochemically as *Salmonella* spp. should be confirmed as described in Chapter 6.

5.4.5 Interpretation and reporting

The only samples, which pose a problem, are those from external biliary drainage—'the T-tube bile' specimens. In common with external urinary drainage, the presence of a foreign body, the catheter, ensures ready colonization with coliforms, *Pseudomonas*, enterococci, and occasionally anaerobes. Just as for catheter urine samples, antibiotic therapy is inappropriate unless the patient shows signs of infection; the catheter is to be manipulated (removed or changed) or something is to be injected up the catheter such as X-ray contrast material for a T-tube cholangiogram. There are two approaches the laboratory can take: first, to perform sensitivity testing and inform the clinicians that this has been done, but not to report the results unless directly asked to do so; secondly, to perform sensitivity testing, report the results, and rely on the clinicians not to use the antibiotics unless they are needed. The best approach depends on local circumstances and each laboratory must decide individually.

5.5 Liver abscesses

5.5.1 Type of sample

Pus or other material from a liver aspirate is usually received. Blood cultures are often helpful.

5.5.2 Expected organisms

Bacterial isolates are frequently multiple. The commonest organisms are *Streptococcus milleri*, other streptococci including enterococci, anaerobes, *E. coli*, other Enterobacteriaceae. *S. aureus*, and group A β-haemolytic streptococci may occur secondary to a bacteraemia.

Protozoal causes include *Entamoeba histolytica* (amoebic abscesses) and *Echinococcus granulosus* (hydatid cysts). These are not discussed further here.

In immunocompromised individuals infection with fungal pathogens, particularly *Candida* spp. may occur.

5.5.3 Processing methods

(a) Perform an urgent Gram stain and telephone the findings to the clinician.

(b) Process basically as for pus (Section 2.1), but pay special attention to anaerobic technique and use prolonged culture (up to seven days), Section 3.2.

(c) Direct sensitivity testing may be set up; choose antibiotics with reference to the Gram stain and those listed in Section 5.1.4.

5.5.4 Identification methods and sensitivity testing

(a) All isolates must be identified to species level. Identify and carry out sensitivity testing on streptococci and *S. aureus* as described in Sections 4.1.4 and 4.1.5, anaerobes as described in Sections 3.3 and 3.4.

(b) Identify and carry out sensitivity testing on Enterobacteriaceae and other aerobic Gram-negative bacilli as described in Sections 5.1.3 and 5.1.4, but identify biochemically to species level.

5.5.5 Interpretation and reporting

This is straightforward, since any isolate must be considered significant, identified, and appropriate sensitivities reported. Antibiotic therapy alone may be successful when micro-abscesses are present, but drainage (either at laparotomy or percutaneously under X-ray guidance), combined with antibiotics, offers the best chance of success.

5.6 Abscesses

Perianal, ischiorectal, and post-anal abscesses are discussed here.

5.6.1 Types of samples and expected organisms

Although pus is preferable a swab is usually sent. Most are mixed infections involving anaerobes, especially *Bacteroides fragilis* group, and aerobic Gram-negative bacilli, usually *E. coli*. Other anaerobic bacteria, streptococci including enterococci, *Proteus* spp., and other Enterobacteriaceae may also be encountered. *S. aureus* may rarely occur, particularly in diabetic patients.

5.6.2. Processing and identification methods and sensitivity testing

(a) Process as described in Section 2.1. No special techniques are necessary.

(b) Identify and carry out sensitivity testing on *E. coli* and aerobic Gram-negative bacilli as described in Sections 5.1.3 and 5.1.4, anaerobes as described in Sections 3.3. and 3.4, and streptococci and *S. aureus* as described in Sections 4.1.4 and 4.1.5.

5.6.3 Interpretation and reporting

Surgical drainage of the abscess alone is sufficient in most cases. Antibiotic therapy is needed only in patients with cellulitis or who appear bacteraemic. The most practical approach for the laboratory is to report the results of limited sensitivity testing in the knowledge that they will rarely be of value.

6 Gynaecological and post-partum infections

6.1 Post-operative infections

Wound infections and pelvic abscesses are the most frequent infections encountered. Swabs are nearly always sent, including vaginal swabs, but occasionally pus is received.

6.1.1 Expected organisms

These are *E. coli*, other Enterobacteriaceae, *Bacteroides fragilis* group, other anaerobes, group B streptococci, and other streptococci including enterococci and occasionally *Staphylococcus aureus*.

6.1.2 Processing and identification methods and sensitivity testing

(a) Process as described in Sections 2.1 and 2.2. No special techniques are necessary.

(b) Identify and carry out sensitivity testing on *E. coli* and aerobic Gram-negative bacilli as described in Sections 5.1.3 and 5.1.4, anaerobes as described in Sections 3.3 and 3.4, and streptococci and *S. aureus* as described in Sections 4.1.4 and 4.1.5.

6.1.3 Interpretation and reporting

As in all wound infections, the presence of cellulitis or pus is the main guide to treatment. Post-operative vaginal swabs are extremely difficult to interpret unless a heavy growth of a likely pathogen is found.

6.2 **Tubo-ovarian sepsis**

Clinical conditions encountered are salpingitis, tubal abscess, ovarian abscess, pelvic inflammatory disease.

6.2.1 Type of sample and expected organisms

A sample of pus taken at operation is the most useful specimen. Free peritoneal fluid or a peritoneal swab are sometimes helpful. Cervical, urethral, and rectal swabs are useful adjuncts in the diagnosis of gonococcal infection, as are cervical swabs in chlamydial infection. *Neisseria gonorrhoeae*, group B streptococci, *S. aureus*, *B. fragilis* group and other anaerobes, and *Chlamydia trachomatis* may be encountered.

6.2.2 Processing methods

Culture media must include both selective and non-selective media for *N. gonorrhoeae* (see Chapter 4) as well as media for wound swabs. Special methods are required for detection/culture of *Chlamydia trachomatis* (see Chapter 4).

6.2.3 Identification methods and sensitivity testing

Identify and carry out sensitivity tests on *N. gonorrhoeae* as described in Chapter 4 and anaerobes as described in Sections 3.3 and 3.4.

6.2.4 Interpretation and reporting

This should pose few problems when samples are taken at operation. Problems arise when the only specimens available in cases of pelvic inflammatory diseases are cervical or vaginal swabs, and these do not yield *N. gonorrhoeae* or *C. trachomatis*; interpretation is then very difficult.

6.3 **Infection associated with intrauterine contraceptive devices (IUCDs)**

An association between pelvic inflammatory disease and IUCD use has been reported but appears to be less clear cut than previously documented (29). Contamination of the endometrial cavity at insertion causes an excess of infections in the first few months. After this time, many infections result from sexually transmitted infections and not the IUCD itself, although ascending infections can occur. The risk of actinomycosis infection of the pelvis increases with the time the IUCD has been in place.

6.3.1 Type of sample and expected organisms

Cervical swabs are acceptable but the IUCD should be cultured whenever possible. Anaerobes, particularly the *Bacteroides fragilis* group are the most common isolate. *Actinomyces* spp., especially *A. israelii*, may be found, particularly in IUCDs that have been in place for more than two years.

6.3.2 Processing and identification methods and sensitivity testing

(a) Culture swabs and IUCDs for anaerobes as described in Section 3.2.

(b) Culture IUCDs and cervical swabs for actinomycetes as described in Protocol 7. In practice many laboratories will simply culture the surface of the IUCD.

(c) Identify and carry out sensitivity testing on anaerobes as described in Sections 3.3 and 3.4. Identify *A. israelii* presumptively on the basis of microscopic and colonial morphology as described in Section 4.5.

Protocol 7

Procedure for the culture of IUCDs and cervical swabs for actinomycetes (adapted from ref. 30)

Equipment and reagents

- IUCD
- Anaerobic broth
- Blood agar plates containing 5% metronidazole

Method

1. Swab the IUCD to remove all the pus and debris.

2. Immerse the swab in 5 ml of a fresh anaerobic broth. Agitate it and squeeze all the excess broth from the swab before removing.

3. Make four appropriate 10-fold dilutions in further 5 ml quantities of the broth.

4. Culture 100 µl of each dilution as a lawn on blood agar plates containing 5% metronidazole to suppress strict anaerobes.

5. Incubate at 37 °C anaerobically.

6. Examine at 5 and 10 days.

6.3.3 Interpretation and reporting

Anaerobes and actinomycetes should be reported with sensitivities. The prevalence of actinomycetes in the vaginal flora of healthy women without IUCDs is very low, but prevalence increases with the amount of time an IUCD is left in place.

In symptomatic women, if actinomycetes are detected on a smear, the IUCD should be removed and cultured for actinomyces. If *A. israelii* is found it should be treated. However, in many women actinomycetes detected on a PAP smear seem to be present only as superficial colonizers of the endometrium, causing no symptoms. In these asymptomatic women the role of the organisms in the development of pelvic infection has not been fully established (31). Furthermore, the correlation between positive smear microscopy and culture is extremely variable. Removal of the IUCD is not recommended unless an equally suitable means of contraception is available.

6.4 Post-partum infections

Endometritis, infected episiotomy wounds, and infected Caesarian section wounds are the commonest clinical conditions. Post-abortion sepsis and clostridial myometritis are uncommon but serious infections.

6.4.1 Types of samples and expected organsisms

Cervical or high vaginal swabs and swabs from the episiotomy or abdominal wounds are usually received. Occasionally lochia or endometrial curettings are sent. Blood cultures can be helpful in endometritis.

Commonly the same organisms are found here as in post-operative gynaecological infections (Section 6.1). Rarely *S. aureus*, group A streptococci, and *Clostrium perfringens* are encountered. The latter organism causes urterine gas gangrene, a very serious infection.

6.4.2 Processing and identification methods and sensitivity testing

(a) Process lochai and endometrial curettings as pus (Section 2.1). An urgent Gram stain may be helpful in certain clinical conditions. No special techniques are necessary.

(b) Identify and carry out sensitivity testing on *E. coli* and aerobic Gram-negative bacilli as described in Sections 5.1.3 and 5.1.4, anaerobes as described in Sections 3.3 and 3.4, and streptococci and *S. aureus* as described in Sections 4.1.4 and 4.1.5.

6.4.3 Interpretation and reporting

The interpretation of the significance of *E. coli* and the Enterobacteriaceae from post-partum wounds is just as difficult as for any other wound. High vaginal swabs can also pose similar problems in interpretation. Swabs from the cervical os are easier to interpret, there being less chance of contamination with normal vaginal flora at this site. Organisms isolated from the cervix in the presence of pus or a fluid discharge must be considered to be potentially pathogenic. *C. perfringens*, group A streptococci, and *S. aureus* must always be reported promptly. *Clostridium perfringens* can be present in the perineum or vagina as a result of faecal contamination or colonization and is not necessarily treated in the absence of clinical signs of infection, but if isolated the clinicians should be informed and its significance discussed.

7 Infections of the skeletal system

7.1 Acute osteomyelitis

7.1.1 Types of samples

Pus obtained from direct aspiration at surgery gives the best results. Swabs of pus may be received but should be discouraged. Blood cultures may yield the organism and should always be taken.

7.1.2 Expected organisms

S. aureus is the most common organism isolated. Less commonly group A β-haemolytic streptococci and *Streptococcus pneumoniae* may be found. In children aged three months to five years *Haemophilus influenzae* may cause acute osteomyelitis, but is rare since the introduction of widespread vaccination programs. In infants *S. aureus* is still the most common organism, although Gram-negative bacilli, particularly *E. coli*, and group B streptococci may also be encountered.

Osteomyelitis associated with vascular insufficiency may be seen, particularly in patients with diabetes mellitus. In this situation multiple organisms may be isolated including, *S. aureus*, coagulase negative staphylococci, streptococci, particularly enterococci, Gram-negative bacilli, and anaerobes.

Rare causes include, *Salmonella* spp. (especially in children with haemoglobinopathies), and *Pseudomonas aeruginosa*.

7.1.3 Processing samples

(a) Process samples as for pus (Section 2.1).

(b) Perform urgent Gram stains. These are usually positive and should be telephoned to the clinician.

(c) Additional culture plates may be set up for neonates (CLED or MacConkey for Enterobacteriaceae) and infants and children (chocolate agar for *H. influenzae*).

7.1.4 Identification methods

All organisms isolated must be fully identified to species level: specimen contamination by skin commensals is very rare.

(a) Identify *S. aureus* (Section 4.1.4), β-haemolytic streptococci (Section 4.1.4), *Streptococcus pneumoniae* (Chapter 3), and *H. influenzae* (Chapter 3). Identify all Gram-negative bacilli as described in Section 5.1.5, but with full identification to species level. If anaerobes are present these should be fully identified to species level as described in Section 3.3.

(b) Telephone the culture reports to the clinician, particularly if a Gram-negative bacillus is isolated since these will not be covered by the usual empirical antibiotic regimen of flucloxacillin and fusidic acid.

7.1.5 Sensitivity testing, interpretation, and reporting

Direct sensitivity testing may be set up; the antibiotics tested being chosen on the basis of the Gram stain and with reference to the list below. The clinicians will start antibiotic treatment on the basis of the Gram stain or empirically in the knowledge that the majority of cases are due to *S. aureus*. Commonly used empirical regimens are flucloxacillin or erythromycin, with or without fusidic acid. In children cefotaxime may be given instead of flucoxacillin to treat possible *H. influenzae*, although given its increasing rarity this is not commonly indicated. Antibiotic regimens are continued or changed on the basis of culture results and sensitivity testing.

Any antibiotic which the patient is on and any to which the organism is resistant should be tested and reported unless they are inappropriate.

(a) *S. aureus* test and report as described in Section 4.1.5.

(b) Streptococci and *S. pneumoniae*, test and report as described in Section 4.1.5.

(c) *Haemophilus influenzae*, test ampicillin, augmentin, clarithromycin, cefuroxime, and cefotaxime, and report all on local antibiotic policy.

(d) Aerobic Gram-negative bacilli (Enterobacteriaceae including *Salmonella* spp.), test and report as described in Section 5.1.4.

(e) *Pseudomonas aeruginosa*, test and report as described in Section 5.1.6.

7.2 Chronic osteomyelitis

7.2.1 Types of samples

Wound swabs from the discharging sinus overlying the area of osteomyelitis are commonly received, but are of limited value (32). The best material for culture is granulation tissue or pus from the site of bone infection. Blood cultures are not helpful or of value as most patients will not be septicaemia.

7.2.2 Expected organisms

The organisms isolated from tissue specimens of patients with chronic osteomyelitis have changed during the last thirty years. *S. aureus* has become less frequent and the Gram-negative bacilli more frequent. Anaerobes are now recognized because culture techniques have improved. This changing pattern reflects nosocomial infection in trauma patients, many of whom have had open operative intervention or internal fixation of fractures.

The following organisms are found: *Staphylococcus aureus*, *Pseudomonas aeruginosa*, *E. coli*, *Proteus mirabilis* and other Enterobacteriaceae, *Bacteroides* spp., *Propionobacterium acnes*, and anaerobic cocci.

Mixed infections are common, usually *S. aureus* with Gram-negative bacilli. Osteomyelitis caused by *M. tuberculosis* and *Brucella* spp. is uncommon, but should be considered in undiagnosed cases of chronic osteomyelitis.

7.2.3 Processing and identification methods

Process pus as in Section 2.1 and tissue as in Section 2.4. Identify *S. aureus* as described in Section 4.1.4, Gram-negative bacilli to species level as described in Section 5.1.4, and anaerobes to species level as described in Section 3.3.

7.2.4 Sensitivity testing, reporting, and interpretation

S. aureus should be tested and reported as described in Section 4.1.5, Gram-negative bacilli as described in Section 5.1.4, and anaerobes as described in Section 3.4.

The results of swabs are difficult to interpret due to colonization of the sinus tract with Gram-negative bacilli and skin flora: comparisons of sinus tract and operative specimens show significant disparities (32). Any isolate from tissue or pus should be assumed to be significant. Antibiotics combined with surgical debridement of dead bone can be successful.

8 Joint infections

8.1 Prosthetic joint infections

Infections in prosthetic joints are discussed here. Acute septic arthritis is discussed in Chapter 2.

8.1.1 Types of samples and expected organisms

Usually a swab is taken from the re-opened joint, and sent to the laboratory, preferably with a sample of granulation tissue and fluid from the joint.

Isolates resemble those from infections in other prostheses (e.g. prosthetic heart valves, ventriculo-atrial/peritoneal shunts). The organisms are predominantly skin commensals introduced at the time of surgery, but any bacteraemia may induce infection of a prosthetic joint by haematogenous spread.

Coagulase negative staphylococci are most frequently encountered, but *S. aureus*, streptococci (viridans, β-haemolytic, and anaerobic), Gram-negative bacilli, and diphtheroids may be seen.

8.1.2 Processing and identification methods and sensitivity testing

(a) Process swabs, tissues, and fluid as described in Section 2. Direct microscopy can confirm the presence of organisms but is of limited value in directing therapy since the causative organisms often have unpredictable sensitivities.

(b) Identify and carry out sensitivity testing of all isolates. The identification and sensitivity testing of coagulase negative staphylococci, diphtheroids, and other such organisms as described in Chapter 2.

8.1.3 Interpretation and reporting

This is essentially the same as for other foreign body associated infections, and the reader is referred to Chapter 2 for details.

9 CNS infections

9.1 Cerebral abscess

Meningitis will not be covered here; see Chapter 2 for details. The only acceptable sample from a cerebral abscess is pus collected at operation.

9.1.1 Expected organisms

The majority of brain abscesses arise by direct spread from a nearby focus of infection such as the mastoids, middle ear, paranasal sinuses, or teeth. The remainder arise either as a result of haematogenous spread from distant sites of infection (most commonly the liver or lungs) or following trauma/neurosurgery. The organisms found reflect the underlying condition.

Streptococci (anaerobic, microaerophilic, or aerobic) are the most commonly isolated bacteria, and infections are frequently mixed. Other bacterial pathogens encountered include:

(a) Common: *B. fragilis* group, *Prevotella melaninogenica*, other *Bacteroides* spp.

(b) Less common: Enterobacteriaceae, *Pseudomonas aeruginosa*, *S. aureus*, *H. influenzae*, *Fusobacterium* spp.

(c) Rare: *Actinomyces* spp.

In immunocompromised patients other organisms, including *Aspergillus* spp., *Candida* spp., *Nocardia* spp., *Toxoplasma gondii*, and *Mycobacterium tuberculosis* may also occur.

9.1.2 Processing methods

(a) Make an urgent Gram stain and phone the results to the clinician.

(b) Process the pus as described in Section 2.1, with special attention to anaerobic culture methods as described in Section 3.2. Incubate plates for a minimum of 14 days before accepting a negative result.

(c) Set up direct sensitivity tests, aerobic and anaerobic, based on the organisms seen in the Gram stain and the antibiotic suggested in Section 9.1.3.

9.1.3 Identification methods and sensitivity testing

All isolates should be fully identified to species level. Help with identification of anaerobes may be obtained from reference laboratories. Streptococci which are not β-haemolytic can be identified biochemically (e.g. with the API Strep, bioMerieux).

Streptococci should be tested against penicillin, ampicillin, third-generation cephalosporins and clindamycin. Anaerobes should be tested against metronidazole as well. Other isolates should be tested against the appropriate antibiotics, but in particular the β-lactams which penetrate the CNS well.

9.1.4 Interpretation and reporting

All isolates with sensitivities should be reported as soon as possible. Sensitivities should be reported without waiting for full identification. Intravenous antibiotics are used, and those with good penetration into brain tissue such as the β-lactams, metronidazole are most appropriate. Surgical drainage is complementary to chemotherapy and should be performed as soon as the lesion has been localized.

10 Eye infections

10.1 Acute conjunctivitis

Infection is usually mild, often resolving spontaneously or responding well to empirical antibiotics. However, if some rarer cases are not diagnosed and adequately treated extensive infection of the eye may result.

10.1.1 Types of samples

Whilst direct inoculation of plates at the beside is preferable, swabs from cases of acute conjunctivitis are the most frequently received ophthalmic specimens. In severe infections scrapings may be taken from the conjunctiva.

Identification of *Chlamydia trachomatis* requires swabs to be placed in special transport medium (see Chapter 4). For trachoma conjunctival scrapings from the upper lid are required.

10.1.2 Expected organisms

The most commonly isolated bacteria are *S. aureus*, *Streptococcus pneumoniae*, *H. influenzae*, and *Neisseria gonorrhoeae*. The most likely organisms encountered depends largely on age. In neonate *Chlamydia trachomatis* and *N. gonorrhoeae* are common causes. *Neisseria cinerea* can cause infections that may be mistaken for gonococcus (33). In young children *Haemophilus influenzae* may be associated with severe conjunctivitis. *H. influenzae* biogroup *aegyptius* causes outbreaks of acute conjunctivitis in children particularly in hot climates (34). More rarely β-haemolytic streptococci, Enterobacteriaceae, *Neisseria meningitidis*, *Pseudomonas aeruginosa*, and *Moraxella* spp. (especially *Moraxella lacunata*) are encountered.

Viruses, particularly adenoviruses, are common causes of acute conjunctivitis, and their diagnosis should be considered, especially when no bacterial pathogen is isolated.

10.1.3 Processing, identification, and sensitivity testing

(a) Examine a Gram stain of the swab or scrapings. Stain for chlamydia if appropriate (Chapter 4).

(b) Inoculate blood agar and chocolate agar plates and incubate in 5% CO_2 for 24 hours. If no growth occurs re-incubate for a further 24 hours. In neonates selective media for the isolation of *Neisseria gonorrhoeae* should be inoculated.

(c) Identify and carry out sensitivity testing on *S. aureus* and β-haemolytic strep-tococci as described in Section 4.1, *Streptococcus pneumoniae* and *H. influenzae* as described in Chapter 3, and *N. gonorrhoeae* as described in Chapter 4.

10.1.4 Interpretation and reporting

This should pose few problems, as genuinely pathogenic bacteria are usually present in large numbers. In the absence of foreign material, coagulase negative staphylococci, diphtheroids, and viridans streptococci should be regarded as contaminating skin flora. It is usual to report only sensitivities to appropriate topical antibiotics.

10.2 Endophthalmitis

This is a serious infection which may be restricted to certain structures of the globe or involve all of the intraocular contents. Pain in the eye with corneal ulceration, inflammation, and pus in the anterior chamber (hypopyon) are typical features. It is most frequently seen following ocular surgery but can also result from penetrating trauma to the eye. Rarely it can arise from haematogenous spread of bacteria to the eye. Superficial swabs are of no value and every attempt should be made to obtain anterior and/or vitreous aspirates.

10.2.1 Expected organisms

Most cases of bacterial endophthalmitis develop after intraocular surgery, usually following lens implantation. *Staphylococcus aureus* and coagulase negative staphylococci are by far the commonest pathogens (35). Rarely *Pseudomonas aeruginosa* and Enterobacteriaceae are encountered, often as a result of peri-operative nosocomial infection. A huge range of bacteria have been described in post-traumatic endophthalmitis, but *Bacillus cereus* is increasingly recognized as a cause of severe disease (36). Metastatic endophthalmitis is caused by bacteria such as *H. influenzae*, *N. meningitidis*, *Nocardia* spp., and various fungi. *Candida* spp. occur particularly in intravenous drug users.

10.2.2 Processing, identification, and sensitivity testing

(a) Process aspirates in the same way as pus (see Section 2.1) and include a chocolate agar plate incubated in 5% CO_2 and a Sabouraud's agar for fungi. Remember to telephone the Gram film result.

(b) See Section 4.1.4 for details of the identification and sensitivity testing of *S. aureus* and coagulase negative staphylococci, and other less frequently encountered bacteria in the appropriate section of this book. Aerobic, Gram-positive bacilli, often forming characteristic large rough colonies after 24 hours incubation, should be assumed to be *B. cereus*. It is β-haemolytic, produces a lecithinase with a wide zone on egg yolk agar, is resistant to penicillin, and produces spores that do not swell the cell. Clindamycin, the aminoglycosides, and possibly imipenem are the preferred treatment, so test all of these.

(c) As only certain antibiotics can be given sub-conjunctivally (e.g. aminoglycosides, vancomycin, ciprofloxacin, ceftazidime) remember to test these agents, as many antibiotics do not penetrate the eye from systemic or topical administration.

10.2.3 Interpretation and reporting

Any growth is likely to be significant (except perhaps some enrichment culture results), and because of the severity of the condition, results should be reported by telephone followed by a written result. Because of the rarity of the condition and the limited number of useful antibiotics, restricted sensitivity reporting is not appropriate.

10.3 Periocular infections

These include infections of the eyelids (blepharitis, stye, and chalazion), lacrimal duct/sac (canaliculitis/dacryocystitis), and orbital cellulitis. In the first two conditions swabs or scrapings should be obtained; in orbital cellulitis a blood culture must be obtained, as infection is usually haematogenous. Extension of periorbital infection into the cavernous sinus will produce thrombosis with characteristic clinical signs and a high mortality.

10.3.1 Expected organisms

Cannalicultis is often caused by the anaerobic Gram-positive filamentous organisms, *Propionobacterium propionicus*, and *Actinomyces* spp.

Dacryocystitis may be caused by *S. aureus*, β-haemolytic streptococci, *Pseudomonas aeruginosa*, and *Streptococcus pneumoniae*. *Chlamydia trachomatis* causes a recurrent infection. Mixed infections are common.

The same bacteria that cause conjunctivitis, particularly *S. aureus* often cause infections of the lid.

Periorbital cellulitis is commonly caused by *S. aureus*, group A β-haemolytic streptococci, and *Streptococcus pneumoniae*. *Haemophilus influenzae* was previously a common cause of periorbital and orbital cellulitis in children under five years of age. Since the introduction of vaccination against *H. influenzae* type B, infections due to this organism are now rare (37).

10.3.2 Processing, identification, and sensitivity testing

(a) Gram stain all specimens. *Actinomyces* spp. and *Propionobacterium propionicus* will be seen as Gram-positive branching filaments.

(b) Process specimens from canaliculitis and dacryocystitis as pus (Section 2.1) and perform identification and sensitivity tests accordingly.

(c) Process specimens from lid infections as conjunctival swabs (Section 10.1.2) and further tests as in Section 10.1.3.

Periorbital infections are difficult to diagnose, as the only specimen obtained other than a conjunctival swab (which is usually unhelpful) is a blood culture; process as described in Chapter 2. If operative material is obtained treat it as pus.

10.3.3 Interpretation and reporting

Generally moderate or heavy growth of bacteria will be significant. Those with sensitivities to systemic and topical agents should be reported if appropriate.

173

Occasionally, colonizing bacteria such as coagulase negative staphylococci will be encountered as in conjunctival swabs; these should be ignored.

References

1. Newell, P. M. and Norden, C. W. (1988). *J. Clin. Microbiol.*, **26**, 401.

2. Roelofsen, E., van Leeuwen, M., Meijer-Severs, G. J., Wilkinson, M. H., and Degener, J. E. (1999). *J. Clin. Microbiol.*, **37**, 3041.

3. Rantakokko-Jalava, K., Nikkari, S., Jalava, J., *et al.* (2000). *J. Clin. Microbiol.*, **38**, 32.

4. Knox, C. M., Cevallos, V., Margolis, T. P., and Dean, D. (1999). *Am. J. Ophthalmol.*, **128**, 511.

5. Redkar, R., Kalns, J., Butler, W., Krock, L., McCleskey, F., Salmen, A., *et al.* (2000). *Mol. Cell. Probes*, **14**, 163.

6. Sunamen, P., Baron, E. J., and Citron, D. M. (ed.) (1993). *Wadsworths anaerobic bacteriology manual*, 5th edn. Belmont Star Publishing.

7. Holdeman, L. V., Cato, E. P., and Moore, W. E. P. (ed.) (1977). *Anaerobe laboratory manual*, 4th edn. Virginia Polytechnic Institute and State University, Blacksburg, VA.

8. Loesche, W. J. (1968). *Appl. Microbiol.*, **18**, 723.

9. Ganguli, L. A., Turton, L. J., and Tillotson, G. S. (1982). *J. Clin. Pathol.*, **35**, 458.

10. Allen, D. S., Siders, J. A., and Marler, L. M. (1995). *Clin. Lab. Med.*, **15**, 333.

11. Murray, P. R., Baron, E. J., Pfaller, M. A., Tenover, F. C., and Yolken, R. H. (1995). *Manual of clinical microbiology*, 6th edn. American Society for Microbiology, Washington DC.

12. Baron, E. J. and Citron, D. M. (1997). *Clin. Infect. Dis.*, **25**, Suppl. 2, S143.

13. Whaley, D. N., Wiggs, L. S., Miller, P. H., Srivastava, P. V., and Miller, J. M. (1995). *J. Clin. Microbiol.*, **33**, 1196.

14. Koneman, E. W., Allen, S. D., Janda, W. M., Schreckenberger, P. C., and Winn, W. C. Jr. (ed.) (1997). *Colour atlas and textbook of diagnostic microbiology*, 5th edn. Lippincott, Williams–Wilkins, Philedelphia, PA.

15. Willis, A. T. (1997). *Anaerobic bacteriology: clinical and laboratory practice*, 3rd edn. Butterworths, London and Boston.

16. Marler, L. M., Siders, L. A., Wolters, L. C., Pettigrew, Y., Skitt, B. L., and Allen, S. D. (1991). *J. Clin. Microbiol.*, **29**, 874.

17. Aldridge, K. E., Ashcroft, D., Combre, K., Pierson, C. L., Jenkins, S. G., and Rosenblatt, J. G. (2001). *Antimicrob. Agents Chemother.*, **45**, 1238.

18. Forbes, B. A., Sahm, D. F., and Weissfeld, A. S. (ed.) (1998). *Bailey and Scotts diagnostic microbiology*, 10th edn. CV Mosby Co, St Louis.

19. Luijendijk, A., van Belkum, A., Verbrugh, H., and Kluytmans, J. (1996). *J. Clin. Microbiol.*, **34**, 2267.

20. van Griethuysen, A., Bes, M., Etienne, J., Zbinden, R., and Kluytmans, J. (2001). *J. Clin. Microbiol.*, **39**, 86.

21. Tilson, L. D., Midolo, P. D., and Kerr, T. G. (2001). *J. Clin. Microbiol.*, **39**, 4221.

22. Petts, D. N. (1984). *J. Clin. Microbiol.*, **19**, 432.

23. Beall, B., Facklam, R., and Thompson, J. (1996). *J. Clin. Microbiol.*, **34**, 953.

24. Smyth, R. W., Kahlmeter, G., Liljequist, B., and Hoffman, B. (2001). *J. Hosp. Infect.*, **48**, 103.

25. Brenner, D. J., Hollis, D. G., Fanning, G. R., and Weaver, R. E. (1989). *J. Clin. Microbiol.*, **27**, 231.

26. Hawkey, P. M., Malnick, H., Glover, S., Cook, N., and Watts, J. A. (1984). *J. Clin. Pathol.*, **37**, 1066.

27. Evans, E. G. V. and Richardson, M. D. (ed.) (1989). *Medical mycology: a practical approach*. IRL Press, Oxford.

28. Gillespie, S. H. and Hawkey P. M. (ed.) (1995). Medical parasitology: a practical approach. OUP, Oxford.

29. Centers for Disease Control and Prevention, Atlanta, GA. (1997). *MMWR*, **46**, 969.

30. Traynor, R. M., Parratt, D., Duguid, H. L. D., and Duncan, I. D. (1981). *J. Clin. Pathol.*, **34**, 914.

31. Fiarino, A. S. (1996). *Obstet. Gynecol.*, **87**, 142.

32. MacKowiak, P. A., Jones, S. R., and Smith, J. W. (1978). *J. Am. Med. Assoc.*, **239**, 2772.

33. Dolter, J., Wong, J., and Janda, J. M. (1998). *J. Infect.*, **36**, 49.

34. Brazilian Purpuric Fever Study Group. (1987). *Lancet*, **2**, 757.

35. Endophthalmitis Vitrectomy Study. (1996). *Am. J. Ophthalmol.*, **122**, 830.

36. Reynolds, D. S. and Flynn, H. W. Jr. (1997). *Curr. Opin. Ophthalmol.*, **8**, 32.

37. Ambati, B. K., Ambati, J., Azar, N., Stratton, L., and Schmidt, E. V. (2000). *Ophthalmology*, **107**, 1450.

Chapter 6

Bacteriology of intestinal disease

Stephen Pedler and Clive Graham

Department of Microbiology, Royal Victoria Infirmary,
Queen Victoria Road, Newcastle upon Tyne NE1 4LP, UK.

1. Introduction

There is a formidable list of bacteria which are known or suspected to cause gastrointestinal infection in human beings. This list is not unchanging; organisms are sometimes added to it, while the status of other organisms varies with the passage of time. In the first edition of this book, for example, examination for enteropathogenic *E. coli* was recommended for all specimens from children aged three years or under, while current practice in many laboratories is not to examine specimens for these organisms routinely. Conversely, the criteria for examining specimens for Verocytotoxic *E. coli* have been expanded so that many more specimens are now routinely examined for this organism. Since the first edition antibiotic treatment has been increasingly recognized as useful in certain gastrointestinal (GI) infections, and with that the problem of antibiotic resistance in pathogenic bacteria has increased in importance.

Certain bacteria, such as salmonellae, shigellae, and campylobacters, are found so commonly that they are included in the shorter list of bacteria that are looked for routinely in every specimen from a patient with GI infection, while other organisms are looked for only in certain circumstances. Since no laboratory could possibly examine all specimens for all potential pathogens, deciding which organisms to look for is of crucial importance. Also, it is recognized that there may be a difference between specimens sent from the community or on acute admission to hospital and those from patients who have been hospitalized for some time. The latter patients are more likely to be infected with *Clostridium difficile* than any other organism, unless they are part of a hospital outbreak, and a case might be made on the grounds of cost-effectiveness to look only for *C. difficile* toxin in specimens from patients who have been hospitalized for more than an arbitrary period, such as 72 hours (1).

While simple culture of faeces is straightforward, the further processing of a specimen after incubation may appear complex and confusing, particularly to the trainee in microbiology. The purpose of this chapter therefore is to discuss culture media and technical methods available for faeces bacteriology, and how a specimen of faeces may be processed in the routine laboratory. Numerous media and methods have been developed for this purpose, and it is not possible to discuss all of them. The exclusion of a particular medium or method does not necessarily imply that it is regarded as unsatisfactory; rather that those methods which are included have been found to be satisfactory in the experience of the authors and editors.

Finally, it should be remembered that other organisms, such as protozoa and viruses, may also cause gastrointestinal infection and viruses in particular may be commoner than bacterial infections. Examination for these organisms does not form part of the scope of this book, but it is important not to forget non-bacterial pathogens when processing faecal specimens.

2 Bacterial enteric pathogens

Table 1 presents a list of those bacteria known or strongly suspected of causing human GI infection. A problem sometimes encountered is in deciding when to examine a specimen for one of the less commonly encountered pathogens, and guidance is given in the table for this purpose.

A discussion of the clinical syndromes and epidemiology of these infections is beyond the scope of this chapter, but will be found elsewhere (2).

3 Culture media

A considerable number of selective media are now available for the isolation of pathogenic bacteria from faeces. The aim of this section is to discuss the advantages and disadvantages of the more frequently used media together with the appearance of organisms which grow on them. It should be realized that the stated reactions apply to the majority of strains of a particular species, but that exceptions may occasionally be seen. In addition to selective plating media, liquid enrichment media and media for identification are also discussed in this section. Further details of media and practical techniques can be found in the references (3).

3.1 Media for the isolation of salmonellae and shigellae

These media are presented in order of increasing selectivity in Table 2. Enrichment media are discussed in Section 3.1.1.

In addition to the media listed in Table 2, *Salmonella* spp. (and *E. coli* 0157) possess certain specific enzymatic activities and these can be demonstrated with fluorogenic or chromogenic substrates in the primary inoculation medium. Potentially significant colonies can be more easily detected, improving accuracy, facilitating rapid detection of these organisms, and reducing the need for processing 'suspect' colonies which turn out to be other Enterobacteriaceae. These

Table 1 Examination of faeces for bacterial pathogens

Category of examination	When to examine
1. Routine examination, all specimens	
Salmonella spp., including *S. typhi*	Routinely
Shigella spp.	Routinely
Campylobacter spp.	Routinely
2. Examination when specific criteria met	
Verocytotoxic *E. coli*	Diarrhoeal[a] specimens; cases of bloody diarrhoea; haemolytic–uraemic syndrome
Vibrio cholerae 01/0139; non-01 *V. cholerae*	Travellers from those parts of the world where these organisms are endemic or epidemic
Vibrio parahaemolyticus	Travellers returning from the far east; food poisoning associated with shellfish consumption
Yersinia enterocolitica	Clinical details suggestive of *Yersinia* infection
Clostridium difficile	Recent antibiotic treatment; antibiotic-associated diarrhoea; pseudomembranous colitis; patients who have been hospitalized for three days or more
3. Outbreaks of food-borne infection	
Clostridium perfringens	Food-borne outbreaks potentially due to one of these organisms
Staphylococcus aureus	
Bacillus cereus	
4. No examination in normal circumstances	
Enteropathogenic *E. coli*	Outbreaks in children now rare in the UK, but remain common in Third World countries
Enterotoxigenic *E. coli*	A major cause of traveller's diarrhoea, but examination for enterotoxin is difficult for non-reference laboratories
Aeromonas hydrophila	Significance in gastrointestinal infection is uncertain
Plesiomonas shigelloides	Significance in gastrointestinal infection is uncertain
Edwardsiella tarda	Significance in gastrointestinal infection is uncertain

[a] Defined as semi-formed or liquid stools.

agar are however significantly more expensive than traditional media and are yet to be widely adopted.

3.1.1 Enrichment media for the isolation of salmonellae and shigellae

(a) *General principles.* Because salmonellae and shigellae may be present in faeces specimens in very small numbers, the routine use of a selective enrichment

Table 2 Selective media for the isolation of salmonellae and shigellae

Medium	Components	Colonial morphology	Comments
Deoxycholate-citrate agar (DCA)	*Selective agent*: sodium deoxycholate. *Indicator system*: lactose + neutral red. H_2S detection system: sodium thiosulfate + ferric ammonium citrate.	Lactose fermenters: small, deep pink colonies. Late fermenters: pale pink or colourless. Non-fermenters: colourless, translucent colonies which may be over-looked if small (esp. shigellae). H_2S producers: (*Proteus*, *Citrobacter*, and most salmonellae) have black-centred colonies.	Relatively low selectivity; this is useful for shigellae which may be inhibited by more selective media.
Xylose-lysine-deoxycholate agar (XLD)	*Selective agent*: sodium deoxycholate. *Indicator system*: sugars: lactose, xylose, and sucrose amino acid: lysine pH indicator: phenol red (pH <6.8 yellow, 6.8–8.4 red, and >8.4 red/purple). H_2S detection system as for DCA.	Organisms that neither decarboxylate lysine nor ferment the sugars produce colourless, translucent colonies, e.g. shigellae and some *Proteeae*. Organisms that do not decarboxylate lysine but ferment one or more of the sugars produce bright yellow colonies, e.g. *E. coli* and *Klebsiella*. Salmonellae decarboxylate lysine but only ferment xylose resulting in colonies which may initially be yellow but are usually red after 24 h incubation. H_2S producers yield black-centred colonies.	Less inhibitory than DCA. Colour change depends on acid produced by sugar fermentation and alkali produced by lysine decarboxylation. This medium is particularly useful for the detection of shigellae.
Hektoen enteric agar (HEA)	*Selective agent*: bile salts. *Indicator system*: sugars: lactose, sucrose, and salicin pH indicator: thymol blue (reacts with the dye acid fuchsin to produce a yellow colour in acid conditions). H_2S detection system as for DCA.	Salmonellae and shigellae do not ferment any of the sugars (apart from rare strains) and produce green or blue/green colonies. Organisms fermenting one or more of the sugars such as *E. coli* produce yellow or orange/yellow colonies. H_2S producers yield black-centred colonies. *Proteus* strains produce small transparent colonies.	Bile salts in relatively high concentrations retard the growth of many coliforms and make this media more selective.

Bismuth sulfite agar (Wilson and Blair's medium)	*Selective agents*: bismuth sulfite and brilliant green. *Indicator system*: glucose and ferrous citrate. When glucose is fermented sulfite is reduced to sulfide, leading to the precipitation of iron sulfide. This gives black colonies and discoloration of the underlying medium.	Shigellae and most Enterobacteriaceae except salmonellae do not grow on this medium. *Salmonella typhi* produce black colonies with a metallic sheen due to H_2S production, the underlying media is often brown or black. Most other salmonellae produce grey/black, grey, or green colonies, larger than those of *S. typhi*. The discoloured zone under the colony may be absent. If the strain is an H_2S producer a metallic sheen is noted.	Used for the isolation of *Salmonella typhi* and other salmonellae, particularly atypical strains such as the Arizona group. It has a short shelf-life (24–36 h) after preparation.
Statens serum institut enteric medium (SSI)	*Selective agents*: sodium deoxycholate and sodium dodecyl benzene sulfonate. *Indicator system*: sugars: lactose and neutral red phenylalanine deaminase: ferric citrate indole: Ehrlichs reagent in lid rough transformation in *S. sonnei*: high concentration of Mg^{2+} and Ca^{2+}.	Salmonellae pale grey with black centre and metallic sheen. *S. typhi* less black, flatter colony. Shigellae flat pale colonies with spreading and irregular edge. Lactose fermenting Enterobacteriacae pink confined to colony because of deoxycholic acid, *Proteus* black centre to colony with brown colour in medium below.	Detection of *Salmonella/Shigella* reported to be marginally superior to XLD and HEA with 100% recovery of *Yersinia* (4).

medium which allows the multiplication of these organisms while inhibiting that of unwanted bacteria is recommended.

(b) *Choice of medium*. Selenite broth is probably the most widely used enrichment medium, containing sodium selenite as the selective ingredient. It permits the growth of most strains of salmonellae, but some strains of shigellae are inhibited. In an attempt to overcome this problem, Gram-negative broth has been used, which contains a low concentration of sodium deoxycholate as the selective agent. However, this medium is probably insufficiently selective for routine use. Tetrathionate broth is a third possibility, but is much too inhibitory for shigellae. Some strains of salmonellae are also inhibited, particularly if brilliant green is included in the formulation. Selenite broth is therefore recommended for general use.

(c) *Subculture of enrichment media*. Enrichment media should be subcultured to a selective solid medium after incubation. In order to isolate shigellae, a medium of relatively low selectivity should be used; DCA or XLD is recommended. If it is desired only to isolate salmonellae (as in a search for *S. typhi*) a more selective medium can be used, such as bismuth sulfite medium.

3.2 Screening identification media for salmonellae and shigellae

Clearly, whichever media are used, the bacteriologist will still be left with a varying number of bacterial isolates which might or might not be pathogens. To identify each one of these isolates to species level would be time-consuming, expensive, and unnecessary. Consequently, a method is needed to screen out organisms not regarded as pathogenic; the small number of organisms which remain may then be identified fully. One approach is to inoculate a short series of biochemical tests with the suspect organism. A suitable range of tests is given in Table 3. If many specimens are being processed the use of individually tubed tests may prove inconvenient. Various composite media have been developed which attempt to carry out several of these tests in one or two tubes. Three of the most widely used of these are described below.

Methods to detect preformed enzymes have also been developed to facilitate rapid diagnosis and reduce the number of isolates requiring further analysis. *Salmonella* spp. possess a C_8 esterase activity not present in other lactose non-fermenting Enterobacteriaceae. Enzyme activity can be determined either as a spot test (see Section 4.4.2 and Protocol 4) or by using a novel chromogenic ester agar (5).

3.2.1 Kligler's iron agar (KIA) and triple sugar iron agar (TSI)

(a) *General principles*. These two composite media are very similar, differing only in that while Kligler's medium contains two sugars (glucose and lactose), TSI also contains sucrose. The pH indicator is phenol red, and a detection system for hydrogen sulfide (H_2S) is included. These media are poured as agar slopes, with the total depth of the medium being between 5 cm and 8 cm. The butt

Table 3 Screening biochemical tests for salmonellae and shigellae

Test	Media	Positive result
O-nitrophenyl galactosidase (ONPG) activity	Tube of O-nitrophenyl galactose broth	Colour change from colourless to yellow
Urease activity	Urea slope: peptone agar plus urea and phenol red	Colour change from pale yellow to bright pink
Indole production	Incubate in a tube of peptone water and after 4–6 h add Kovac's reagent	Red ring produced on top of the peptone water
Hydrogen sulfide production	(i) Tube of peptone water. Insert lead acetate paper between cap and tube	Blackening of paper due to formation of lead sulfide
	(ii) Triple sugar iron agar	Ferric sulfide produced, blackening the medium
Carbohydrate fermentation	Peptone water and fermentable carbohydrate plus pH indicator	Colour change due to acid production (depends on indicator used)

(the deep section of the medium) is inoculated by stabbing with a straight wire, while the surface of the slope is inoculated by streaking.

(b) *Culture results.* Organisms which ferment glucose produce acid which initially turns the whole medium yellow. Degradation of protein in the medium leads to the production of alkaline amines, but since this requires the presence of oxygen it occurs only in the sloped section, which is exposed to the air, and not in the butt. After 24 hours, organisms which ferment only glucose produce an acid butt and an alkaline (red) slope. Lactose (and sucrose if present) are present in excess; if either is fermented, sufficient acid is produced to turn the whole medium yellow, regardless of amine production. The production of H_2S will turn the medium black. It is also possible to detect gas production from glucose in these media. This may manifest itself as bubbles of gas in the agar, separation of the agar from the wall of the tube, or in some cases complete disruption of the medium. These media cannot readily distinguish salmonellae and shigellae from many strains of the *Proteeae* ; for this reason they should be read in conjunction with a test for urease production or the presence of phenylalanine deaminase. Typical reactions in these media are shown in Table 4.

3.2.2 Kohn's composite media

This is a two tube medium.

Tube 1 contains glucose, mannitol, and urea, and is poured as a slope similar to TSI and KIA. The pH indicator is phenol red. Organisms which ferment only

Table 4 Reactions in Kliger's iron agar and triple sugar iron agar

Butt	Slope	H$_2$S	Interpretation
Acid	Acid	No	*E. coli*, *Klebsiella* spp., *Enterobacter* spp., some *Citrobacter* strains
Acid	Acid	Yes	Some *Citrobacter* strains
Acid	Alkaline	No	*Shigella* spp., some *Proteeae*, occasional *Citrobacter* strains
Acid	Alkaline	Yes	*Salmonella* spp., *Proteeae*, some *Citrobacter* strains
Alkaline	Alkaline	No	Non-fermenters such as *Pseudomonas aeruginosa*

glucose turn the butt acid (yellow) whilst those which also ferment mannitol (which is present in excess) turn the slope yellow as well. This is the reaction seen with many of the Enterobacteriaceae, including *E. coli*, *Citrobacter*, *Enterobacter*, and *Salmonella*. Most strains of *Shigella* also produce this reaction, with the exception of *S. dysenteriae* types 1–10, which do not ferment mannitol. Regardless of sugar fermentation, those organisms which hydrolyse urea (*Proteus* spp., *Morganella morganii*, and *Providencia rettgeri*) produce a uniform bright pink colour due to the production of ammonia.

Tube 2 contains sucrose and salicin, the pH indicator is bromothymol blue, and sodium thiosulfate is included as a sulfur source. The tubed agar is allowed to set vertically, not as a slope. After inoculation, paper test strips for H$_2$S and indole production are suspended from the top of the tube by wedging them between the wall of the tube and the plug. Fermentation of sucrose and/or salicin (not fermented by the majority of *Salmonella* or *Shigella* strains) turns the blue/green medium yellow. Hydrogen sulfide production turns the appropriate indicator paper black, while the production of indole turns the other paper pink (from pale yellow).

It should be noted that neither tube contains lactose, and it is recommended that a test for ONPG activity is set up in conjunction with these tubes.

3.3 Media for the isolation of *Escherichia coli* 0157, *Yersinia enterocolitica*, and other commonly encountered gastrointestinal pathogens

Table 5 presents details of media for the isolation of these organisms.

4 Routine specimen processing

In this section methods and techniques are discussed for the processing of a specimen of faeces for salmonellae, shigellae, and campylobacters, which are the three groups of organisms looked for routinely in a patient with a gastrointestinal infection. Methods for other bacteria are found in Section 5.

Table 5 Media and enrichment broths for the isolation of *Escherichia coli* 0157, *Yersinia enterocolitica*, and other commonly encountered gastrointestinal pathogens

Medium	Components	Colonial morphology	Comments
Sorbitol MacConkey agar (SMAC)	*Selective agent*: bile salts. *Indicator system*: d-sorbitol plus neutral red pH indicator.	95% of *E. coli* ferment sorbitol and produce pink colonies. Most *E. coli* 0157 do not ferment sorbitol (within 24 hours of incubation) and produce small, round grey/colourless colonies. Other non-sorbitol fermenting organisms include *Escherichia hermanii*, *Proteus* spp., *Morganella* spp., and *Pseudomonas* spp.	Cefixime, tellurite, or rhamnose may increase selectivity. *E. coli* 0157 does not ferment rhamnose. Cefixime inhibits growth of *Proteus* spp. Tellurite inhibits non-0157 *E. coli*
Modified tryptone soya broth (MTSB)		Not applicable.	Improves isolation of 0157 from convalescent and contact specimens.
Campylobacter medium	*Blood agar base. Selective agents*: vancomycin, polymyxin B, and trimethoprim. Incubation at 43°C increases selectivity.	Most other bacteria will not grow on this medium. *Campylobacter* spp. produce large, flat, glistening grey colonies, often with the long axis of the colony lying along the inoculation streak.	
Thiosulfate-citrate-bile salt-sucrose agar (TCBS)	*Selective agents*: bile salts, sodium thiosulfate, and sodium citrate, pH 8.6, high sodium chloride content. *Indicator system*: sucrose plus thymol blue/bromothymol blue as pH indicators. H$_2$S detection system.	Most strains of Enterobacteriaceae are inhibited; some *Proteeae* may grow as yellow colonies if sucrose is fermented, with black centres if H$_2$S is produced. *Vibrio cholerae* ferments sucrose giving flat yellow colonies. *V. parahaemolyticus* does not ferment sucrose and colonies are large, blue, or blue/green.	Note that *Vibrio* spp. do not produce H$_2$S.

Medium	Components	Colonial morphology	Comments
Alkaline peptone water (APW)	Peptone water is rendered alkaline with a phosphate buffer (pH 8.6). Many bacteria are inhibited at this pH; however, inhibition is incomplete and bacteria may grow after 6–8 h incubation.	Not applicable.	May be subcultured to TCBS after 6 or 24 h.
Cycloserine-cefoxitin agar	Blood agar base. *Selective agents*: cycloserine and cefoxitin.	After 48 h incubation *Clostridium difficile* colonies are large (4–8 mm), greyish/white, and flat with a filamentous outline. There is characteristic smell, similar to paracresol.	Examine colonies under Wood's light for the characteristic yellow/green fluorescence.
Mannitol-salt agar	*Selective agent*: sodium chloride in high concentration (7.5%). Indicator system: mannitol plus phenol red as pH indicator.	Almost all bacteria except staphylococci and halophilic vibrios are inhibited. *Staphylococcus aureus* ferments mannitol to produce yellow zones around the colony.	Suspect colonies should be identified using standard laboratory methods.
Cefsoludin-irgasan-novobiocin (CIN) agar	*Selective agent*: sodium deoxycholate, irgasan (a disinfectant) and two antibiotics, cefsoludin and novobiocin. Indicator system: mannitol plus neutral red as pH indicator.	Most bacteria do not grow on this medium. *Y. enterocolitica* produce medium-sized deep pink colonies (due to mannitol fermentation). *Citrobacter*, *Enterobacter*, and *Serratia* may produce similar colonies.	
Bacillus cereus selective medium (PEMBA)	*Selective agent*: polymyxin B. Indicator system: mannitol plus pH indicator. Egg yolk to detect lecithinase production.	*Bacillus cereus* colonies are large and flat with an irregular outline; they are surrounded by an opaque zone of precipitated egg yolk. *Bacillus cereus* does not ferment mannitol and does not produce an acid reaction.	*B. subtilis* or *B. licheniformis* may also be detected.

4.1 Specimen collection

4.1.1 Types of specimen and transport to the laboratory

Rectal swabs are not a suitable alternative to a specimen of faeces. Whilst there may be difficulties in obtaining specimens from some patients (notably young children and the elderly) there can be no justification for sending rectal swabs from patients with diarrhoea and such specimens should not be accepted.

The specimen can be collected after passing into a suitable container such as a bedpan. For transport to the laboratory, the most appropriate specimen container is a wide-mouthed, screw-capped plastic pot, containing a small plastic or wooden spoon which fits into the pot when closed. If the faeces is liquid, the pot may be filled to one-third full (no more, in order to avoid spillage when opened); if solid, the spoon is used to collect one spoonful of faeces. Enthusiastic clinicians or nurses who send the entire contents of the bedpan should be discouraged.

Once collected, the specimen may be forwarded to the laboratory by the routine local transport. However, a delay in reaching the laboratory of more than three to four hours will result in the development of an acid pH which will rapidly decrease the viability of any shigellae in the specimen.

4.2 Microscopy

Other than a search for parasites (see *Medical parasitology: a practical approach*, OUP) this is not usually done, but occasionally the laboratory may be asked to look for pus cells in the specimen. The following procedure may be used.

Protocol 1

Microscopy for pus cells in faeces

Reagents

- Methylene blue stain

Method

1 If pus or mucous exudate is present on a solid specimen, mix a small portion with a drop of methylene blue on a slide. A liquid specimen may be examined directly.

2 Cover the drop with a coverslip and examine under the ×10 and ×40 objectives.

When appropriate, faeces may also be examined for mycobacteria. Methods are the same as for other types of specimen (see Chapter 3).

4.3 Culture

4.3.1 Choice of media

Culture media for these organisms is discussed in Section 3. Which of these media are chosen is, to a great extent, a matter of personal preference, but it should be noted that no one medium can be regarded as entirely satisfactory for isolating all strains of salmonellae or shigellae. At least two media should be used; suitable combinations would be DCA plus XLD or XLD plus one of the other media listed in Table 5. In addition a tube of selenite broth and a selective medium for campylobacters (Table 5) should be inoculated. If there is a desire or need to examine specifically for *S. typhi* (for example, during an outbreak) bismuth sulfite agar should be added to the set of media used.

4.3.2 Culture technique

Inoculate a liquid specimen using a bacteriological loop, wooden stick, or cotton-tipped swab. If a solid specimen is received, first make a thick emulsion of the specimen in peptone water. Either a liquid specimen or the thick emulsion may then be inoculated into the chosen enrichment medium (use about 1 ml of specimen per 20 ml of broth). Incubate all plates (with the exception of the campylobacter plate) in air at 37 °C. Incubate the campylobacter medium under the special atmosphere required, i.e. 5% O_2, 10% CO_2, and 85% N_2. This mixture can be achieved in an anaerobic jar either by the use of a pre-mixed gas supply or a gas generating kit designed especially for this purpose (e.g. the CampyPak, Becton Dickinson, Oxford, UK). It is occasionally recommended that an ordinary anaerobic gas generating kit be used without putting a catalyst in the jar. This must not be done as potentially explosive mixtures of oxygen and hydrogen may be generated. Candle jars are also inadequate for culturing campylobacters. The plate may be incubated at 37 °C but the selectivity of the medium may be increased by incubating at 42 °C which the authors recommend if an incubator is available for this purpose.

4.4 Reading the plates

This section describes how to examine the culture plates after incubation and the setting up and interpreting of screening identification tests. When reading the plates and carrying out further tests it is essential that all results are recorded on the worksheet accompanying the specimen. This is, of course, good bacteriological practice with any specimen; but it is perhaps the least interesting part of any investigation and is sometimes overlooked, with dire consequences. In addition, it cannot be emphasized too strongly that when picking colonies for further identification only isolated single colonies are chosen. Many of the problems which may be encountered stem from a failure to inoculate tests with a pure strain of an organism. If purity cannot be guaranteed, subculture the colony to MacConkey agar and proceed with further investigation the next day. Remember that it is not necessary to be an expert bacteriologist to process a faeces specimen correctly but it is essential to be a careful one.

4.4.1 The campylobacter plate

i. *Examination*

Protocol 2

Examination of the campylobacter plate

1 After overnight incubation examine this plate for colonies suggestive of *C. jejuni/coli* (see Table 5). If none are found, re-incubate the plate for a further 24 h.

2 If suggestive colonies are found, Gram stain them and look for the typical curved or S-shaped Gram-negative bacilli. Perform an oxidase test (see Chapter 4). Oxidase positive organisms which grow at 42 °C under micro-aerophilic conditions and which show typical microscopic morphology can be presumptively identified as a *Campylobacter* spp. and a report issued to this effect.

---

ii. *Confirmation of identity*

Most general laboratories do not identify these organisms further, but if it is desired to do so, the tests in Table 6 may be used. Note that hippurate hydrolysis may be used to distinguish between *C. jejuni* and *C. coli*. A commercial latex agglutination test (Oxoid Ltd., Basingstoke, England) is available for the identification of campylobacters (6). A DNA probe has also been produced, but this technique is unlikely to be available to most routine laboratories.

iii. *Sensitivity testing*

When antibiotic treatment is required for campylobacter enteritis, erythromycin or ciprofloxacin is the drug of choice. Gentamicin has been used successfully for the treatment of the occasional systemic infection with *C. jejuni/coli*. Carry out sensitivity testing at 37 °C on blood agar in the appropriate gaseous environment.

4.4.2 Media for salmonellae and shigellae

i. *Enrichment medium*

Subculture the selenite broth (or other enrichment medium) to a DCA or XLD plate. Examine this plate after overnight incubation.

Table 6 Identification of *Campylobacter jejuni/coli*

Organism	Growth at 25 °C	Growth at 42 °C	Catalase	Oxidase	Urease	H$_2$S	Hippurate hydrolysis
C. jejuni	−	+	+	+	−	−	+
C. coli	−	+	+	+	−	−	−

STEPHEN PEDLER AND CLIVE GRAHAM

ii. *Examination of solid media*

Protocol 3

Examination of solid media for salmonellae and shigellae

1 Examine these plates for organisms showing colonial morphology and/or colour reactions suggestive of salmonellae or shigellae (see Table 2).

2 For each colonial type of suspect colony inoculate one of the following sets of screening tests:
   (a) A short series of biochemical tests (see Table 3).
   (b) Kligler's iron agar (or Triple Sugar Iron agar) plus a test for urease production.
   (c) Kohn's tubed composite media plus a test for ONPG activity.
   (d) For salmonellae only, suspect colonies may be screened with the fluorescent MUCAP test.

See Section 3.2 for a discussion of Kligler's and Kohn's media. Inoculate KIA or TSI by stabbing the butt and streaking the slope. Inoculate Kohn's medium 1 in this way, and inoculate medium 2 by stabbing.

The MUCAP test comprises a reagent (4-methylumbelliferyl caprilate) which is formed from an ester containing eight carbon atoms conjugated with umbelliferone. A C_8 esterase enzyme present in salmonellae releases umbelliferone which fluoresces in ultraviolet light at 366 nm (Wood's light). This test is very sensitive and highly specific for salmonellae; greater than 99% specificity has been reported (7). The test method is described in Protocol 4.

Protocol 4

The MUCAP test

Reagents

• MUCAP reagent (4-methylumbelliferyl caprilate) (Biolife Italiana Srl, Milan)

Method

1 Add 5 μl of MUCAP reagent to each suspect colony type.

2 Wait for 3–5 min and examine the colonies under Wood's light (366 nm) in a semi-darkened room. A positive result is denoted by fluorescence within 5 min of adding the reagent.

3 Subculture positive colonies to blood or nutrient agar for final identification and serotyping. The reagent does not affect the viability of the colony.

If one of the composite media is chosen, use the remains of the colony to inoculate a purity plate. We have found it useful to use a Petri dish divided in two by a plastic divider (Sterilin Ltd., Stone, England), with one-half of the plate containing blood agar and the other MacConkey agar. Growth on the blood agar may be used for slide agglutination tests if necessary. Setting up a purity plate at this stage will avoid confusion in the interpretation of results later on and also avoids the possibility of discarding a potential salmonella or shigella due to contamination with another organism.

iii. *Reading the screening tests*
If KIA or TSI and a urease test were used, first examine the purity plate. If the culture is not pure results of biochemical tests are meaningless and should be repeated using a single colony of each non-lactose fermenter on the plate. If the culture is pure, examine the test for urea hydrolysis; organisms giving a positive result cannot be a salmonella or shigella and may be discarded. Then examine the KIA/TSI slope. Interpretation of the possible reactions may be carried out using Table 4.

When using Kohn's tubes, check the purity of the culture as above, then examine medium 1 for evidence of urea hydrolysis. If this is absent, read the remaining biochemical reactions and interpret them using Table 7.

It must be understood that the screening tests described here do not confirm the identity of the organism. For that, further tests are needed as described in Sections 4.5 and 4.6.

4.5 Serotyping of salmonellae and shigellae
4.5.1 Salmonella serotyping
The final identification of a salmonella can be regarded as consisting of confirmation of identity by biochemical testing plus determination of serotype. Neither method is adequate when used alone; biochemical tests merely confirm that the organism is a salmonella, but provide no useful information for epidemiological purposes. Serological identification must always be confirmed with biochemical tests due to the presence of similar antigens in other members of the Enterobacteriaceae. This section describes practical techniques for salmonella serotyping, but makes no attempt to discuss the theoretical basis of classification by the Kauffman–White scheme. The reader is referred elsewhere for this (8).

i. *Choice of antisera*
Only a limited number of serotypes are encountered regularly in a general laboratory, and consequently no such laboratory need possess more than a basic set of antisera, as shown in Table 8.

ii. *Initial screening tests*
Test all suspect organisms by slide agglutination (see Protocol 5) against polyvalent O and polyvalent H (specific and non-specific phases). If the organism does

Table 7 Biochemical reactions of some enteric Gram-negative bacilli

	E. coli	Enteroinvasive	Klebsiella pneumoniae	Enterobacter cloacae	Citrobacter freundii	Yersinia enterocolitica	Proteus mirabilis	Proteus vulgaris	Morganella morganii	Salmonella typhi	Salmonella spp.	Shigella dysenteriae	Shigella flexneri	Shigella boydii	Shigella sonnei	Vibrio cholerae	Vibrio parahaemolyticus
Motility	+	−	−	+	+	−ᵃ	+	+	+	+	+	−	−	−	−	+	+
VP reaction	−	−	v	v	−	−	v	−	−	−	−	−	−	−	−	+	−
Simmons' citrate	−	−	+	+	+	−	v	v	−	−	+	−	−	−	−	+	+
Urease	−	−	+	−	−	+	+	+	+	−	−	−	−	−	−	−	−
H₂S	−	−	−	−	+	−	+	+	v	+	+	−	−	−	−	−	−
Indole	+	v	−	−	v	v	−	+	+	−	−	v	v	v	−	+	+
LDC	+	−	+	−	−	−	−	−	−	+	+	−	−	−	−	+	+
ODC	v	v	−	+	v	+	+	−	+	−	+	−	−	−	+	+	+
PPA	−	−	−	−	−	−	+	+	+	−	−	−	−	−	−	−	−
ONPG	+	v	+	+	+	+	−	−	−	−	−	−	−	−	+	+	−
Gas from glucose	+	−	+	+	+	−	+	+	+	−	+	−	−	−	−	−	−
Acid from																	
dulcitol	v	v	−	−	−	−	−	−	−	−	+	−	−	−	−	−	−
mannitol	+	+	+	+	+	+	−	−	−	+	+	−	+	+	+	+	+
salicin	v	v	+	+	−	v	−	v	−	−	−	−	−	−	−	−	−
sorbitol	+	v	+	+	+	+	−	−	−	+	+	v	v	v	−	−	−
sucrose	v	v	+	+	v	+	+	+	−	−	−	−	−	−	−	+	−

Key:
+ = 90% or more reactions positive.
− = 10% or fewer reactions positive.
v = 11–89% of reactions positive.
ᵃ Motile at 22 °C.

Table 8 Antigenic structure of and antisera for the identification of *Salmonella* serotypes seen in the UK and USA

Common serotypes	Antigenic structure (O: phase 1 h: phase 2 h)
S. typhi	9, 12 (Vi): d
S. paratyphi B	1,4,5,12: b: 1,2
S. enteritidis	1,9,12: g,m: 1,7
S. typhimurium	1,4,5,12: i: 1,2
S. dublin	1,9,12: g,p

O antisera	H antisera
Polyvalent O, groups A–G	Polyvalent H, specific and non-specific phases Polyvalent H, non-specific phase
Monovalent O antisera: 2; 4; 6,7; 8; 9; 3,10; 15; 19 Vi antiserum	Monovalent H antisera: a; b; c; d; e,h; f,g; g,m; i;k; l,v; m,t; r

not agglutinate with polyvalent O, test it again with Vi antiserum. Vi is a surface antigen and if present may mask the underlying O antigens.

Protocol 5

Slide agglutination tests

Reagents

- Polyvalent or monovalent antisera

Method

When performing these tests, never use colonies growing on a selective medium, as erroneous results may be obtained.

1 Pick a small amount of growth from a pure culture on a nutrient or blood agar plate and make a smooth, dense suspension in saline on a glass slide. There must be no clumps or particles visible in the suspension.

2 To this, add a small loopful of antiserum and mix the two by rocking the slide gently backwards and forwards.

3 Look for visible clumping occurring within 60 sec of mixing the suspension and the antiserum which indicates agglutination. This is best seen if the slide is held against a dark background such as a black tile.

4 Remember that this is a live culture, therefore discard the slide into the bench disinfectant pot.

In the UK an organism which does not agglutinate with the polyvalent O antiserum groups A–G or with Vi is unlikely to be a salmonella, even if it agglutinates with polyvalent H antiserum (the frequency of cross-reactions with H antisera is high). However, members of rare serogroups not included in the polyvalent O antisera are occasionally seen. If full biochemical identification still indicates that the organism is a salmonella, it should be sent to a reference laboratory for identification. Conversely, the Vi antigen is also possessed by other members of the Enterobacteriaceae and O antisera occasionally cross-react with organisms other than salmonellae; again, biochemical testing is useful. Negative polyvalent H agglutination may occur with rare serotypes not included in the polyvalent sera, or the strain may be non-motile (no H antigens present).

iii. *Determination of serogroup (O antigens)*

If the organism agglutinates in polyvalent O antiserum, re-test it with monovalent sera to determine the serogroup. If polyvalent O agglutination was negative but Vi agglutination was positive, the Vi antigen may be removed and the strain re-tested (see Protocol 6).

Protocol 6

Inactivation of Vi antigen

Reagents

• Saline

Method

1 Make a heavy suspension of the organism in 1 ml saline and heat it for 30 min at 100 °C min.

2 Centrifuge the suspension in a microcentrifuge at 12 000 g and resuspend the pellet of bacteria in 0.5 ml saline.

3 Use this suspension to repeat the O agglutination tests.

Slide agglutination is usually sufficient to determine the O group, but if there is the slightest doubt about the result (e.g. a weak or slow reaction) confirm it with a tube agglutination test (see Section 4.5.1.vi).

iv. *Determination of serotype (H antigen)*

If the organism agglutinates in polyvalent H (specific and non-specific) anti-serum, test it with polyvalent H non-specific antiserum. If there is no agglutination (or the reaction is very weak) the organism is in the specific phase and may then be tested with individual antisera or the Rapid Diagnostic Sera (see below). Since the serogroup has already been determined it is not necessary to test every H antiserum straight away—start with those known to occur in that particular serogroup. If there is strong agglutination with polyvalent H (non-specific) antiserum the organism is in the non-specific phase and must be changed to the specific phase before the serotype can be determined (see Section 4.5.1.vii). Because cross-reactions with motile organisms other than salmonellae are common with H antisera, all positive slide agglutination tests for H antigens must be confirmed with a tube agglutination test.

Rapid diagnostic sera (RDS) contain a mixture of antisera to various H antigens, and the pattern of reactions which occurs may be used to determine the serotype. This removes the need to test multiple individual antisera. Different combinations may be available from different commercial sources; a popular combination obtainable from Murex (Murex, Dartford, UK) is as follows:

(a) RDS 1: antisera to b, d, r, and the E complex.

(b) RDS 2: antisera to b, k, the E complex, and the L complex.

(c) RDS 3: antisera to d, k, the E complex, and the G complex.

Note that antiserum to H antigen 'i' is not included and this must therefore be tested separately. This is important because *S. typhimurium*, one of the commonest serotypes seen in the UK and USA, possesses this H antigen. The reaction patterns which occur may be interpreted using Table 9.

v. *Colour latex agglutination tests*

An alternative to conventional slide agglutination tests are commercial kits using coloured latex particles (Wellcolex Salmonella, Murex, Dartford, UK). The two reagents in this kit each contain latex particles of three different colours. Each group of coloured particles is coated with antibody to one or more group-specific O antigens of salmonellae. Before adding an antigen, the suspension of particles is a grey/brown colour, but if agglutination takes place agglutinated coloured particles can be seen and the background colour changes correspondingly. The pattern of colour changes which takes place can be used to determine the serogroup (9).

The manufacturer's instructions should be used to carry out this test and interpret the results.

Table 9 Interpretation of reactions using RDS antisera

Agglutination with RDS			Indicates H antigen
1	2	3	
+	+	+	E complex
+	+	−	b
+	−	−	r
−	+	+	k
−	−	+	G complex
−	+	−	L complex
+	−	+	d

vi. *Tube agglutination tests*

These are used to confirm the results of slide tests. The aim is to show that the antiserum will agglutinate a suspension of the test organism at a dilution equal to or greater than that stated on the antiserum package. Cross-reactions with other organisms will usually give agglutination only at lower titres than that stated on the bottle. The method is given in Protocol 7.

Protocol 7

Method for tube agglutinations for salmonellae

Equipment and reagents

- Agglutination tubes
- 50 °C water-bath
- Salmonella antisera

Method

1 Preparation of antigens.
   (a) O antigens: suspend the growth from a nutrient or blood agar plate in 2 ml saline. Heat the suspension for 10 min at 100 °C, which denatures the flagellae.
   (b) H antigens: add a few drops of formalin to an overnight broth culture to kill the organism.
   (c) Vi antigen: suspend the growth from a plate culture in saline (note: this is a live antigen preparation and must be handled with care).

2 For each antiserum to be tested, first make a 1/10 dilution of the antiserum in saline, then set up a rack of seven agglutination tubes.

3 To tubes 2–7, add 200 µl of saline, and to tubes 1 and 2 add 200 µl of the diluted antiserum. Prepare a series of doubling dilutions of antiserum in tubes 2–6, by taking 200 µl from tube 2 and adding it to tube 3. Repeat this process down to tube 6, and discard 200 µl from this tube.

4 Finally, add 200 µl of antigen to each tube. Tubes 1–6 now contain a series of doubling dilution of antiserum from 1/20 to 1/640, while tube 7 is a negative control with no antiserum.

5 Incubate the tubes at 50 °C in a water-bath, and read them after 4 h. If the results are negative, incubate the tubes at room temperature overnight and read them again the next day.

6 Read the tubes in a good light against a dark background. Agglutination appears as a clumping of the bacteria which form a deposit on the bottom of the tube, with clearing of the supernatant. It may be necessary to use a hand lens to detect fine traces of agglutination. The result is defined as the highest dilution of antiserum giving visible agglutination.

vii. *Method for changing the phase of a salmonella from non-specific to specific phase*

Two methods are given in Protocol 8.

Protocol 8

Changing the phase of a salmonella

Equipment and reagents

- 30 ml sterile bottle containing a small inner tube (method B)
- Polyvalent H non-specific phase antisera

A. Bridge plate method (see Figure 1)

(This is the simpler of the two methods given here.)

1 Using a sterile scalpel blade, cut a trough 1 cm wide across a fresh, moist, blood or nutrient agar plate.

2 Inoculate one-half of the plate with the non-specific phase culture.

3 Bridge the trough with a strip of moistened sterile filter paper (see Figure 1).

4 Place a drop of polyvalent H non-specific phase antiserum on the bridge (point A on Figure 1) and incubate the plate overnight at 37 °C.

5 Motile organisms will migrate across the bridge, but those in the non-specific phase will be immobilized by the antiserum. Subculture the organism from growth on the other half of the plate (point B on Figure 1).

6 The subcultured organisms should now be in the specific phase, but the process may need to be repeated if the organism is still in the non-specific phase.

B. Craigie tube method (see Figure 2)

1 Prepare 10 ml semi-solid (0.5%) nutrient agar and mix the agar with three drops of polyvalent H non-specific phase antiserum.

2 Pour the agar into a sterile 30 ml bottle, taking care that the upper end of the small inner tube (a length cut from a disposable Pasteur pipette is ideal for this purpose: see Figure 2) is above the surface of the agar. Take care not to disturb the tube, or the motile salmonella in the non-specific phase will by-pass the agar and not be immobilized.

3 Inoculate the tube at point A on Figure 2 and incubate overnight at 37 °C.

4 Organisms in the non-specific phase will be immobilized by the antiserum, but those in the specific phase will migrate down the inner tube and up onto the surface of the agar, from where they can be subcultured (point B on Figure 2).

5 Repeat the procedure if the organism is still not in the specific phase.

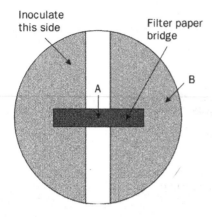

Figure 1 Changing the phase of salmonella: bridge plate method.

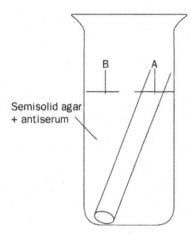

Figure 2 Changing the phase of salmonella: Craigie tube method.

viii. *Problems encountered in salmonella serotyping*

Difficulties and apparent anomalies are sometimes seen when attempting to determine the serotype of a suspected salmonella. Some of the commoner problems and possible solutions are listed in Table 10.

4.5.2 Shigella serotyping

i. *Choice of antisera*

A general laboratory should at least possess polyvalent antisera to the four species of *Shigella*, that is polyvalent *S. dysenteriae* 1–10, polyvalent *S. flexneri*, polyvalent *S. boydii* 1–15, and *S. sonnei* antigenic phase 1 and 2. Laboratories which deal with large numbers of faeces specimens may also find it useful to keep individual antisera to *S. dysenteriae* types 1 and 2, and a panel of antisera to *S. flexneri* serotypes.

198

Table 10 Problems in the serotyping of salmonellae

O agglutination	H agglutination	Possible reasons
+	−	(i) The organism is non-motile (e.g. *S. pullorum*)
		(ii) The strain is poorly motile. Select the motile subpopulation by subculturing to a semi-solid (0.5%) agar plate, incubate, and subculture from the spreading edge of the growth obtained.
		(iii) The strain is an H serotype not included in the antisera available. Send the strain to a reference laboratory for typing.
		(iv) The organism is not salmonella; cross-reactions with other members of the Enterobacteriaceae sometimes occur. Check the biochemical identification of the organism.
−	+	(i) The organism is not salmonella; a non-specific antigen–antibody reaction may rarely occur due to the incomplete removal of antibodies from the antiserum other than those directed against the specific H antigens. Check the biochemical identification of the organism.
		(ii) The strain belongs to an unusual O serotype not included in the available antisera. Send the strain to a reference laboratory for typing.
		(iii) Vi antigen is masking the O antigen. Check agglutination with Vi antiserum. If agglutination occurs, remove the Vi antigen (see Protocol 6) and repeat the O agglutination tests.
−	−	(i) This is a rare occurrence and implies that the organism is not a salmonella. Check the biochemical identification of the organism.
		(ii) A combination of some of the circumstances listed above could also give rise to negative agglutination reactions.
More than one O antiserum positive	+ or −	(i) The organism may possess O antigens shared between O groups, or a non-specific antigen–antibody reaction may be occurring. In either case, tube agglutinations should determine the O group to which the organism belongs.
		(ii) The organism is not salmonella. Check the biochemical identification of the organism.

ii. *Colour latex agglutination tests*

As with salmonellae, commercial kits using coloured latex particles (Wellcolex Shigella, Murex, Dartford, UK) are available. The two reagents in this kit contain latex particles of different colours, and each group of coloured particles is coated with polyvalent antibody to one species of shigella. The test works as described in Section 4.5.1.

iii. *Determination of serotype*

Test suspect organisms by slide agglutination against the polyvalent antisera, starting with antisera to *S. sonnei*, as this is the commonest species encountered in the UK and USA. If the organism agglutinates with one of the polyvalent antisera, the serotype of the identified species may be determined by slide agglutination with monovalent antisera, if available. The method for slide agglutination is the same as for salmonellae (see Section 4.5.1). Tube agglutinations are not usually necessary, but should be performed if there is any doubt about the slide agglutination result, or if biochemical identification is not clear-cut (cross-reactions in slide agglutination tests are common, especially with strains of *E. coli*, some of which are biochemically atypical and may resemble shigellae). Prepare the antigen for tube agglutination tests by suspending growth from an agar plate in saline, and adjusting the opacity to the equivalent of about 10^8 organisms/ml with an opacity standard. Kill the culture with a few drops of formalin, and carry out tube agglutinations as described for salmonellae (see Protocol 7).

iv. S. flexneri *serotyping*

The antigenic structure of *S. flexneri* is complex, and determination of serotype may appear confusing. Consequently serotyping of this species merits a section to itself.

There are six main serotypes of *S. flexneri*, which are determined by the presence of a specific type antigen (labelled I to VI). Sub-serotypes are determined by the presence of group antigens, which are shared between the six main serotypes. In addition, there are two variants (X and Y) which do not possess a type antigen but do possess different group antigens. The antigenic structure of *S. flexneri* is shown in Table 11.

Table 11 Antigenic structure of *Shigella flexneri*

Serotype	Sub-serotype	Type antigen	Group antigen
1	1a	I	1,2,4
1	1b	I	1,2,4,6
2	2a	II	1,3,4
2	2b	II	1,7,8
3	3a	III	1,6,7,8
3	3b	III	1,3,4
3	3c	III	1,6
4	4a	IV	1,3,4
4	4b	IV	1,3,4,6
5	–	V	1,7,8
6	–	VI	1,2,4
X variant			1,7,8
Y variant			1,3,4

4.6 Biochemical identification

4.6.1 Introduction

The full identification by biochemical testing of a member of the Enterobacteriaceae is straightforward if the strain exhibits reactions typical of the species, but can be very difficult with atypical strains. As a result, a full treatment of the subject is beyond the scope of this chapter, and the interested reader is referred to standard textbooks (3, 10).

Although the media for biochemical testing may be prepared in the user's own laboratory, most laboratories now find it more convenient to use a commercial kit system for identification of the Enterobacteriaceae. Several such kits are available, but in the authors' experience the API 20E system (BioMerieux SA, France) gives accurate and reproducible results. In this system, a number of tests contained on a plastic strip are inoculated with a suspension of the test organism and after 24 hour incubation the results are combined to produce a seven digit number (the 'API profile') which may then be looked up in a large database to determine the identity of the organism. Should the reader wish to attempt identification of a salmonella or shigella from first principles, Table 7 may be used to determine which tests to set up and the reactions which may be expected. It must be emphasized that the reactions given are those of the majority of strains of a particular species. There will always be some exceptions, and some of the more important of these are discussed below.

4.6.2 Atypical reactions of the salmonellae and shigellae

The reactions given in Table 7 are those seen with the majority of strains of a particular organism. As might be expected, minor differences may be seen, but these do not affect the identification of the organism to genus level. Occasionally more significant variations are seen which might lead to misidentification of an organism, and these will now be described.

i. *Salmonellae*

S. typhi is ODC negative, does not grow on Simmons' citrate, and does not produce gas from glucose. Most strains of *S. paratyphi* A do not produce H_2S; this serovar is also LDC negative and will not grow on Simmons' citrate. *S. pullorum* and *S. gallinarum* are non-motile variants and are citrate negative; in addition *S. gallinarum* is ODC negative and does not produce gas from glucose. The Arizona group (*S. arizonae*; *Salmonella* subgenus III) are ONPG positive, and may appear as lactose fermenters on media containing this carbohydrate. This clearly causes a problem when using such media, as Arizona strains may be inadvertently discarded. In other respects they behave much as typical salmonellae, and if infection with these organisms is considered possible (for example, during an outbreak) a medium such as bismuth sulfite agar may be used as this medium does not rely on failure to ferment lactose as an identifying characteristic.

ii. *Shigellae*

S. dysenteriae type 1 is catalase negative and is thus an exception to the general rule that the Enterobacteriaceae are catalase positive; it also produces a positive ONPG test. The Newcastle and Manchester variants of *S. flexneri* type 6 are atypical in producing gas from glucose, and most strains ferment dulcitol. The Newcastle variant does not ferment mannitol, unlike all shigellae other than *S. dysenteriae*.

iii. E. coli *and* Shigella *spp.*

These two genera are closely related and there is considerable overlap in biochemical and antigenic reactions between certain strains of *E. coli* and the shigellae. Enteroinvasive *E. coli* (EIEC) may appear on initial examination to be a *Shigella*, as they are LDC negative, non-motile, and do not produce gas from glucose. They may be late-or non-lactose fermenters. Further details are given in Table 7.

4.7 Sensitivity testing of salmonellae and shigellae

4.7.1 Choice of antimicrobials

All strains of salmonellae and shigellae should be tested against an appropriate range of antimicrobial agents. For salmonellae, this should at least include amoxycillin, trimethoprim, and ciprofloxacin. The range for shigellae should include amoxycillin, tetracycline, trimethoprim, and ciprofloxacin. Technical methods for sensitivity testing are the same as for other Enterobacteriaceae and are described in Chapter 7.

4.8 Reporting to the clinician

4.8.1 When to report?

The question of when to report the isolation of a salmonella or shigella is sometimes a difficult one. If the report is made too early and subsequently has to be retracted not only will the laboratory's credibility suffer, but inconvenience may have been caused to the patient (unnecessary isolation in hospital, or withdrawal from work in the community) and to medical and nursing staff. Alternatively, if the report is issued only after full identification has been made the patient may not have been isolated or may have continued to work in a sensitive occupation such as food handling, thereby putting others at risk. While hard and fast rules cannot be laid down, each case being judged individually, a report should never be issued on the basis of screening biochemical tests alone, nor on slide agglutination results without the back-up of results from at least some biochemical tests. A provisional report may be issued on the basis of screening tests in composite media plus satisfactory slide agglutinations; to wait for full identification might delay the report for at least one more day. The price which must be paid for early reporting is the recognition that occasional false positive reports will be issued. Such reporting should therefore always be done direct to the clinician or the consultant in communicable disease control by telephone or a visit to the ward and it should be stressed that the report is provisional and subject to confirmation.

4.8.2 What to report?

The isolation of a salmonella from faeces will be provisionally reported as *'Salmonella* sp. isolated—further identification to follow'. A further report will be issued later (possibly several days later, or even longer) when the full identity and serotype of the strain is known. This must be determined and reported in all cases if the fact of isolation is to be of any use for epidemiological purposes, and some common serotypes may also need to be phage-typed. However, all laboratories should be capable of distinguishing *S. typhi* from other serovars and reporting the fact without needing to refer the strain to a reference laboratory before a report is issued.

When reporting the isolation of a shigella, a species name may usually be given on the basis of slide agglutination tests with polyvalent antisera. However, full serotyping of the strain may need the services of a reference laboratory.

It used to be thought that antimicrobial therapy was generally not useful in the treatment of gastrointestinal infections. However, current opinion holds that for salmonella infection appropriate treatment may lead to a shorter period of illness and reduce the period during which the organism is excreted in faeces. The authors recommend that appropriate antibiotic sensitivities (e.g. ciprofloxacin and trimethoprim in the first instance) are therefore reported to the clinician. For shigella, the picture is less clear. Most cases of infection due to *S. sonnei* are mild and will probably not benefit from antibiotic treatment; therefore, reporting of antibiotic sensitivities is probably not helpful. However, infection with one of the other species of *Shigella* will require treatment and the same antibiotic sensitivities as for salmonellae should be reported.

5 Specimen processing for organisms other than salmonellae, shigellae, and campylobacters

5.1 *Escherichia coli*

Five groups of *E. coli* are associated with gastrointestinal disease:-

(a) Enterotoxigenic *E. coli* (ETEC).

(b) Enteropathogenic *E. coli* (EPEC).

(c) Enteroinvasive *E. coli* (EIEC).

(d) Enterohaemorrhagic (or Verocytotoxic) *E. coli* (EHEC/VTEC).

(e) Enteroaggregative *E. coli* (EaggEC).

VTEC infection is an important cause of haemolytic–uraemic syndrome and haemorrhagic colitis which carries a significant risk of morbidity and mortality. To permit prompt recognition of this pathogen laboratory methods have evolved and the diagnosis of infection due to other pathogenic *E. coli* become less important. We will therefore concentrate in this section on laboratory diagnosis of VTEC.

5.1.1 *E. coli* and haemorrhagic colitis

i. *Background*

E. coli (particularly serotype 0:157 H:7) has been associated with sporadic cases and outbreaks of haemorrhagic colitis and haemolytic–uraemic syndrome (HUS). One unusual characteristic of this serotype is that unlike most other strains of *E. coli* and many other Enterobacteriaceae it does not ferment sorbitol; suspect strains may therefore be screened for sorbitol fermentation before serotyping. A differential medium, consisting of MacConkey agar without lactose but with 10 mg/litre of sorbitol has been described for the isolation of non-sorbitol fermenting organisms from faeces. Selective agents such as tellurite and cefixime may be added to the agar as may rhamnose (60% of non-sorbitol fermenting *E. coli* belonging to serogroups other than 0157 ferment rhamnose). Enrichment culture using a modified tryptone soya broth improves isolation rates especially from contacts or convalescent specimens; immunomagnetic separation has also been used (11).

Most 0157 VTEC strains do not produce β-glucuronidase and this can be determined by using 4-methyl umbelliferyl-β-D-glucuronide and visualizing under ultraviolet light (12).

ii. *Identification*

Emulsify suspect colonies in saline on a glass slide and attempt to agglutinate the suspension with *E. coli* 0157 antiserum or by using latex particles coated with 0157 antiserum. A positive test is indicated by rapid agglutination and clearing of the suspension; appropriate negative controls should be performed in parallel. Non-sorbitol fermenting colonies which agglutinate in 0157 antiserum must be confirmed as *E. coli* by further biochemical testing. Send suspect isolates to a reference laboratory to confirm Verocytotoxin production (either by cell culture or DNA probe) and for epidemiological typing.

VTEC infection may also be diagnosed serologically in those patients in whom there is strong clinical suspicion but stool culture is negative. It is performed using an ELISA with confirmatory immunoblotting when required. Non-0157 strains have been shown to cause HUS and may be commonly encountered in certain countries such as Germany. In such cases it is important to consider screening faeces for the presence of *E. coli*, both sorbitol fermenting and non-fermenting strains, and to look for the presence of Verocytotoxin directly in faecal specimens.

5.1.2 Enteropathogenic *E. coli*

EPEC causes infantile diarrhoea. The incidence of EPEC-associated outbreaks in the developed world has fallen dramatically but it remains common in the developing world. It rarely causes disease in children over one year and most cases occur in children less than six months of age. Some authors have suggested that in the UK routine screening is not worthwhile (13).

Attempt isolation of EPEC using routine enteric media such as MacConkey agar and screening representative lactose fermenting colonies by slide agglutination with polyvalent antisera for EPEC-associated O antigens. Perform slide and then tube agglutinations; identify isolates as *E. coli* and submit them to a reference laboratory for confirmation and determination of the H antigen. Other detection methods include ELISA and the FAS test in which a Filamentous Actin Stain is used to identify the 'attaching and effacing' lesions produced by EPEC in cell culture. DNA probes can also be used to detect the presence of the *eaeA* gene (13).

5.1.3 Enterotoxigenic *E. coli*

Enterotoxigenic strains of *E. coli* (ETEC) are now regarded as a common cause of traveller's diarrhoea and infant diarrhoea in developing countries. ETEC may produce one or both of two different enterotoxins, referred to as heat stable (ST) and heat labile (LT) respectively.

Detection of LT and ST is complicated and mainly performed in reference laboratories. Diagnosis of infection with ETEC is best accomplished by the direct demonstration of toxin in faeces, or by demonstrating the ability of strains of *E. coli* isolated from the patient to produce enterotoxin. This may be accomplished by several methods including enzyme-linked immunosorbent assay, co-agglutination using *Staph. aureus*, or by gene probes. Unfortunately, these methods are either not yet generally available or are expensive, and until this situation changes the most practical method for a general laboratory is a tissue culture assay.

5.1.4 Enteroinvasive *E. coli* and enteroaggregative *E. coli*

Neither of these organisms are routinely looked for in clinical specimens at the present time.

5.2 *Yersinia enterocolitica*

5.2.1 Isolation

The isolation of *Y. enterocolitica* from faeces is problematical, partly because the organism grows slowly and may be overgrown by other organisms. Selective culture for this organism is only indicated when the specimen is accompanied by appropriate clinical details such as abdominal pain, as routine culture of all specimens carries a low yield. Although a number of isolation methods have been described, the most commonly used is the selective medium CIN agar (see Table 5). Incubate the inoculated plate at 28–30 °C, the optimum growth temperature for *Y. enterocolitica*, for 48 hours.

Another approach which has been used to isolate the organism is cold enrichment; make a suspension of faeces in phosphate-buffered saline, and store it at 4 °C. After seven days subculture the suspension onto CIN; this can be repeated at weekly intervals for up to six weeks. However this method is not likely to be of use to the individual patient, and is not recommended for routine diagnostic use.

5.2.2 Identification

Suspect colonies may be identified by biochemical testing as for other Enterobacteriaceae; typical reactions are given in Table 7, which gives reactions obtained at 37 °C. Results with *Y. enterocolitica* may vary at lower incubation temperatures (for example, the organism is motile at 22 °C but not at 37 °C). It is recommended that all identified strains be sent to a reference laboratory for confirmation of identity and serotyping.

5.3 *Vibrio cholerae* and *V. parahaemolyticus*

5.3.1 Isolation

Enrichment culture has been shown to increase the diagnostic yield; inoculate specimens both onto TCBS agar and into 20 ml alkaline peptone water (APW). Subculture the APW onto TCBS after either 6 or 24 hours. Subculturing after 6 hours offers no increase in diagnostic yield but may carry significant resource implications for the diagnostic laboratory (14). After overnight incubation examine the TCBS plates. The colonial morphology and colour reactions of *V. cholerae* and *V. parahaemolyticus* are described in Table 5.

5.3.2 Identification of *V. cholerae*

Gram stain suspected colonies on the TCBS plate. If they are Gram-negative bacilli (they may not always have the curved shaped typical of *Vibrio*), make a heavy subculture to blood agar. This is essential because neither slide agglutination tests nor an oxidase test should be made using growth on TCBS, as erroneous reactions may occur. Six to eight hours later there should be sufficient growth on the blood agar for further tests to be made. Carry out an oxidase test, and test the strain by slide agglutination with antiserum to *V. cholerae* 01. An oxidase positive Gram-negative bacillus which grows on TCBS agar with sucrose fermentation and which agglutinates in the above antiserum is presumptively identified as *V. cholerae* 01 (i.e. a potential epidemic strain). The clinician, local public health laboratory and (in the UK) the Consultant in Communicable Disease Control must be informed immediately.

It was previously believed that non-01 strains did not cause epidemic cholera, but the recent recognition of the 0139 strain has shown that this is not completely true and agglutination using antisera to this strain must also be performed. If the strain does not agglutinate in 01 or 0139 antiserum but otherwise fulfils the criteria for presumptive identification, it may be a non-01/0139 strain of *V. cholerae*. An additional useful test at this stage is the 'string' test. Suspend a colony in 0.5% sodium deoxycholate in saline on a glass slide and *Vibrio* spp. will lyse, releasing DNA which can be pulled up like a piece of string.

Biochemical identification may also be carried out in the general laboratory with the media and tests used for the Enterobacteriaceae (results are shown in Table 7). Kit systems such as the API 20E may be used, although this system is not specifically intended for use with *Vibrio*. *V. cholerae* non-01/0139 strains are biochemically identical to *V. cholerae* 01/0139, and may be reported as 'Non-cholera vibrio' even though this is not taxonomically correct. *V. cholerae* 0139 are biochemically similar to the El Tor strain *of V. cholerae* 01.

All strains of *V. cholerae* should be sent to a reference laboratory for confirmation of identity, biotyping, and serotyping.

5.3.3 Identification of *V. parahaemolyticus*

Subculture suggestive colonies on TCBS to blood agar and CLED (cystine lactose electrolyte-deficient) medium. *V. parahaemolyticus* is oxidase positive but will not grow on CLED because it is a halophilic (salt requiring) organism. Organisms meeting these criteria may be fully identified by biochemical testing (Table 7). Because this species is halophilic it may not grow in media used for the Enterobacteriaceae unless sodium chloride is added to a concentration of 1%. Such modified media is also suitable for the Enterobacteriacaeae avoiding the need for duplicate sets of media. When using a kit identification system, the inoculum should be prepared in sterile saline rather than distilled water as growth of *V. parahaemolyticus* may otherwise be very poor.

5.4 *Clostridium difficile*

5.4.1 Introduction

C. difficile is the major cause of antibiotic-associated diarrhoea and pseudomembranous colitis. The incidence of infection is increasing especially among elderly patients in hospitals and nursing homes. To confirm the clinical diagnosis, demonstration of the presence of *C. difficile* cytotoxin is usually all that is required by the diagnostic laboratory. Isolation of the organism (described below) cannot produce a result quickly enough for it to be clinically useful, and the occurrence of toxin negative strains may lead to misdiagnosis if isolation alone is performed. It is still performed in reference centres and research units where sensitivity testing and epidemiological typing may be carried out.

5.4.2 Isolation of *C. difficile*

Inoculate the specimen onto cycloserine–cefoxitin containing medium and incubate anaerobically for 48 hours. Examine the plate for the characteristic irregular colonies of *C. difficile* (see Table 5). Cultures may also have a powerful and characteristic odour due to the production of paracresol and isocaproic acid. A Gram stain of suggestive colonies should reveal Gram-positive or Gram-variable bacilli. Colonies of *C. difficile* fluoresce yellow/green (chartreuse) under Wood's lamp (UV light at 360 nm). Confirmatory identification may be carried out by latex agglutination with *C. difficile* somatic antigen, but biochemical testing is expensive and rarely necessary. Sensitivity testing and typing may be performed.

5.4.3 Demonstration of cytotoxin in faeces

Cell culture remains the 'gold standard' and detects toxin B, the *C. difficile* cytotoxin. The method is given in detail in Protocol 9. It is positive in over 90% of patients with pseudomembranous colitis and it is important to realize that a negative test does not rule out *C. difficile* as the cause of diarrhoea. Follow-up testing of asymptomatic patients is not recommended.

Many laboratories do not have cell culture facilities and use enzyme immunoassay (EIA) to look for the presence of enterotoxin (toxin A), cytotoxin (toxin B), or both. It should be noted that a number of toxin A negative/B positive strains occur and that testing for toxin A alone may result in a false negative report. EIA is rapid and inexpensive when performed in batches; it is highly specific but sensitivity results vary from 70–95%.

Latex agglutination detects the presence of glutamate dehydrogenase, not toxin A, and may produce false positive results due to non-toxigenic strains of *C. difficile* and other bacteria that produce this enzyme. Sensitivity is similar to EIA but specificity is lower.

Protocol 9

Method for the detection of *Clostridium difficile* cytotoxin in faeces

Equipment and reagents

- HeLa, human embryonic lung fibroblasts, or Vero cell monolayers
- Antiserum to *C. sordellii* toxin, diluted 1/50 in phosphate-buffered saline (PBS)

Method

1 Centrifuge a liquid stool or an extract of formed stool (at 2000 g for 20 min or 10 000 g for 10 min). Discard the deposit, and use the supernatant for the test.

2 Mix 0.1 ml of the cell-free supernatant with 0.1 ml of PBS and add this mixture to a tissue culture tube.

3 For each batch of tests set up positive and negative controls.

4 Incubate the tubes at 37 °C overnight.

5 Examine the tubes for the typical cytopathic effect (CPE) of *Clostridium difficile* cytotoxin, seen as rounding up and separation of the cells. If human embryonic lung fibroblasts are used there may also be filamentous projections from the cells.

6 Re-test specimens in which a CPE has been observed, this time after the addition of 0.1 ml of antiserum to *C. sordellii* toxin to each tube. Examination of the tubes should reveal complete neutralization of the CPE.

The titre of the toxin may be determined using 10-fold dilutions of the supernatant. However, the titre is not correlated with the severity of the disease although it may decline with successful treatment. It is not recommended as a routine procedure.

5.5 'Food poisoning' due to *Clostridium perfringens*, *Staphylococcus aureus*, and *Bacillus cereus*

5.5.1 Introduction

When investigating an outbreak of food poisoning, it is necessary to obtain both epidemiological and laboratory data in order to identify the source and route of transmission of the agent responsible. There are of course numerous potential causes of 'food poisoning', not all of which are bacterial (or even microbial) in origin. If the nature of the outbreak suggests that the cause may be *Clostridium perfringens*, *Staphylococcus aureus*, or *Bacillus cereus*, the laboratory should attempt the isolation of these organisms from faeces. Other specimens may also be collected such as vomit, swabs from utensils, specimens from food handlers, and the food itself. Methods for processing these specimens are beyond the scope of this chapter, but procedures are given below for the treatment of faeces specimens.

Since all of these organisms produce disease by the production of an enterotoxin, either in the food or in the intestine, methods for the demonstration of toxin in food or faeces may eventually replace culture methods. At the present time such methods should be regarded as reference laboratory or experimental procedures.

5.5.2 Isolation and identification of *Clostridium perfringens*

Strains of *Clostridium perfringens* implicated in food poisoning outbreaks were originally described as heat resistant and non- or weakly haemolytic, but subsequently classical strains have also been associated with the disease. Since almost all of the healthy population carry this organism as part of the normal bowel flora, simple isolation of the organism from faeces is of little help. Therefore a semi-quantitative determination of a spore count can be performed; this is described in Protocol 10. Isolates should be retained for serotyping and faecal specimens may also be tested in a reference laboratory for the presence of *C. perfringens* enterotoxin. If still available, isolation of the organism from suspected food should also be attempted. Confirmation that an outbreak of food poisoning is due to *C. perfringens* is obtained if one (preferably more) of the criteria below is satisfied:

(a) Isolation of the same serotype from the faeces of affected individuals and from food.

(b) Faecal spore counts of $>10^5$ organisms per gram.

(c) Detection of enterotoxin in faeces.

Protocol 10

Isolation of *Clostridium perfringens* from faeces in suspected food poisoning outbreaks

Reagents

- Neomycin-FAA: fastidious anaerobe agar containing 75 mg/litre of neomycin
- Phosphate-buffered saline (PBS)
- 95% (v/v) ethanol in distilled water

Protocol 10 continued

Method

1 Prepare a 1:5 dilution of faeces in PBS (minimum 0.1 g of faeces in 0.5 ml of PBS).

2 Add an equal volume of 95% (v/v) ethanol in distilled water, and shake. Leave the suspension to stand for 30 min at room temperature.

3 From this 1:10 dilution prepare two further 10-fold dilutions in PBS (i.e. dilutions of 1:100 and 1:1000).

4 Inoculate 0.1 ml aliquots of the 1:100 and 1:1000 dilutions onto neomycin-FAA and incubate anaerobically at 35–37 °C overnight.

5 Perform a colony count to determine the spore count in the original specimen.

6 A vegetative cell count may be determined by omitting stages 2 and 3, simply diluting the faeces in PBS to 1:10 and 1:100 dilutions and inoculating onto neomycin-FAA.

C. perfringens enterotoxin may be detected by either ELISA and RPLA (reverse passive latex agglutination). It is particularly useful in hospitalized patients who often have elevated *C. perfringens* spore counts in the absence of symptoms.

5.5.3 Isolation of *Staphylococcus aureus*

Faeces should be inoculated onto a selective medium such as mannitol-salt agar (see Table 5). Suspect colonies may be identified by standard laboratory methods.

Staphylococcus aureus may be isolated from the faeces of healthy individuals so isolation *per se* has little meaning. In cases of infection *S. aureus* is usually present in large numbers and quantitative culture may be performed. Strains from the faeces of patients, from food, and from food handlers should be phage typed and tested for enterotoxin production by a reference laboratory. Enterotoxin-producing strains of identical phage types when isolated from the above sources can be assumed to be the cause of the outbreak. Note that *S. aureus* produces enterotoxin in food, not in the intestinal tract, and if the food is subsequently heated the organism may be killed but the toxin left intact; this may still be detected by immunoassay. Thus the failure to isolate enterotoxigenic strains of *S. aureus* from faeces does not exclude staphylococcal food poisoning.

5.5.4 Isolation of *Bacillus cereus*

As with *Clostridium perfringens* and *Staphylococcus aureus*, *Bacillus cereus* can be isolated (usually in small numbers) from the stools of a proportion of the healthy population. A semi-quantitative culture method is therefore necessary, together with isolation from the suspected food.

Liquid specimens may be used directly, otherwise make a heavy suspension of the specimen in peptone water. Prepare 1/10 serial dilutions of the specimen in PBS and plate 0.1 ml of each dilution onto a selective medium for *B. cereus* (see Table 5). After overnight incubation obtain a viable count of presumptive colonies of *B. cereus*.

Strains of suspected *B. cereus* isolated from faeces and food may be sent to a reference laboratory to determine if they are the same strain (by serotype, biotype, phage type, plasmid type, etc.). An outbreak is probably due to *B. cereus* if one or more of the criteria below is satisfied.

(a) The viable count of *B. cereus* obtained from food is greater than 10^4 per gram.

(b) *B. cereus* is isolated from both food and faeces, and the isolates are of the same type.

5.6 *Helicobacter pylori*

The role of *Helicobacter pylori* in gastrointestinal disease is complex. It can be regarded as part of the 'normal' flora with carriage resulting in a chronic gastritis that is often asymptomatic. Carriers have an increased risk of peptic ulcer disease, adenocarcinoma of the antrum and body of the stomach, and primary non-Hodgkin's lymphomas of the stomach. Screening for and eradication of *H. pylori* in such cases is clearly worthwhile, but the benefit of treating patients with non-ulcer dyspepsia (which has a variety of causes) is not clear-cut. Some strains of *H. pylori* may be protective against oesophageal disease, and therefore eradication of asymptomatic carriers is inappropriate as they may simply alter their disease risk.

Initial diagnosis may be made by a number of methods (15):

(a) *Rapid urease test.* A gastric mucosal biopsy is added to a commercial kit containing urea substrate and a pH-sensitive marker. If sufficient numbers of *H. pylori* are present (certain agents may reduce the bacterial load) then urea is broken down to ammonia altering the pH and resulting in a visible colour change. Positive results are often apparent before the patient is discharged.

(b) *Histology.* Specimens are usually sent for histology when urease tests are negative or malignancy is suspected. If chronic active gastritis is present in an untreated patient infection is likely, but presence of intestinal metaplasia or gastric atrophy may make the diagnosis difficult, as may prior treatment.

(c) *Serology.* Serum IgG levels are a sensitive and specific method for diagnosing infection but analysis of isolated serum samples have limited use in the post-treatment period. Some authors have suggested that quantitative enzyme-linked immunosorbent assays on acute and convalescent specimens can be used to confirm eradication but only when performed in parallel.

(d) *Urea breath test.* This test determines production of urea by *H. pylori* urease. An isotope-labelled urea is ingested, urease liberates carbon dioxide into the bloodstream that can be measured on exhalation. The test is more expensive than serology but cheaper than endoscopy and probably has a role when it is necessary to confirm eradication.

(e) *Stool antigen enzyme immunoassay*. This recently described technique is used to detect active infection and hence has an advantage over serology in the initial assessment of patients. It may also be used to assess response to eradication therapy.

It is sometimes necessary to perform sensitivity testing and typing of *H. pylori* strains and culture for the organism may therefore be required.

Protocol 11

Culture and sensitivity testing of *H. pylori*

Reagents

- Non-selective culture medium (10% blood agar or chocolate agar)
- *H. pylori* selective medium (contains vanco-mycin, cefsulodin, and amphotericin B)

Method

1 Transport specimens to the laboratory in a humid atmosphere (i.e. near the neck of a bijou with 0.2 ml of sterile normal saline) or immersed in normal saline if a significant delay is expected.

2 Smear the biopsy sample onto a non-selective medium and onto *H. pylori* selective medium.

3 Promptly incubate the agar plates in a microaerobic atmosphere (6% O_2, 10% CO_2) as delays of more than 30 min may result in failure to culture *H. pylori*.

4 Small (1–2 mm) domed translucent colonies appear from 48 h onwards, but cultures should continue for seven days.

5 Isolates are urease positive, oxidase and catalase positive, and have similar morphol-ogy to *Campylobacter* on Gram staining.

6 Resistance to amoxycillin and tetracycline is rarely encountered but test these antibi-otics plus clarithromycin and metronidazole. Perform disc testing on chocolate agar with a Columbia agar base and *H. pylori* NCTC 127822 as a sensitive control. E-testing is more reliable for metronidazole as low level resistance is often encountered (minimum inhibitory concentration approx. 8 mg/litre).

References

1. Valenstein, P., Pfaller, M., and Yungbluth, M. (1996). *Arch. Pathol. Lab. Med.*, **120**, 206.
2. Mandell, G. L., Bennett, J. E., and Dolin, R. (ed.) (2000). *Principles and practice of infectious diseases*, 5th edn. Churchill Livingstone, New York.
3. Murray, P. R., Baron, E. J., Pfaller, M. A., Tenover, F. C., and Yolken, R. H. (ed.) (1999). *Manual of clinical microbiology*, 7th edn. ASM Press, Washington DC.

4. Blom, M., Meyer, A., Gerner-Smidt, P., Gaarslev, K., *et al.* (1999). *J. Clin. Microbiol.*, **37**, 2312.

5. Cooke, V. M., Miles, R. J., Price, R. G., and Richardson, A. C. (1999). *Appl. Environ. Microbiol.*, **65**, 807.

6. Nachamkin, I. and Barbagallo, S. (1990). *J. Clin. Microbiol.*, **28**, 817.

7. Ruiz, J., Sempere, M. A., Varela, M. C., and Gomez, J. (1992). *J. Clin. Microbiol.*, **30**, 525.

8. Old, D. C. and Threlfall, E. S. (1998). In *Topley and Wilson's microbiology and microbial infections*, 9th edn. (ed. L. Collier, A. Balows, and M. Sussman), Vol. 2, p. 969. Edward Arnold, London.

9. Bouvet, P. J. M. and Jeanjean, S. (1992). *J. Clin. Microbiol.*, **30**, 2184.

10. Barrow, G. I. and Feltham, R. K. A. (ed.) (1993). *Cowan and Steel's manual for the identification of medical bacteria*, 3rd edn. Cambridge University Press, Cambridge.

11. Chapman, P. A. and Siddons, C. A. (1996). *J. Med. Microbiol.*, **44**, 267.

12. Smith, H. R. and Scotland, S. M. (1993). *J. Clin. Pathol.*, **46**, 10.

13. Morris, K. J. and Gopal Rao, G. (1992). *J. Hosp. Infect.*, **21**, 163.

14. Lesmana, M., Richie, E., Subekti, D., Simanjuntak, C., and Walz, S. E. (1997). *J. Clin. Microbiol.*, **35**, 1856.

15. McNulty, C. A. M. and Wyatt, J. I. (1999). *J. Clin. Pathol.*, **52**, 338.

Chapter 7

Antimicrobial susceptibility testing

Derek F. J. Brown
Cambridge Laboratory, Health Protection Agency, Addenbrooke's
Hospital, Hills Road, Cambridge CB2 2QW, UK.

Jenny Andrews
Department of Microbiology, City Hospital NHS Trust,
Birmingham B18 7QH, UK.

Trevor Winstanley
Department of Microbiology, Royal Hampshire Hospital,
Glossop Road, Sheffield S10 2JF, UK.

Alasdair P. MacGowan
Department of Medical Microbiology, Southmead Hospital,
Bristol B10 5NB, UK.

1 Introduction

In vitro antimicrobial susceptibility testing is undertaken in clinical laboratories to predict the likely *in vivo* response of the infecting organism to a selected range of antimicrobial agents. Susceptibility tests are designed to give a result interpreted as susceptible (sensitive, S), intermediate (moderately susceptible, moderately resistant, I), or resistant (R). A patient infected with a susceptible organism should respond to treatment with the manufacturer's recommended dosage regimen, whereas one infected with a resistant organism is unlikely to respond. For an organism categorized as intermediate there is uncertainty whether or not the patient will respond to standard doses, but they will be more likely to respond to higher doses or if the agent is concentrated at the site of the infection, such as in the urinary tract. However, intermediate is a term which clinicians find unhelpful, and in practice the intermediate and resistant categories are combined and reported as resistant.

Susceptibility breakpoints are the concentrations of antimicrobial agents or, for disc diffusion tests, zone diameters which distinguish the different categories of susceptibility. Minimum inhibitory concentration (MIC) breakpoints are based on pharmacodynamics, MIC distributions, resistance mechanisms, and clinical experience of the use of a particular agent. In standardized disc diffusion methods, zone diameter breakpoints are based on correlation of zone sizes with MICs, the distribution of zone diameters for different species, and clinical experience. With antimicrobial agents which exhibit a bimodal distribution of susceptibility, for example tetracycline, choosing a breakpoint to differentiate between susceptible and resistant populations is easily achieved by any method. Unfortunately, with many agents a bimodal distribution is not seen and differentiation of susceptible and resistant populations is unclear. Consequently the choice of breakpoints can be difficult.

The ideal test of performance of any *in vitro* susceptibility test is the correlation of results with clinical outcome. This is tenuous, however, as with *in vitro* testing it is difficult to take account of the variability in pharmacological factors such as absorption, distribution, metabolism, excretion, protein binding, interaction of the chosen agent with other prescribed agents, and patient-related factors such as the site and severity of infection, mixed infections, associated illness, immune status, and recovery unrelated to treatment.

Local data accumulated over fixed time periods on the prevalence of resistance for different species forms the basis for empirical therapy when patients are treated before laboratory results are available. In addition, testing is of value for surveillance purposes in order to monitor changes in susceptibility over time. The susceptibility pattern may also help in identification of the infecting organism, and antimicrobial susceptibility may be a useful phenotypic characteristic in typing organisms for epidemiological purposes.

2 Disc diffusion methods for antimicrobial susceptibility testing

Disc diffusion methods are the most widely used in the UK for routine antimicrobial susceptibility testing. The methods are convenient, technically simple, and, if correctly performed, reasonably reliable.

The surface of an agar plate is evenly inoculated with the test organism and filter paper discs containing defined amounts of the agents are applied to the plate. After incubation, usually overnight at 35–37 °C, a circular zone of inhibition of growth is formed as a result of diffusion of the agent into the agar. The size of the zone of inhibition is an indication of the susceptibility of the organism, more resistant organisms giving smaller zones. The size of the zone of inhibition is, however, influenced by technical variables that must be controlled to produce meaningful results. The theoretical aspects of zone formation developed by Cooper and Linton have been interpreted in relation to more recent diffusion procedures by Acar and Goldstein (1).

2.1 Factors affecting diffusion tests

These have been extensively reviewed (1, 2) and are summarized below.

2.1.1 Medium

The culture medium should support the growth of organisms normally tested without being antagonistic to the activity or diffusion of agents. Some of the factors influencing the activity of various agents are shown in Table 1. For defined methods the medium used is specified whereas for the comparative methods various media may be used.

Supplementation is necessary for some organisms and the supplements used depend on the method (3–9). Five per cent horse or sheep blood are commonly used to supplement media for the growth of streptococci and anaerobes. With some methods, for *Neisseria* spp. and *Haemophilus* spp. 5% heated (chocolated) horse blood may be added, whereas for others more complex media may be defined, e.g. 5% horse blood +20 mg/litre NAD for *Haemophilus* spp. in the BSAC method (4). Agents which are highly protein bound, such as fusidic acid, have smaller zones on media containing blood.

The antagonistic effects of thymidine can be avoided by use of a medium low in thymidine. The effects of thymidine can be eliminated by adding lysed horse blood to the medium. Thymidine phosphorylase in the lysed horse blood converts thymidine to thymine, which is about 100 times less antagonistic than thymidine. Excessive thymine can also cause problems, so medium should preferably be low in both.

Several commercial media are produced specifically for antimicrobial susceptibility testing, and these should be used for routine tests. Standardized methods

Table 1 Factors affecting antimicrobial activity in culture media

Factor	Agents affected	Effect on activity
Thymidine	Sulfonamides Trimethoprim	Reduced
Raised pH	Aminoglycosides Macrolides Lincosamides Nitrofurans	Increased
Lowered pH	Tetracycline Methicillin Fusidic acid Novobiocin	Increased
Monovalent cations (e.g. Na^+)	Bacitracin Fusidic acid Novobiocin	Increased against staphylococci
	Penicillin	Increased against *Proteus*
Divalent cations (e.g. Mg^{2+} and Ca^{2+})	Tetracycline Aminoglycosides Polymyxins	Reduced Reduced against *Pseudomonas* spp.

specify particular media, e.g. Mueller–Hinton for the NCCLS method (6) and Iso-Sensitest agar for the BSAC method (4).

2.1.2 Depth of medium

Zones of inhibition increase as the depth of agar decreases, and the effects are more marked with very thin plates. Plates should have a consistent level depth of 4 mm.

2.1.3 Inoculum density

Increasing the inoculum reduces zone sizes with all antimicrobial agents to some extent. Variation in inoculum size is one of the main sources of error in susceptibility testing. Some disc diffusion methods require an inoculum resulting in semi-confluent growth of colonies (3, 4). This has the advantage that an incorrect inoculum can be seen and the test repeated. The inoculum is generally acceptable if the density is between almost confluent and colonies separated so that they do not touch. Other methods use a confluent inoculum standardized against a 0.5 McFarland standard (6).

2.1.4 Pre-incubation and pre-diffusion

Pre-incubation of inoculated plates before discs are applied reduces zone sizes, and pre-diffusion of antimicrobial agents prior to incubation has the opposite effect. Although a set pre-diffusion time of 30–60 minutes may improve reproducibility of tests, standardization of pre-diffusion and pre-incubation present practical difficulties, so they should be avoided.

2.1.5 Antimicrobial discs

Commercially produced filter paper discs are almost universally used. Although problems with the discs are occasionally due to manufacturing failures, most faults are related to inadequate handling of discs in the laboratory. High temperatures and humidity lead to more rapid deterioration of labile agents, especially β-lactams. Discs should therefore be stored and handled as in Table 2.

It is essential to use the disc contents recommended for the method in use. Discs should be in close even contact with the medium to avoid impaired diffusion

Table 2 Handling and storage of antimicrobial discs

1.	Store discs, including those in dispensers, in sealed containers in the dark. This is especially important for light-susceptible agents, e.g. metronidazole, rifampicin, chloramphenicol, and the quinolones.
2.	Containers must include an indicating desiccant.
3.	Store stocks at −20 °C to 8 °C. Store working supplies of discs at <8 °C.
4.	To minimize condensation on discs, allow them to warm to room temperature before opening containers.
5.	Leave discs in sealed containers at room temperature during the day rather than repeatedly transfer them from <8 °C to room temperature.
6.	Do not use discs beyond the expiry date given by the manufacturer.

of agents into the medium. No more than six agents should be tested on a 9 cm plate to avoid unacceptable overlap of zones.

2.1.6 Incubation

Most plates are incubated at 35–37 °C in air unless another atmosphere is required for growth. An atmosphere containing additional CO_2 should be avoided unless specified for fastidious organisms, e.g. *Haemophilus* spp. Oxacillin susceptibility tests on staphylococci are incubated at 30 °C in some methods (4). Stacks of plates should be as small as possible as plates in the middle of stacks may take longer to warm to incubator temperature than those at the top or bottom.

2.1.7 Reading of zones

With clear medium, plates may be read from the upper surface or through the medium. If the medium contains blood, plates must be read from the upper surface with the lid removed. Zones of inhibition should be circular, unless there is antagonism or synergy between adjacent agents or problems in testing.

Reproducibility of reading zones is related to clarity of zone edges. Hence reading of tests with sulfonamides and on streptococci tend to be most variable. Generally there is an obvious zone edge. Small colonies or a film of growth at zone edges, swarming of *Proteus* spp. into zones, or haemolytic effects on media supplemented with blood should be ignored. Colonies growing within the zone of inhibition may indicate contamination or a resistant subpopulation, and it may be necessary to subculture, identify, and re-test any such colonies. Any growth within the zone of inhibition may indicate resistance with staphylococci tested against methicillin/oxacillin, and staphylococci and enterococci tested against vancomycin.

If the method requires semi-confluent growth there should be no individual colonies and the growth should not be completely confluent. If the growth is too heavy or too light, the test should be repeated.

If it is necessary to measure zones, calipers (preferably) or a ruler should be used. For standardized methods that translate zone sizes into a category of susceptibility on the basis of fixed zone size breakpoints, a template may be used. When using templates the plate is placed over the template and zones interpreted according to the zone diameter breakpoints marked on the template. With media containing blood, the template, printed on a transparent sheet, is placed over the plate. A program for preparation of templates is available from the BSAC web site (http://www.bsac.org.uk).

Several reader systems are commercially available for measuring zone diameters. These include the Aura Image (Oxoid), the BioMIC (Giles Scientific), the Mastascan Elite (Mast), the Osiris (Bio-Rad), and the Sirscan (i2a). The readers take an image of the susceptibility plate with a camera or scanner and use image analysis software to calculate zone sizes. Zone readers should improve reproducibility of reading zones, reduce error in transcription of results, and provide automatic interpretation of zone diameters. Readers include epidemiological packages that facilitate detailed examination of accumulated data and electronic transfer of data for regional or national resistance surveillance. Some readers include expert software which can improve quality by checking results according to a set of rules (see Section 8). The readers appear to perform reasonably well. They differ in the way plates are handled, the way test information is entered into the system, the way results are reported, and the sophistication of the epidemiological and expert systems.

2.2 Methods of disc diffusion susceptibility testing

Methods in current use have developed from different directions, and involve different controls and interpretation. There are several methods world-wide (10) and it is likely that most of these will give reasonably reliable results if correctly performed. Few attempts have been made to compare the performance of different methods, but no major differences in reliability have been demonstrated.

In the USA, the Kirby–Bauer method has been developed into a standardized method by the National Committee for Clinical Laboratory Standards (NCCLS) method (6). The method is the most widely used world-wide and is the recommended by the World Health Organisation (WHO). Following the recommendations of the WHO-sponsored International Collaborative Study of Susceptibility Testing (11), standardized methods have also been developed in several European countries. Although there are slight variations in methodology, generally following national guidelines, the control of variation in all the standardized methods is based on rigid standardization of all aspects of the technique. Interpretation is by reference to tables of zone size breakpoints based largely on statistical correlation of zone sizes with minimum inhibitory concentrations. Zone size breakpoints are related to MIC breakpoints established in the individual country.

Comparative methods were developed in the UK (3) and have a fundamentally different approach to standardized methods. They allow some variation in technique and medium, although within individual laboratories the method is likely to be closely defined. It is assumed that variation in the test will be controlled by the method of interpretation, which involves comparison of test zone sizes with the zone sizes of specified control organisms set up at the same time as the test and under identical conditions. Variation is assumed to affect the test and control organisms in the same way and thus cancel any adverse effect on interpretation. In Stokes' modification of this method, the control is extended by having the control organism on the same plate as the test organism. The criteria for interpretation are not based on any formal evaluation of the relationship of MIC to zone size, but have been developed by relating the results of the tests to clinical effectiveness of the agents, by experience over the years, however there is a correlation between the results of tests done by Stokes' method and MIC (12).

Many laboratories in the UK still use Stokes' method. However, there are limitations to the effectiveness of control by Stokes' method (13), and it has not been updated for some newer, highly active agents or for newer resistance mechanisms. It may be possible to modify interpretation to compensate for these limitations, but the method has not been updated in a consistent way and there is a very wide variation in detail of technique and interpretative criteria in different laboratories. The British Society for Anti-microbial Chemotherapy (BSAC) has recently published a standardized disc diffusion method (4, http://www.bsac.org.uk) in line with those published in other countries, but with breakpoints related to MIC breakpoints established in the UK.

2.2.1 The comparative (Stokes') method

i. Preparation of plates

The method for preparation of plates is given in Protocol 1.

Protocol 1

Preparation of plates

Equipment and reagents

- 90 mm sterile Petri dishes
- Medium

- 5% defibrinated horse blood
- 5% lysed horse blood

Method

1 Prepare and sterilize the medium as directed by the manufacturers.

2 If 5% defibrinated horse blood is added for tests on fastidious organisms allow the medium to cool to 50 °C before adding the blood. If the medium is not free of thymidine add 5% lysed horse blood for tests on sulfonamides and trimethoprim.

3 Pour the medium into 90 mm sterile Petri dishes on a flat horizontal surface to give a depth of 4 mm ± 0.5 mm and allow to set on a level surface.[a]

4 Dry the plates so that there are no visible droplets of moisture on the surface of the agar but do not overdry the plates.[b]

5 Store the plates at ≤8 °C.

[a] Use of a medium dispenser will ensure that the depth of agar remains constant.

[b] Plate drying, storage conditions, and shelf-life should be determined as part of the media quality assurance programme.

---

ii. Preparation of inoculum

The inoculum should give semi-confluent growth of colonies after overnight incubation. Tests with confluent growth or clearly separated colonies should be repeated. The dry swab method of inoculation is commonly used and is described in Protocols 2-4. Other methods of inoculation are given in Protocol 5.

Protocol 2

Preparation of inoculum

Equipment and reagents

- Cotton wool swabs
- Screw-capped jars
- Nutrient broth

A. Test strains

1 Prepare a fully grown broth culture (18 h, or 3–5 h if heavily inoculated).

2 Alternatively emulsify several colonies of the test organism in broth to give a suspension of a similar density to a broth culture.

B. Control strains

1 For preparation of pre-impregnated swabs with control organisms, sterilize cotton wool swabs in screw-capped jars at 160 °C for 2 h.[a]

2 Inoculate the swabs by pipetting a suspension of organisms on the swabs.[b]

3 For *Staphylococcus aureus* NCTC 6571, make a control suspension by adding 0.5 ml of an overnight broth culture to 20 ml nutrient broth. For *Escherichia coli* NCTC 10418 and *Pseudomonas aeruginosa* NCTC 10662, use 0.25 ml of overnight culture in 20 ml.

4 Store sealed containers at 4 °C for up to a week.

5 Use one swab for each plate.

[a] 3 inch (7.5 cm) swabs, 'Q-tips', are available from Cheesborough-Ponds Ltd.
[b] 20 ml of control suspension is enough for a jar containing about 90 swabs.

Protocol 3

Inoculation with control on a separate plate

Equipment and reagents

- Plates
- Rotary plater
- Inoculum
- Sterile swabs

Method

1 Make a single streak of a 4 mm loopful of the inoculum across the diameter of the plate.

2 Spread the inoculum with a sterile dry swab over the entire surface of the medium in three directions, 60° apart. Alternatively use a rotary plater.

Table 3 Control organisms for the comparative methods

Control organism	Group of organisms to be controlled
Escherichia coli NCTC 10418	Coliform organisms
P. aeruginosa NCTC 10662	*Pseudomonas* spp.
E. faecalis NCTC 12697	Enterococci
H. influenzae NCTC 11931	*Haemophilus* spp.
N. gonorrhoeae NCTC 12700	*N. gonorrhoeae*
S. aureus NCTC 6571	Other organisms that grow aerobically
Clostridium perfringens NCTC 11229	*Clostridium* spp.
Bacteroides fragilis 9343	Other anaerobic organisms

Protocol 3 continued

3 Inoculate control organisms on separate plates by the use of pre-impregnated control swabs, again spreading evenly over the entire surface of the medium in three directions.

[a] See Section 3.1.4 and Table 3 for required controls.

Protocol 4

Comparative method with control on the same plate (Stokes' method)

Equipment and reagents

• See Protocol 3

A. Band plating method

1 Apply the control culture[a] in two bands on either side of the plate, leaving a central area uninoculated.[b]

2 Transfer a 4 mm loopful of the broth culture or suspension of the test organism to the centre of the plate and spread this evenly in a band across the centre of the plate with a dry sterile swab.[c]

B. Rotary plating method

1 Place the uninoculated plate on a turntable (Life Sciences International) marked with a circle visible through the medium and 15 mm in from the edge of the plate.

2 Use a pre-impregnated control swab to apply the control organism to the centre of the plate by holding the swab on the surface of the medium and moving the swab slowly across the plate as it rotates on the turntable.[d,e]

3   Transfer a 4 mm loopful of the test organism to the uninoculated edge of the plate and spread the organism evenly with a sterile dry swab as the plate rotates on the turntable.[f]

[a] See Table 3 for required controls.

[b] This is best achieved by the use of pre-impregnated swabs, but a 4 mm loopful of an inoculum prepared as for test organisms may be transferred to both sides of the plate and spread evenly in the two bands with a dry sterile swab.

[c] There should be a gap of 2 mm between the test and control bands.

[d] An uninoculated 15 mm band is left around the edge of the plate.

[e] The same effect may be achieved by transferring a 4 mm loopful of the control organism to the centre of the plate and spreading evenly with a sterile dry swab as the turntable rotates.

[f] There should be a 2 mm gap between the test and control organisms.

iii. Inoculation of plates

Plates may be inoculated with the control organism on a separate plate (Table 5); with the control organism on the same plate, inoculated using the band plating method (Table 6; Figure 1); or with the control on the same plate, inoculated using a rotary plating method (Table 6; Figure 2).

Protocol 5

Alternative methods of standardizing inoculum and inoculating plates

Equipment and reagents

- See Protocol 3
- 0.48 M BaCl$_2$ (1.17%, w/v BaCl$_2$.2H$_2$O)
- 0.18 M H$_2$SO$_4$ (1%, w/v)

A. Standardization with McFarland standard

1   Prepare 0.5 McFarland standard by adding 0.5 ml of 0.048 M BaCl$_2$ to 99.5 ml of 0.18 M H$_2$SO$_4$ with constant stirring. Distribute the standard into tubes of the same size and volume as those used to grow broth cultures or make suspensions of the test organism. Seal the tubes tightly to prevent evaporation and store them in the dark at room temperature for up to six months. Vigorously vortex mix the standard before use.[a]

2   Inoculate several test colonies into sterile distilled water or broth to produce a suspension which matches the turbidity of the 0.5 McFarland standard.

3   Alternatively for non-fastidious organisms transfer colonial growth to broth and grow at 35–37 °C (growth will be more rapid if cultures are shaken) until the turbidity is equivalent to or exceeds that of the 0.5 McFarland standard.

4   Compare the test suspension with the 0.5 McFarland standard against a white background with a contrasting black line and, if necessary, adjust the density of the suspension to that of the standard by adding distilled water.

5   To obtain semi-confluent growth, dilute the prepared suspension in sterile distilled water before inoculation as follows:

1:100	1:10	No dilution
Haemolytic streptococci	*Staphylococcus* species	*N. gonorrhoeae*
Enterococci	*S. pneumoniae*	
Enterobacteriaceae	*N. meningitidis*	
Pseudomonas species	*M. catarrhalis*	
Acinetobacter species		
Haemophilus species		

6   Use the adjusted suspension within 15 min to inoculate plates.

7   Dip a dry sterile cotton swab into the suspension and remove excess fluid by turning the swab against the inside of the tube. Spread the inoculum evenly over the surface of the agar plate by swabbing in three different directions. Alternatively, use a rotary plater.

8   Allow the medium to dry before applying discs.

B. Standardization with spectrophotometer

1   Suspend colonies evenly in 3 ml distilled water or broth in a $4 \times \frac{1}{2}"$ glass tube to give just visible turbidity. Do not leave the organisms standing in water.

2   Zero the spectrophotometer with sterile water or broth at a wavelength of 500 nm.

3   Measure the absorbance of the bacterial suspension.

4   Select the volume to transfer (with appropriate fixed volume micropipette) to 5 ml sterile distilled water as below.[c]

Organisms	Absorbance reading at 500 nm	Volume (μl) to transfer to 5 ml sterile distilled water
Enterobacteriaceae	0.01–0.05	250
Enterococci	>0.05–0.1	125
Pseudomonas species	>0.1–0.3	40
Staphylococcus species	>0.3–0.6	20
	>0.6–1	10
Haemophilus species	0.01–0.05	500
Haemolytic streptococci	>0.05–0.1	250
Miscellaneous fastidious	>0.1–0.3	125
organisms	>0.3–0.6	80
	>0.6–1	40

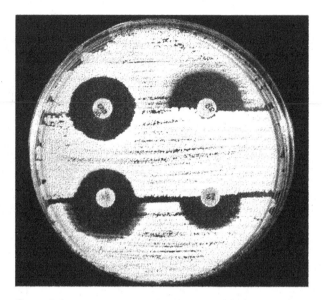

Figure 1 Comparative sensitivity test (Stokes' method) inoculated by the band plating method. The control organism is the two outer bands.

Protocol 5 continued

5   Use the adjusted suspension within 15 min to inoculate plates.

6   Dip a dry sterile cotton swab into the suspension and remove excess fluid by turning the swab against the inside of the tube. Spread the inoculum evenly over the surface of the agar plate by swabbing in three different directions.[d]

7   Allow the medium to dry before applying discs.

[a] The 0.5 McFarland standard is available commercially (e.g. bioMérieux, Basingstoke, UK).

[b] This method may be used with any organisms but is the method of choice for fastidious organisms.

[c] Different spectrophotometers may differ slightly so it may be necessary to adjust the dilutions slightly to achieve semi-confluent growth with any individual set of laboratory conditions.

[d] Alternatively, use a rotary plater.

iv. Control organisms

The original descriptions of Stokes' method recommended using *S. aureus* NCTC 6571 as control for isolates from systemic infections and *E. coli* NCTC 10418 for isolates from urinary tract infections, with all *Pseudomonas* spp. being controlled with *Ps. aeruginosa* NCTC 10662. However, many laboratories now use control strains typical of the isolate rather than based on the source of the isolate and these are detailed in Table 3. Additional control strains may be used in particular situations, and details are included in relevant sections. A methicillin-resistant

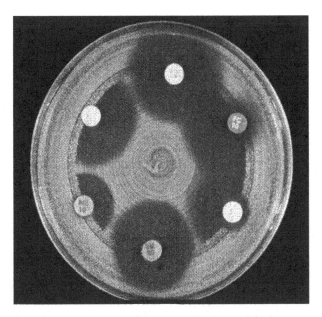

Figure 2 Comparative sensitivity test (Stokes' method) inoculated by the rotary plating method. The control organism is the inner area.

strain of *Staphylococcus aureus* NCTC 12493 may be used to improve control of methicillin/oxacillin susceptibility tests. *Enterococcus faecalis* NCTC 12697 may be used to check that the thymidine and thymine content of media are not too high for sulfonamide and trimethoprim tests. A β-lactamase-producing strain of *E. coli* (NCTC 11560) may be used to control discs containing both a β-lactam agent and a β-lactamase inhibitor.

There is concern that with some newer agents the comparative methods tend to report strains falsely resistant because disc contents may be inappropriately high and/or control organisms are too susceptible. These problems are yet to be resolved.

v. Application of discs

Discs should be applied to plates as follows:

(a) Ensure that the inoculum has dried.

(b) Use discs with contents as in Table 4.

(c) Apply discs to the medium with forceps or a dispenser, ensuring that there is close even contact of discs with the medium.

(d) Do not relocate discs on plates as agents begin to diffuse immediately on contact with the agar.

(e) When the control is on the same plate (Stokes' method), apply the discs on the line between the test and control organisms. Four discs can be accommodated on a 9 cm plate inoculated by the band method. With the rotary plating method and when the control is on a separate plate, use up to six discs.

Table 4 Disc contents (µg except where units stated) for comparative methods

Agent	Organisms from sites other than the urine	Organisms from urine
Amikacin	30	30
Ampicillin/amoxicillin		
Enterobacteriaceae and enterococci	10	25
Haemophilus, Branhamella, staphylococci	2	2
Amoxicillin–clavulanate		
Enterobacteriaceae and enterococci	20/10	20/10
Haemophilus, Branhamella, staphylococci	2/1	2/1
Azithromycin	15	—
Carbenicillin	100	
Cephaloridine	5	30
Cefotaxime	30	30
Ceftazidime	30	30
Cefuroxime	30	30
Cephalothin	30	30
Cephalexin	30	30
Cephradine	30	30
Chloramphenicol		
Enterobacteriaceae	30	—
Haemophilus, pneumococci, meningococci	10	—
Ciprofloxacin	1	1
Clarithromycin	10	—
Clindamycin	2	—
Colistin	10	—
Co-trimoxazole	25	25
Erythromycin	10	—
Fusidic acid	10	—
Gentamicin	10	10
Imipenem	10	10
Kanamycin	30	30
Methicillin	5	—
Mupirocin	5	—
Nalidixic acid	—	30
Neomycin	30	—
Netilmicin	10	10
Nitrofurantoin	—	50
Ofloxacin	1	1
Oxacillin	1	—
Penicillin		
Staphylococci	2 Units	2 Units
Str. Pneumoniae, N. meningitidis, N. gonorrhoeae	0.25 Units	—
Piperacillin	30	30
Rifampicin	5	—

Table 4 (*Continued*)

Agent	Organisms from sites other than the urine	Organisms from urine
Spectinomycin	100	—
Sulfafurazole		
Enterobacteriaceae and enterococci	100	100
N. meningitidis	25	—
Teicoplanin	30	30
Tetracycline	10	30
Ticarcillin–clavulanic acid	75/10	75/10
Tobramycin	10	10
Trimethoprim	1.25	5
Vancomycin	5	5

vi. Incubation of plates

Incubate test and control organisms at 35–37 °C. 30 °C may be used for methicillin/oxacillin tests on staphylococci (see Section 2.4.2).

vii. Reading of tests

If test zones are obviously larger than the control or give no zone at all, it is not necessary to make any measurement. If there is any doubt, zones should be measured with calipers or a ruler.

(a) *Control on a separate plate.* Zone diameters should be measured when possible. If not, measurements should be taken from the edge of the zone to the edge of the disc, in which case adjustment should be made to the criteria for interpretation.

(b) *Control on the same plate (Stokes' method).* Measure from the edge of the disc to the edge of the zone. As the control and test are adjacent, the difference between the respective zone sizes can be easily seen.

viii. Interpretation of zone sizes

A scheme for interpretation of zone sizes is given in Table 5.

2.2.2 The BSAC standardized disc diffusion method

Many of the details are similar to those in Section 2.2.1 but the method is standardized and no variation from the defined technique is allowed (4).

i. Preparation of plates

Prepare Iso-Sensitest agar plates (ISA) (Oxoid CM471 or equivalent medium shown to have the same performance as ISA) as in Protocol 1. The media specified for different organisms is as in Table 6. In order to reduce the number of different

Table 5 Interpretation of zone sizes for comparative methods

Control on a separate plate	
Susceptible	Zone diameter equal to, wider than, or not more than 6 mm smaller than the control.
Intermediate	Zone diameter greater than 10 mm but smaller than the control by more than 6 mm.
Resistant	Zone diameter 10 mm or less.
Control on the same plate (Stokes' method)	
Susceptible	Zone size (zone edge to disc) equal to, wider than, or not more than 3 mm smaller than the control.
Intermediate	Zone size greater than 2 mm but smaller than the control by more than 3 mm.
Resistant	Zone size 2 mm or less.
Exceptions to standard interpretation	
Penicillinase-producing staphylococci	Isolates showing heaped up, clearly defined zone edges against β-lactams should be reported resistant irrespective of zone size.
Polymyxins	Polymyxins diffuse poorly in agar so that zones are small and the above criteria cannot be applied—the intermediate category is not used and in the case of control on a separate plate an isolate is defined as resistant if the zone diameter is >6 mm smaller than the control.
Co-amoxiclav	When the control is on a separate plate replace 6 mm with 10 mm when the 30 μg disc is used and replace 6 mm with 20 mm when the 3 μg disc is used. When the control is on the same plate replace 3 mm with 5 mm when the 30 μg disc is used and replace 3 mm with 10 mm when the 3 μg disc is used.
Teicoplanin with staphylococci	Any strain showing a zone smaller than the control should be tested by an MIC method.
Ciprofloxacin and ofloxacin	When the control is on a separate plate, replace 6 mm with 14 mm if the control strain is *S. aureus* NCTC 6571 or *Ps. aeruginosa* NCTC 10662, and replace 6 mm with 20 mm if the control strain is *E. coli* NCTC 10418 or *H. influenzae* NCTC 11931. When the control is on the same plate, replace 3 mm with 7 mm if the control strain is *S. aureus* NCTC 6571 or *Ps. aeruginosa* NCTC 10662, and replace 3 mm with 10 mm if the control strain is *E. coli* NCTC 10418 or *H. influenzae* NCTC 11931.

media used, ISA + 5% whole horse blood + 20 mg/litre NAD may be used for all fastidious organisms listed in Table 6.

ii. Preparation of inoculum

The inoculum used should give semi-confluent growth of colonies after overnight incubation. The means by which the correct inoculum is achieved is not critical as long as semi-confluent growth is obtained. The alternative methods described in Protocol 5 have been shown to work well.

iii. Inoculation of plates

Evenly inoculate plates as described in Protocol 5.

Table 6 Media for the BSAC standardized method

Species	Medium
Enterobacteriaceae	ISA
Pseudomonas species	ISA
Staphylococci (agents other than methicillin/oxacillin)	ISA
Staphylococci (methicillin/oxacillin testing)	Columbia agar with 2% NaCl
Enterococci	ISA
Streptococcus pneumoniae	ISA +5% whole horse blood
β-haemolytic streptococci	ISA + 5% whole horse blood
M. catarrhalis	ISA +5% whole horse blood
Neisseria meningitidis	ISA +5% whole horse blood
Haemophilus species	ISA +5% whole horse blood +20 mg/litre NAD
N. gonorrhoeae	ISA +5% whole horse blood

iv. Application of discs
Disc contents are as specified for the BSAC method (4) and are listed in Table 7. Apply discs as in Section 2.2.1.v.

v. Incubation of plates
Incubate plates within 15 minutes of disc application. Incubation conditions are as in Table 8.

Enterococci should be incubated for 24 hours before reporting a strain as susceptible to vancomycin or teicoplanin as small colonies within zones may not be visible with shorter incubation.

vi. Reading of plates
Use a ruler, calipers, or automated zone reader to measure diameters of zones of inhibition. Alternatively, a template can be used to interpret susceptibility without measuring zones (see Section 2.2.1.vii).

vii. Interpretation of zone sizes
Interpret zone diameters by reference to published tables of breakpoints (4). The latest version of the breakpoints is on the BSAC web site (http://www.bsac.org.uk).

viii. Quality control
Specified control strains (Table 9) should be tested daily and it should be confirmed that zones of inhibition for the control strain fall within the acceptable range (4, http://www.bsac.org.uk). See also Section 2.5.

Table 7 Disc contents (μg) for the BSAC standardized disc diffusion method

Agent	Isolates from sites other than urine	Isolates from urine
Amikacin	30	
Ampicillin		
Enterobacteriaceae and enterococci	10	25
M. catarrhalis and *Haemophilus* spp.	2	
Azithromycin	15	
Aztreonam	30	
Carbenicillin	100	
Cefaclor	30	
Cefamandole	30	
Cefepime	30	
Cefixime	5	
Cefoperazone	30	
Cefotetan	30	
Cefotaxime		
Enterobacteriaceae	30	
Other organisms	5	
Cefoxitin	30	
Cefpodoxime		
Enterobacteriaceae	5	
Str. pneumoniae	1	
Cefpirome	20	
Ceftazidime	30	
Ceftibuten	10	
Ceftizoxime	30	
Ceftriaxone	30	
Cefuroxime		
Enterobacteriaceae	30	
Other organisms	5	
Cephalothin	30	
Cephalexin	30	30
Cephradine	30	
Chloramphenicol	10	
Ciprofloxacin	1	1
Pseudomonas spp.	1 or 5	
Clarithromycin		
Staphylococci	1	
Haemophilus spp.	5	
Other organisms	2	
Clindamycin	2	
Co-amoxiclav		
Enterobacteriaceae	20/10	20/10
Other organisms	2/1	

Table 7 (*Continued*)

Agent	Isolates from sites other than urine	Isolates from urine
Colistin	25	
Co-trimoxazole	25	
Doxycycline	30	
Erythromycin	5	
Fosfomycin	200/50	
Fusidic acid	10	
Gatifloxacin	2	
Gemifloxacin		
Pseudmonas spp.	5	
Other organisms	1	
Gentamicin		
Enterococci	200	
Other organisms	10	
Imipenem	10	
Levofloxacin		
Pseudmonas spp.	5	
Other organisms	1	
Linezolid	10	
Mecillinam		
Enterobacteriaceae		10
Staphylococci		50
Meropenem	10	
Methicillin	5	
Moxifloxacin		
Pseudmonas spp.	5	
Other organisms	1	
Mupirocin	5	
Nalidixic acid	30	30
Neomycin	10	
Netilmicin		
Pseudmonas spp.	30	
Other organisms	10	
Nitrofurantoin		200
Norfloxacin		2
Ofloxacin		
Pseudmonas spp.	5	
Other organisms	1	
Oxacillin	1	
Penicillin	1U	
Piperacillin	75	
Piperacillin–tazobactam	75/10	
Quinupristin/dalfopristin	15	
Rifampicin		

Table 7 (*Continued*)

Agent	Isolates from sites other than urine	Isolates from urine
Str. pneumoniae	5	
Other organisms	2	
Spectinomycin	25	
Streptomycin	10	
Sulfamethoxazole	100	
Teicoplanin	30	
Tetracycline		
Enterobacteriaceae	30	
Other organisms	10	
Ticarcillin–clavulanic acid	75/10	
Tobramycin	10	
Trimethoprim		2.5
Enterobacteriaceae	2.5	
Staphylococci and *Haemophilus* spp.	5	
Vancomycin	5	

Table 8 Incubation conditions for the BSAC standardized disc diffusion method

Organisms	Incubation conditions
Enterobacteriaceae	35–37 °C in air for 16–20 h
Pseudomonas species	35–37 °C in air for 16–20 h
Staphylococci (agent other than methicillin/oxacillin)	35–37 °C in air for 16–20 h
Staphylococci (methicillin/oxacillin)	30 °C in air for 24 h
M. catarrhalis	35–37 °C in air for 16–20 h
Haemolytic streptococci	35–37 °C in air for 16–20 h
Enterococci	35–37 °C in air for 24 h
N. meningitidis	35–37 °C in 4–6% CO_2 in air for 16–20 h
S. pneumoniae	35–37 °C in 4–6% CO_2 in air for 16–20 h
H. influenzae	35–37 °C in 4–6% CO_2 in air for 16–20 h
N. gonorrhoeae	35–37 °C in 4–6% CO_2 in air for 16–20 h

2.3 Selection of agents for routine testing

Agents should be grouped according to the identity of the organism, e.g. Enterobacteriaceae, *Pseudomonas* spp., staphylococci, and streptococci. The choice of agents for testing will differ from one laboratory to another, depending on local preferences. However, similar agents will probably have similar susceptibilities, so only one member of the group need be tested. If one agent in a group is

Table 9 Control strains for the BSAC standardized disc diffusion method

Control organism	Strain
Escherichia coli	NCTC 12241 (ATCC 25922) or NCTC 10418
S. aureus	NCTC 12981 (ATCC 25923) or NCTC 6571
S. pneumoniae	NCTC 12977 (ATCC 49619)
E. faecalis	NCTC 12697 (ATCC 29212)
P. aeruginosa	NCTC 12934 (ATCC 27853) or NCTC 10662
H. influenzae	NCTC 12699 (ATCC 49247) or NCTC 11931
N. gonorrhoeae	NCTC 12700 (ATCC 49226)

frequently used locally, it would be reasonable to test that in place of the agents listed below, with the exception of anti-staphylococcal β-lactams.

(a) Penicillin G is representative of all penicillinase-sensitive penicillins when testing staphylococci.

(b) Methicillin or oxacillin are representative of all penicillinase-resistant penicillins and cephalosporins when testing staphylococci.

(c) Ampicillin is representative of amoxicillin and ampicillin esters.

(d) Combinations of a β-lactam agent and a β-lactamase inhibitor should be tested by use of discs containing both the inhibitor and the β-lactam agent.

(e) Cefaclor, cefadroxil, cephalexin, and cephradine are similar and only one need be tested.

(f) Tetracycline is representative of all tetracyclines (a few tetracycline-resistant strains of *S. aureus* and Enterobacteriaceae are susceptible to minocycline).

(g) Clindamycin is representative of lincomycin. Inducible resistance to these agents will not be detected in the absence of erythromycin.

(h) Sulfafurazole or sulfamethoxazole are representative of all sulfonamides.

(i) Colistin is representative of polymyxin B.

2.4 Specific problems in testing

2.4.1 Tests with anaerobic organisms

The reliability of diffusion tests on many anaerobic organisms is questionable. The comparative methods permit testing of rapidly growing anaerobes, the BSAC standardized method includes tentative criteria for a very limited range of tests (5) and requires others to be done by an MIC method, and the NCCLS method requires all tests on anaerobes to be done with an MIC method.

2.4.2 Methicillin susceptibility tests with staphylococci

The expression of resistance is markedly affected by test conditions, particularly with coagulase negative staphylococci, and there are marked differences among strains. The BSAC recommend the following (14).

(a) Use Columbia agar with 2% NaCl. Mueller–Hinton with 2% NaCl may be used for tests on *S. aureus* but Columbia agar with 2% NaCl is superior for coagulase negative staphylococci.

(b) Use a semi-confluent inoculum (see Section 2.2.2.ii).

(c) Use methicillin 5 μg or oxacillin 1 μg discs.

(d) Incubate tests for 24 h at 30 °C in air.

(e) Examine zones carefully in good light to detect colonies, some of which may be very small, within zones. Resistance may appear as a reduced zone size, gradual reduction in colony size up to the disc, a film of growth within zones, or isolated colonies of various sizes within zones.

(f) Interpretation of zone diameters for both methicillin 5 μg or oxacillin 1 μg discs is: susceptible ≥15 mm, resistant <14 mm.

(g) *S. aureus* NCTC 12493 is a methicillin-resistant strain that can be used to check that conditions are favourable for the detection of resistance.

(h) Some hyper-producers of penicillinase may produce small zones of inhibition, <15 mm in diameter, whereas the greater majority of true methicillin/oxacillin-resistant strains produce no zone of inhibition. If in doubt such strains should be tested by a PCR method (15) or a latex agglutination method to detect PBP2a (16).

2.4.3 Rapid β-lactamase testing

Rapid biochemical tests may be used to detect β-lactamase production by *Haemophilus* spp., *Neisseria* spp., and *Morexella catarrhalis*. Several methods have been used (17). The most widely used are the acidometric and chromogenic substrate methods. The first is described in Chapter 4, and the second in Protocol 6. Commercial kits are available for these methods.

Protocol 6

Chromogenic substrate test for β-lactamase activity in *Haemophilus* spp., *Neisseria* spp., and *Morexella catarrhalis*

Equipment and reagents

- Microwell tray
- Nitrocefin (GSK)

- Dimethyl sulfoxide
- 0.05 M phosphate buffer pH 7.0

Method

1 Dissolve nitrocefin in dimethyl sulfoxide to a concentration of 10 g/litre and dilute the solution to 500 mg/litre in 0.05 M phosphate buffer pH 7.0.[a] Store the solution at 4 °C in the dark for up to a month.

Protocol 6 continued

2 Transfer 50 µl nitrocefin solution to a well in a microwell tray.

3 Make a dense suspension of several colonies of the test organism in a small volume of saline.

4 Add 50 µl test suspension to the well containing nitrocefin.

5 Set up positive and negative controls by the same method.

6 Incubate at 37 °C. A colour change from yellow to red within 30 min indicates production of β-lactamase.

[a] Ready-prepared solution may be purchased from Oxoid Ltd.

2.4.4 Tests for extended spectrum β-lactamases (ESBLs)

Most ESBLs are inhibited by clavulanate and this is the basis of current tests, but no currently available test is completely reliable (18, 19). Some methods practical for routine use are described in Protocol 7.

Protocol 7

Detection of extended-spectrum β-lactamases

Equipment and reagents

* Plates
* Discs

A. The double disc synergy test

1 Inoculate plates as described for the BSAC standardized method (see Sections 2.2.2.ii and 2.2.2.iii).

2 Place discs containing ceftazidime 30 mg, cefotaxime 30 mg, or aztreonam 30 mg at a distance of 30 mm (centre to centre) around a disc of co-amoxiclav 30 mg.[a]

3 Incubate plates as described for the BSAC standardized method (see Section 2.2.2.v).

4 Examine zones for interactions between agents. ESBL-producers show enhanced zones between co-amoxyclav and one or more of the other agents.

B. Etest

1 Set up tests as instructed by the manufacturer.

2 A difference ≥8 in the ratio of ceftazidime or cefotaxime MICs with and without clavulanate indicates ESBL production.

C. Combined disc methods

1 Set up tests as instructed by the manufacturer.

2 Measure zone sizes around ceftazidime, cefotaxime,[b] or cefpodoxime[c] discs, and around discs containing the same agents with clavulanate.

3 Interpret differences in zone diameters between discs with and without clavulanate according to the manufacturer's instructions.

[a] Note that the distance between discs is critical. False negatives may occur with *Proteus mirabilis* which give large zones, and with organisms hyper-producing cephalosporinases in addition to producing EsβLs.

[b] Ref. 17.

[c] Ref. 18.

2.4.5 Penicillin resistance in *Streptococcus pneumoniae*

To detect intrinsic resistance to penicillin in *Streptococcus pneumoniae* oxacillin 1 μg discs should be used. Strains appearing resistant in this screening test should be tested by an MIC method to confirm resistance.

2.4.6 Glycopeptide intermediate *Staphylococcus aureus* (GISA)

S. aureus with vancomycin MICs >4 mg/litre are rare. Strains which are heterogeneous in susceptibility to vancomycin (hetero-GISA strains) have MICs ≤4 mg/litre by conventional MIC methods but have a resistant subpopulation with a vancomycin MIC of >4 mg/litre and are more common although the clinical significance of such isolates is disputed. Glycopeptide-resistant *S. aureus* cannot be detected by disc diffusion methods. Appropriate methods are as follows (20).

(a) Population analysis is reported to be the most reliable method for detecting heterogeneous resistance to vancomycin. However, such methods are not practical for routine use (21).

(b) For the agar screening test 10 ml of 0.5 McFarland suspension bacteria (10^6 cfu) are spotted on BHI agar containing 6 mg/litre vancomycin. After incubation at 35 °C for 24 and 48 h plates are examined for colonies. The sensitivity of this approach has been reported to be low compared with other methods.

(c) For the Etest screening method use BHI agar, an inoculum adjusted to a 2.0 McFarland standard, and incubation at 35 °C for 48 h. Vancomycin and teicoplanin MICs both ≥8 mg/litre or teicoplanin MICs alone ≥12 mg/litre indicate reduced susceptibility to glycopeptides (20).

(d) If vancomycin resistance is suspected on clinical grounds, or if any of the above tests indicate resistance, the organism should be sent to a reference laboratory for confirmation.

2.5 Quality assurance

2.5.1 External quality assessment

Participation in an external quality assessment scheme provides several benefits:

(a) An independent assessment of performance.

(b) Comparison with other participating laboratories.

(c) Detection of sources of error in testing.

(d) A stimulus to attain and maintain standards.

2.5.2 Internal quality control

This is used to detect day-to-day variation. Control strains (Table 9) should be used with each batch of tests to check the performance of the method, or in the case of Stokes' method, to provide an internal control of variation with every test. Control strains should be handled as follows.

(a) Store working cultures on agar slopes.

(b) Subculture slopes every two weeks.

(c) Replace cultures on slopes every two months, or sooner if contamination is suspected, with fresh cultures from freeze-dried or frozen cultures (−70 °C in glycerol broth).

The degree of control exercised will depend on the interest and resources of the laboratory. If a defined standardized method is used the required control will be specified. A range of tests of increasing complexity is given below.

(a) Briefly examine control zones to ensure that zone sizes are approximately correct. This approach will indicate major problems only and is not acceptable for standardized methods.

(b) Regularly record control zones on a chart, which may be pinned on a notice board in the laboratory. Changes in zone size are more readily seen and trends are obvious.

(c) Establish zone size limits by recording zone sizes for at least 30 sequential observations. Then calculate 95% confidence limits and draw the limits on a chart prepared as in (b) above. Zone sizes should be close to the midpoint of the acceptable range and no more than 1 in 20 observations would be expected to fall outside the limits. Such limits are published for some standardized methods.

In addition to routine control strains, additional tests may be set up to control particular problem areas as follows.

(a) A methicillin/oxacillin heteroresistant strain of *S. aureus* (NCTC 12493) may be set up with new batches of medium to confirm that resistance is detected (colonies should grow up to the disc).

(b) A β-lactamase producing strain of *E. coli* (NCTC 11954 or NCTC 11560) may be used to detect deterioration of the β-lactamase inhibitor in discs containing a combination of a β-lactamase inhibitor and a β-lactam agent. Decrease in zone sizes will be seen if the β-lactamase inhibitor deteriorates.

If control tests indicate a problem with the method then possible sources of error should be investigated. In this situation tests must be interpreted with caution and, depending on the cause of the error, it should be considered whether results should be withheld and/or tests repeated. There are several common errors indicated by control tests.

(a) A gradual decrease in zone sizes may indicate inactivation of labile agents in discs due to improper storage and handling in the laboratory. Test new batches before they are put into routine use.

(b) A general decrease or increase in zone sizes may indicate too heavy or too light an inoculum.

(c) Fluctuating zone sizes may indicate errors in measuring or transcribing zone sizes. In particular, different observers may read zone edges differently. Fluctuating zone sizes may also indicate variation in the depth of the medium.

(d) Larger zones with aminoglycosides and erythromycin, and smaller zones with tetracycline, oxacillin, and fusidic acid may indicate that the pH of the medium is too high. The reverse might occur if the pH is too low. Test new batches of medium before they are put into routine use.

(e) Any alteration in the zone sizes might indicate contamination or mutational changes in the control strain.

2.6 Primary susceptibility tests

These are tests in which the inoculum is the specimen itself. The use of primary tests is discussed by Waterworth and del Piano (22).

The advantages of primary tests are:

(a) Results will be available the next day, 24 hours earlier than tests on pure cultures.

(b) Differences in susceptibility may facilitate isolation from mixed cultures.

(c) Small numbers of resistant variants, which might otherwise be missed, may be seen within zones of inhibition.

Care must be taken to avoid the potential disadvantages of primary tests.

(a) To avoid wasteful tests that show no growth or need to be repeated, carry out primary tests only on specimens from sites that are normally sterile and on urine specimens shown to contain organisms by direct microscopy or by other methods. Direct tests should not be done on specimens that are likely to be heavily contaminated, e.g. from bedsores, ears, varicose ulcers, lesions connected with the large bowel, or on specimens from patients receiving antimicrobial treatment.

(b) The inoculum cannot be controlled, but many pus swabs and urine specimens contain a density of organism such that semi-confluent growth is often achieved if the correct method is used. Tests that are mixed or have incorrect inocula must be repeated.

(c) Take care to avoid reporting the susceptibility of commensal organisms.

Primary tests can be done by the comparative and BSAC methods as described in this chapter except for the method of inoculation.

(a) Evenly streak pus swabs on the plate in place of the methods used on pure cultures.

(b) With urines, a well-mixed specimen replaces the broth culture or suspension of colonies used with pure cultures (as described in Protocol 2). Plates may be inoculated with a loop and swab (Protocol 4) or a wet swab (Protocol 5).

(c) With the comparative methods the control organisms used are *E. coli* NCTC 10418 for organisms from urine and *S. aureus* NCTC 6571 for other specimens. If, after incubation, the control is seen to be inappropriate (see Section 2.1.7), the test should be repeated.

(d) If the inoculum is correct and the culture is pure the zones of inhibition of significant pathogenic organisms can be interpreted as for pure cultures.

3 Methods for determining minimum inhibitory concentrations

3.1 Agar dilution

Minimum inhibitory concentrations (MICs) are used to determine the quantitative activity of antimicrobials. MICs are considered the 'gold standard' for determining *in vitro* activity and are a much used research tool for assessing the activity of new antibiotics. These methods of testing have the advantage that they can be used to investigate the activity of both actively multiplying and slow growing bacteria such as anaerobes and mycobacteria. Most diagnostic laboratories do not perform routine MICs to determine the susceptibility of clinical isolates, however, MICs are used to confirm resistance or to elucidate equivocal results. For results to be meaningful it is essential that a standardized method of testing is used. The following method is based on that recommended by the British Society of Antimicrobial Chemotherapy (BSAC) (4) although other standardized methods are available for example, those described in the NCCLS (6).

3.1.1 Standard material

Standard material should always be obtained from the pharmaceutical company or a reputable supplier (e.g. Sigma Chemicals, Poole, UK). Information on storage, stability, potency, expiry date, solubility, and any other Control of Substances Hazardous to Health (COSHH) information should be obtained. Antibiotic powders may be affected by heat, light, or moisture and are generally stored below room temperature (4–8 °C), over a desiccant (e.g. silica gel), and protected from light (unless otherwise directed by the pharmaceutical company).

3.1.2 Preparation of antibiotic solutions

Stock solutions should be prepared following the manufacturer's instructions using the recommended solvent and making adjustments to the amount of material weighed by correcting for the potency of the antibiotic ('as is' potency expressed as mg per mg of powder).

The following formula can be used to prepare stock solutions making adjustments for potency:

$$\frac{1000}{P} \times V \times C = W$$

where: V = volume of stock solution required (ml); C = final concentration of stock solution (multiples of 1000 mg/litre); P = potency of the standard material (μg per mg); W = weight of antibiotic powder to be dissolved in V (mg).

For example: potency of standard powder 980 mg per mg; volume required 25 ml; final concentration 10 000 mg/litre:

$$\frac{1000}{980} \times 25 \times 10 = 255.1\,mg$$

Most antibiotics can be dissolved in sterile distilled water and because contamination of antibiotic powders is extremely rare, require no further treatment, such as filtration, before use. Antibiotics requiring solvents other than distilled water are shown in Table 10.

Stock solutions of antibiotic in excess of 1000 mg/litre can generally be stored at temperatures below −20 °C for at least one month (should be confirmed by consulting the data sheets provided with the powder). Clavulanate and imipenem are known to be unstable as solutions and therefore it is recommended that fresh solutions of clavulanate be used, and that solutions of imipenem in MOPS buffer should be stored at temperatures of −30 °C or below. Once a stock solution has been frozen and thawed it should be used once and then discarded.

Further dilution of stock solutions from an initial 10 000 mg/litre solution (solution A) are made as follows:

1 ml of 10 000 mg/litre solution +9 ml of diluent =1000 mg/litre (solution B)

100 μl of 10 000 mg/litre solution +9.9 ml of diluent =100 mg/litre (solution C)

Note: diluent is normally water. For exceptions consult Table 10.

These solutions can be prepared using volumetric glassware.

Table 10 Antibiotics requiring solvents other than sterile distilled water for dissolving powders or for further dilution of stock solutions

Antibiotic	Solvent	Diluent
Amoxicillin	DMSO or saturated NaHCO$_3$	Water
Ampicillin	Saturated NaHCO$_3$	Water
Azithromycin	Ethanol	Water
Aztreonam	Saturated NaHCO$_3$	Water
Cefixime	Saturated NaHCO$_3$	Water
Ceftazidime	Saturated NaHCO$_3$	Water
Chloramphenicol	Ethanol	Water
Clarithromycin	DMSO	Water
Clavulanate	0.1 M phosphate buffer pH 6	0.1 M phosphate buffer pH 6
Erythromycin	Ethanol	Water
Fusidic acid	Ethanol	Water
Imipenem	1 M MOPS buffer pH 6.8	1 M MOPS buffer pH 6.8
Gatifloxacin	Water and 0.1 M NaOH dropwise to dissolve	Water
Gemifloxacin	Methanol	Water
Nalidixic acid	Water and 0.1 M NaOH dropwise to dissolve	Water
Nitrofurantoin	DMF	DMF
Norfloxacin	1 ml water + 10 µl glacial acetic acid, after completely dissolved make to volume with water	Water
Ofloxacin	Saturated NaHCO$_3$	Water
Rifampicin	DMSO	Water
Roxithromycin	Ethanol	Water
Sparfloxacin	Water and 0.1 M NaOH dropwise to dissolve	Water
Sulfamethoxazole	Water and 0.1 M NaOH dropwise to dissolve	Water
Tazobactam	Saturated NaHCO$_3$	Water
Teicoplanin	Ethanol	Water
Telithromycin	1 ml water + 10 µl glacial acetic acid	0.07 M phosphate buffer pH 8
Trimethoprim	1 ml water + 10 µl glacial acetic acid, after completely dissolved make to volume with water	Water

3.1.3 Preparation of antibiotic dilution range

The range of antibiotic concentrations which are used to determine MICs are universally accepted to be in doubling dilution steps up and down from 1 mg/litre as required. An example of antibiotic concentrations ranging from 1 mg/litre to 128 mg/litre in a volume of 20 ml agar or broth is as follows, however, other methods for preparing antibiotic dilutions can be used.

(a) Label 11 sterile containers (the container, amount of antibiotic, and volume of agar or broth added can be varied depending on the number of plates required) as follows: 128, 64, 32, 16, 8, 4, 2, 1, 0.5, 0.25, and 0 mg/litre (antibiotic-free control).

(b) From solution A pipette the following amounts with a micropipette:

256 µl into the container labelled 128 mg/litre.

128 µl into the container labelled 64 mg/litre.

64 µl into the container labelled 32 mg/litre.

32 µl into the container labelled 16 mg/litre.

(c) From solution B pipette the following amounts with a micropipette:

160 µl into the container labelled 8 mg/litre.

80 µl into the container labelled 4 mg/litre.

40 µl into the container labelled 2 mg/litre.

(d) From solution C pipette the following amounts with a micropipette:

200 µl into the container labelled 1 mg/litre.

100 µl into the container labelled 0.5 mg/litre.

50 µl into the container labelled 0.25 mg/litre.

3.1.4 Medium

The composition of culture media can affect the activity of antibiotics and it is well recognized that free calcium and magnesium ions can have a marked effect on the activity of aminoglycosides and tetracycline antibiotics (23). Indeed, daptomycin has been shown to require a concentration of free calcium equivalent to that found *in vivo* for *in vitro* activity to be visualized (24). To aid standardization of performance, NCCLS methodology recommends that both Mueller–Hinton broth and agar contain 20–35 mg/litre of Mg^{2+} and 50–100 mg/litre of Ca^{2+}. These concentrations are provided by the manufacturer or can be added after sterilization, by the addition of sterile solutions of $MgCl_2$ and $CaCl_2$ (6). Other substances, for example thymidine, present in culture media have been shown to reduce the activity of folate inhibitor (23). Semi-defined culture media (for example Iso-Sensitest agar Oxoid, Basingstoke, UK) have been developed for susceptibility testing. These provide a nutritional environment for the micro-organism, with minimum 'batch-to-batch' variation, and without the need to add blood to neutralize the effect of inhibitors. For the growth of fastidious organisms media has been supplemented with blood, NAD, or other commercial supplements, however, it must be shown that supplements added to media do not affect the *in vitro* activity of the antibiotics to be tested. Whole defibrinated horse blood with a defined shelf-life is recommended because the performance of media can vary depending on the way in which lysed blood is prepared (freezing and thawing, treatment with saponin, or ultrasonication). To prevent organisms such as *Proteus* species from swarming 50 mg/litre *p*-nitrophenyl glycerol (PNPG) (BDH Merck, Lutterworth, UK) or 350 mg/litre Matexil (Astra Zeneca, Cheshire, UK) have been added to agar or the agar concentration has been increased. All of these adjustments to the medium can affect the activity of some antibiotics and should only be used if essential and with evidence that they do not affect antimicrobial action. For the detection of oxacillin/methicillin resistance in staphylococci it has been shown that media such as Mueller–Hinton agar and Columbia agar with the addition of sodium chloride are preferable (25). In the case of anaerobes, Wilkins and Chalgren agar is the medium of choice.

3.1.5 Preparation of agar dilution plates

Prepare Oxoid Iso-Sensitest agar (ISA) (Oxoid, Basingstoke, UK) or equivalent following the manufacturer's instructions. Cool medium to 50 °C before adding supplements. If the medium is supplemented with NAD ensure that the temperature of the medium does not exceed 42 °C as this has a detrimental effect on NAD.

(a) Add 20 ml of molten agar to each container, including the antibiotic-free control. Mix well before pouring into a 90 mm Petri dish. To minimize the exposure of the antibiotic to a temperature circa 50 °C, add agar, mix, and pour each concentration in turn.

(b) Allow agar to set and then dry the surface of the agar in a fan assisted oven, without UVL, for 10 min or in a still incubator (the time needed for drying will be determined depending on the efficiency of the cabinet).

(c) Store plates at 4–8 °C protected from light until inoculated. Ideally, plates should be used on the day of preparation. If plates are to be stored before use the stability of individual antibiotics in agar should be determined.

3.1.6 Preparation of inoculum

An inoculum of 10^4 cfu/spot is generally used for agar MICs. However, for organisms which produce extracellular β-lactamase a higher inoculum may be needed when testing some β-lactam antibiotics so that strains do not appear falsely sensitive. The inoculum should be prepared by comparison with a 0.5 McFarland standard. See Protocol 5 for methods for aerobic organisms.

3.1.7 Preparation of inoculum for testing anaerobes

i. Anaerobes other than Bacteroides species

Anaerobic organisms have markedly different sizes and shapes and therefore the method described has limitations, but offers a practical procedure for clinical laboratories.

(a) Colonies should be taken from plates where cultures have been grown on blood agar enriched with haemin and menadione.

(b) Colonies should not be more than 72 hours old and should not be left in an aerobic atmosphere for more than 30 minutes before the suspension is prepared.

(c) Prepare a suspension in Wilkins and Chalgren broth (Oxoid) to match a 0.5 McFarland standard.

ii. Bacteroides

(a) Emulsify the growth from a plate which has not been incubated for more than 24 hours in 1 ml of sterile distilled water to match or exceed the 0.5 McFarland standard.

(b) Mix well with a vortex mixer.

3.1.8 Adjustment of the suspension to match the 0.5 McFarland standard

(a) By adding sterile distilled water adjust the density of the organism suspension to match the 0.5 McFarland standard.

(b) To aid comparison, compare the standard and test using a white background with a contrasting black line.

(c) Suspensions should contain between 10^7 and 10^8 cfu/ml depending on genera (6).

3.1.9 Final dilution of suspension before inoculation

Final dilution of organism suspension in sterile distilled water before inoculation. (Table 11).

3.1.10 Quality control

Appropriate control strains must be included with every batch of tests. Recommended control strains available from national collections are shown in Table 12.

3.1.11 Inoculation

(a) Use a multipoint inoculator (e.g. Denley, Mast Diagnostics, Bootle, UK) to deliver 1–2 ml on to the surface of the agar.

(b) Allow the inoculum to be absorbed before incubation.

Table 11 Final dilution of organism suspensions[a]

1:10	No dilution
Haemolytic streptococci	*S. pneumoniae*
Enterobacteriaceae	*M. catarrhalis*
Pseudomonas species	*N. meningitidis*
Acinetobacter species	*N. gonorrhoeae*
Haemophilus species	Anaerobes (not bacteroides)
Enterococci	
Staphylococci	
Bacteroides species	

[a] Organism suspensions should be used within 30 minutes of preparation.

Table 12 Appropriate control strain for agar dilution method, depending on genera

Organism	ATCC control strain		NCTC control strain
	ATCC number	NCTC catalogue number	
Escherichia coli	25922	12241	10418
Staphylococcus aureus	25923	12981	6571
Pseudomonas aeruginosa	27853	12934	10662
Enterococcus faecalis	29212	12697	
Haemophilus influenzae	49247	12699	11931
S. pneumoniae	49619	12977	
N. gonorrhoeae	49226	12700	
B. fragilis			9343

3.1.12 Incubation conditions

Generally, incubation of plates is at 35–37 °C in air for 18–20 hours. With regard to incubation of fastidious organisms such as *Haemophilus influenzae* and *Streptococcus pneumoniae* there is much debate about the atmospheric conditions which are necessary for adequate growth of newly isolated clinical strains. The debate has arisen because an atmosphere enriched with CO_2 significantly reduces the *in vitro* activity of the macrolide antibiotics. However, we would support the need for enriching the atmosphere with CO_2 because 20% of *H. influenzae* and 40% of *S. pneumococci* failed to grow, or grew poorly, on the antibiotic-free control plate after overnight incubation in air (unpublished data). This view is supported by a recent publication proposing that the acid conditions within the respiratory tree may reduce the efficacy of macrolide and azolide antibiotics (26). In the case of anaerobes incubation in a cabinet or jar providing an atmosphere of 10% CO_2, 10% H_2, and 80% N_2 is recommended, however, the duration of incubation depends on individual organism requirements. Recommended incubation conditions are summarized in Table 13.

3.1.13 Reading and interpretation

(a) After incubation ensure that all strains have grown on the antibiotic-free control plate.

(b) Determine the lowest concentration of antibiotic where no visible growth is observed, one or two colonies or a fine film of growth being ignored (MIC mg/litre).

(c) Confirm that the MIC value for the control strain is within plus or minus one two-fold dilution of the expected MIC (see Tables 14 and 15).

3.2 Broth dilution methods

The method cited above can be adapted for macro and micro broth dilution methods. Unlike agar dilution methods, test and control organisms are not in

Table 13 Incubation conditions for MIC plates

Organism	Temperature	Atmosphere	Duration
Enterobacteriaceae	35–37 °C	Air	18–20 h
Pseudomonas spp.	35–37 °C	Air	18–20 h
Staphylococci (other than tests on methicillin/oxacillin)	35–37 °C	Air	18–20 h
Staphylococci (tests on methicillin/oxacillin)	30 °C	Air	24 h
M. catarrhalis	35–37 °C	Air	18–20 h
β-haemolytic streptococci	35–37 °C	Air	18–20 h
Enterococci	35–37 °C	Air	18–20 h
Neisseria spp.	35–37 °C	4–6% CO_2 in air	18–20 h
S. pneumoniae	35–37 °C	4–6% CO_2 in air	18–20 h
Haemophilus spp	35–37 °C	4–6% CO_2 in air	18–20 h
Anaerobes (anaerobic cabinet or jar)	35–37 °C	10% CO_2/10% H_2/ 80% N_2	Dependent on individual organism requirements

precisely the same environment, and broth methods require stringent aseptic technique to avoid contamination. However, broth methods allow the detection of minority resistant populations and minimum bactericidal concentration determinations. A macrodilution method is given in Protocol 8, and a microdilution method in Protocol 9.

Protocol 8

Broth macrodilution MIC method

Equipment and reagents

- Sterile capped 75 × 12 mm tubes
- Broth medium suitable for susceptibility testing
- Lysed blood
- Antibiotic

Method

1 Follow Sections 3.1.1 and 3.1.2, preparing a range of concentrations in a broth medium suitable for susceptibility testing, e.g. Iso-Sensitest broth (Oxoid) one dilution higher than that required to compensate for the addition of an equal volume of inoculum (i.e. if a final range of 0.5, 1, 2, 4, 8, and 16 mg/litre is needed, prepare a range of 1, 2, 4, 8, 16, and 32 mg/litre).

2 If the medium is to be supplemented with blood, use lysed blood to aid visibility.[a]

3 Arrange sufficient sterile capped 75 × 12 mm tubes in duplicate (one row for the test the other for the control) to cover the range of dilutions plus a tube for the antibiotic-free control.

Table 14 Expected MIC values for control strains[a]

Antibiotic	H. influenzae NCTC 11931	H. influenzae ATCC 49247	Ent. faecalis ATCC 29212	S. pneumoniae ATCC 49619	B. fragilis NCTC 9343	N. gonorrhoeae ATCC 49226
Amoxicillin	0.5	4	0.5	0.06	32	0.5
Ampicillin			1	0.06	32	
Azithromycin	2	2		0.12		
Aztreonam			>128		2	
Cefaclor		128	>32	2	>128	
Cefixime	0.03	0.25		1	64	
Cefotaxime		0.25	32	0.06	4	
Cefpirome	0.06	0.5	16		16	
Cefpodoxime	0.12	0.5	>32	0.12	32	
Ceftazidime	0.12		>32		8	
Ceftriaxone			>32	0.06	4	
Cefuroxime	2	16	>32	0.25	32	
Cephadroxil			>32		32	
Cephalexin			>32		64	
Chloramphenicol			4	4	4	
Ciprofloxacin	0.008	0.008	1	1	2	0.004
Clarithromycin	8	4		0.03	0.25	0.5
Clindamycin			8	0.12	0.5	
Co-amoxiclav	0.5	8	0.5	0.06	0.5	0.5
Co-trimoxazole		1	2	4		
Erythromycin	8	8	4	0.12	1	0.5

Table 14 (*Continued*)

Antibiotic	H. influenzae NCTC 11931	H. influenzae ATCC 49247	Ent. faecalis ATCC 29212	S. pneumoniae ATCC 49619	B. fragilis NCTC 9343	N. gonorrhoeae ATCC 49226
Gentamicin			8		128	
Imipenem			0.5		0.06	
Levofloxacin		0.015		0.5	0.5	
Linezolid				2	4	
Mecillinam			>128		>128	
Meropenem			2		0.06	
Metronidazole					0.5	
Moxifloxacin	0.03	0.03	0.25	0.5		0.004
Naladixic acid		1		>128	64	
Nitrofurantoin			8			
Norfloxacin			2		16	
Ofloxacin			2		1	
Oxacillin				1		
Penicillin		4	2	0.5	16	
Piperacillin			2		2	
Quinupristin/dalfopristin			1	0.5	16	
Rifampicin			2	0.03		
Roxithromycin	16	16		0.12	2	
Sparfloxacin		0.002		0.25	1	
Teicoplanin			0.25			
Telithromycin	1	2	0.008	0.008		0.03
Tetracycline		16	16	0.12	0.5	
Ticarcillin					4	
Tobramycin			16			
Trimethoprim		0.25	0.25	4	16	
Vancomycin			2	0.25	16	

[a] Strains tested on Iso-Sensitest agar (*B. fragilis* tested on Wilkins and Chalgren media), supplemented with 5% defibrinated horse blood and 20 mg/litre NAD for testing *N. gonorrhoeae*, *S. pneumoniae*.

Table 15 Expected MIC values for control strains[a]

Antibiotic	E. coli NCTC 10418	E. coli ATCC 25922	Ps. aeruginosa NCTC 10662	Ps. aeruginosa ATCC 27853	S. aureus NCTC 6571	S. aureus ATCC 25923	S. aureus ATCC 29213
Amikacin	0.5	1	2	2	1		2
Amoxicillin	2	4	>128	>128	0.12	0.25	
Ampicillin	2	4	>128	>128	0.06		
Azithromycin					0.12	0.12	0.12
Aztreonam	0.03	0.25	4	2	>128		>128
Carbenicillin	2		32		0.5		
Cefaclor	1	2	>128	>128	1		1
Cefixime	0.06	0.25	16		8	8	16
Cefotaxime	0.03	0.06	8	8	0.5		1
Cefoxitin	4		>128	>128	2		
Cefpirome	0.03	0.03	4	1	0.25		0.5
Cefpodoxime	0.25	0.25	128	>128	1	4	2
Ceftazidime	0.06	0.25	1	1	4		8
Ceftizoxime	0.008				2		
Ceftriaxone	0.03	0.06	8	8	1		2
Cefuroxime	2	4	>128	>128	0.5	1	1
Cephadroxil	8	8	>128	>128	1		2
Cephalexin	4	8	>128	>128	1		4
Cephaloridine			>128	>128	0.06		
Cephalothin	4	8	>128	>128	0.5		0.25
Cephradine			>128	>128	2		

Table 15 (*Continued*)

Antibiotic	E. coli NCTC 10418	E. coli ATCC 25922	Ps. aeruginosa NCTC 10662	Ps. aeruginosa ATCC 27853	S. aureus NCTC 6571	S. aureus ATCC 25923	S. aureus ATCC 29213
Chloramphenicol	2	4	128		2		2
Ciprofloxacin	0.015	0.015	0.25	0.25	0.12	0.5	0.5
Clarithromycin					0.12	0.12	0.12
Clindamycin					0.06	0.12	0.06
Co-amoxiclav	2	4	>128	128	0.12	0.12	0.25
Colistin	0.5		2		128		
Co-trimoxazole	0.25	0.25					2
Dirythromycin					1		1
Erythromycin					0.12	0.5	0.25
Farapenem	0.25	0.12	>128	>128	0.12		
Fleroxacin	0.06		1		0.5		
Flucloxacillin			>128	>128	0.06		
Fosfomycin	4		>128	>128	8		
Fusidic acid	>128				0.06	0.12	0.06
Gatifloxacin	0.015				0.03		
Gentamicin	0.25	0.5	1	1	0.12	0.25	0.25
Imipenem	0.06	0.12	2	1	0.015		0.015
Kanamycin	1		1		2		
Levofloxacin	0.03	0.03	0.5	0.5	0.12	0.25	0.25
Linezolid					0.5	1	
Mecillinam	0.12	0.12	8		8		64
Meropenem	0.015	0.008	2	0.25	0.03	0.06	0.06

Methicillin	2		>128	1	2	2
Mezlocillin	0.03		8	0.5		
Moxalactam	0.03		8	8		
Moxifloxacin	0.03		2	0.06	0.06	0.06
Mupirocin				0.25	0.25	0.12
Naladixic acid	2	4	>128	>128	128	128
Neomycin			32	0.12		
Nitrofurantoin	4	8		8		16
Norfloxacin	0.06	0.06	1	0.25		1
Ofloxacin	0.06	0.03	1	0.25		0.5
Oxacillin			>128	0.25	0.25	0.5
Penicillin		>128	>128	0.03	0.03	0.12
Piperacillin	0.5	2	4	0.25		1
Quinupristin/ dalfopristin				0.12	0.25	0.25
Rifampicin	16			0.004	0.015	0.004
Roxithromycin				0.25	0.5	0.5
Rufloxacin	0.5		8	1		
Sparfloxacin	0.015		0.5	0.03		
Sulfonamide	16		>128	64		
Teicoplanin				0.25	0.5	0.5
Telithromycin				0.03	0.06	0.06
Temocillin	2		>128	128		
Tetracycline	1	2	32	0.06		0.5

Table 15 (*Continued*)

Antibiotic	E. coli NCTC 10418	E. coli ATCC 25922	Ps. aeruginosa NCTC 10662	Ps. aeruginosa ATCC 27853	S. aureus NCTC 6571	S. aureus ATCC 25923	S. aureus ATCC 29213
Ticavcillin plus fixed 4 mg/litre clavulanate			32	16			
Ticarcillin	1		16		0.5		
Tobramycin	0.25	0.5	0.5	0.5	0.12		0.5
Trimethoprim	0.12	0.25	32		0.25		0.5
Vancomycin					0.5	0.5	1

[a] Strains tested on Iso-Sensitest agar.

4   Add 1 ml of each antibiotic dilution in broth and antibiotic-free broth to the two rows of tubes.

5   Retain the antibiotic dilutions and antibiotic-free broth not dispensed and incubate to check for sterility.

6   Prepare organism suspensions in broth as cited in (Protocol 5) including the appropriate control strain (see Table 12).

7   To obtain a final inoculum of 10^5 cfu/ml dilute a suspension equivalent to a McFarland 0.5 standard 1:100 in broth for the following organisms: haemolytic streptococci, staphylococci, Enterobacteriaceae, *S. pneumoniae*, *Pseudomonas* spp., *M. catarrhalis*, *Acinetobacter* spp., *Neisseria* spp., *Haemophilus* spp., and enterococci.

8   Add 1 ml of the test organism suspension in broth to one set of tubes and 1 ml of the control organism suspension to the other set of tubes. Mix and incubate at 35–37 °C in air for 18–20 h.

9   After incubation examine the antibiotic-free control tube to ensure that the medium supports the growth of the test and the control.

10 Read the MIC end-point as the lowest concentration of antibiotic inhibiting the visible growth of the organism.

11 Ensure that the MIC for the control strain is within plus or minus one doubling dilution step of the expected MIC value (see Tables 14 and 15).

[a] The performance of lysed blood may vary and therefore individual laboratories should confirm the suitability of the blood used as part of the laboratory QC programme.

Protocol 9

Broth microdilution MIC method

Equipment and reagents

- See Protocol 8
- 96-well sterile microtitre tray

Method

1   Follow Sections 3.1.1 and 3.1.2 preparing a range of concentrations in a broth medium suitable for susceptibility testing, e.g. Iso-Sensitest broth (Oxoid) one dilution higher than that required to compensate for the addition of an equal volume of inoculum (i.e. if a final range of 0.5, 1, 2, 4, 8, and 16 mg/litre is needed, prepare a range of 1, 2, 4, 8, 16, and 32 mg/litre).

2   If the medium is to be supplemented with blood, use lysed blood to aid visibility.[a]

Protocol 9 continued

3   Label a 96-well sterile microtitre tray with the appropriate antibiotic concentrations.

4   Add 75 μl of each antibiotic dilution and the antibiotic-free control broth to two rows of wells.

5   Retain the antibiotic dilutions and antibiotic-free broth not dispensed and incubate to check for sterility.

6   Prepare the organism suspension as above.

7   Dispense 75 μl of the test organism into one row of wells and 75 μl of the control organism into the second row of wells.

8   Cover with a lid or plate sealing film and incubate at 35–37 °C in air for 18–20 h.

9   Read the MIC end-point as the lowest concentration of antibiotic inhibiting the visible growth of the organism.

10 Ensure that the MIC for the control strain is within plus or minus one doubling dilution step of the expected MIC value (see Tables 14 and 15).

[a] The performance of lysed blood may vary and therefore individual laboratories should confirm the suitability of the blood used as part of the laboratory QC programme.

3.3 Etest

The Etest is an alternative method of determination of MICs (27). It consists of a plastic strip 6 × 0.5 cm in size, with an exponential antimicrobial gradient dried on one side and an MIC scale printed on the other. The range corresponds to 15 two-fold dilutions in a conventional MIC method.

Tests are set up in a similar way to disc diffusion tests except that the disc is replaced with the Etest strip. The details of media, inocula, incubation conditions, and reading vary with the test and are specified by the manufacturer (AB Biodisk). On incubation an elliptical zone is formed and the MIC is read at the point of intersection of the zone with the strip. For most tests the Etest gives similar results to the agar dilution method. The method is useful in routine laboratories for confirmation of unusual resistances, checking equivocal results, for testing slower-growing organisms, and for organisms where a quantitative result is desirable, such as in cases of endocarditis.

4 Breakpoint methods

The categories of susceptibility commonly used in interpretation and reporting of tests are susceptible, intermediate, and resistant. These categories are distinguished by *in vitro* breakpoint concentrations of agents. The breakpoint method is an abbreviated MIC method where isolates are tested only against the fixed concentrations chosen as breakpoint concentrations between the categories of susceptibility. Agar incorporation is the method usually used, with plates inoculated with a multipoint inoculator (28).

The recommended breakpoints are those published by the Susceptibility Testing Working Party of the British Society for Antimicrobial Chemotherapy (4, http://www.bsac.org.uk). Tests are set up as described in Protocol 10.

Protocol 10

Susceptibility testing by the agar breakpoint method

Equipment and reagents

- Agar plates, with and without antibiotics
- Multipoint inoculator with sterile inoculator pins
- Medium
- Inoculum

Method

1 Prepare medium containing agents as described for agar dilution MIC tests (Section 3.1.5).[a]

2 Dry plates so that there are no droplets of moisture on the surface of the agar.

3 Prepare inocula as described in Section 3.1.8 so that the inoculum delivered to the plates is 10^4 cfu/spot. Plate organisms from suspensions to ensure that inocula are pure.

4 Transfer inocula to sterile inoculum wells of the replicating device and use a multipoint inoculator with sterile inoculator pins to transfer inoculum to test plates.[b] Inoculate first a control plate without antibiotic followed by plates containing antimicrobial agents.

5 Incubate plates under conditions appropriate for the organisms (Table 8).

6 Examine purity plates and if cultures are mixed repeat the tests. Examine the control plate without antimicrobial agents to ensure that growth is adequate. Examine plates for growth or the absence of growth. Disregard single colonies or a faint haze produced by the inoculum.

7 Consider the organism as susceptible if there is no growth on the plate containing the agent and adequate growth on the control plate. Consider the organism as resistant if it has grown on the plate containing antibiotic.

[a] Antimicrobial agents solutions may be made from pure antibiotic powders or from commercial freeze-dried agents in vials. Alternatively, tablets commercially prepared for breakpoint testing may be used. Note that the shelf-life of labile agents, such as imipenem and clavulanate combinations such as co-amoxiclav and ticarcillin–clavulanate is short.

[b] The number of test organisms per plate will depend on plate size and the format of the inoculator pins.

Breakpoint methods have several advantages over disc diffusion:

(a) They are suitable for mechanization of inoculation and reading.

(b) They can be combined with agar incorporation identification tests.

(c) They are economical for testing large numbers of isolates.

(d) They usually have clear end-points.

The main limitations are as follows:

(a) Lack of standardization among laboratories.

(b) The all-or-none result which masks finer degrees of susceptibility. To some extent this can be overcome by the inclusion of additional plates to widen the range tested beyond the breakpoint concentrations.

(c) The difficulty in effectively controlling tests because standard control strains may have MICs several dilutions away from breakpoint concentrations.

Approaches to control include the following:

(a) Bioassay of agar plugs taken from breakpoint plates although this will detect only gross errors.

(b) Comparison of the performance of new batches of plates with in-use batches.

(c) Testing new batches of plates with a battery of strains chosen to have MICs just above and below the breakpoint concentrations tested.

5 Serum bactericidal tests and determination of minimum bactericidal concentrations

Serum bactericidal tests (SBTs) have been used to assess antibacterial effect in a number of conditions such as oesteomyelitis, cystic fibrosis, neutropenic fever, and most often infective endocarditis. Minimum bactericidal concentrations (MBCs) have been mainly measured in the context of infective endocarditis and much less commonly in other conditions. The most recent guidance on the antimicrobial therapy of infective endocarditis does not recommend the use of either MBCs or SBTs in the management of such patients (29).

Theoretically SBTs should be of value in the prediction of therapeutic and bacteriological outcome in conditions like infective endocarditis and there are data to support a relationship between the SBT and outcome on a population basis, however the value of the SBT in individual patient prediction is much less clear and perhaps most importantly very few laboratories in the United Kingdom are able to perform SBTs in such a way as to be able to identify penicillin tolerance. The important technical factors related to good performance of SBT are shown on Table 16 (30).

Table 16 Factors related to acceptable or poor performance of SBT with alpha haemolytic streptococci

---

Factors related to acceptable performance

---

1. Sonication of broth prior to counting (prevents chaining).
2. Knowing the size of the inoculum added in cfu/ml (allows clear definition of cidal end-point as 99.9% kill of initial inoculum).
3. Use of 4–8 broth cultures to make inoculum (allow inoculum to be in log phase).
4. Incubation of recovery plates for >36 h (allow identification of 'persisters').
5. Use of calibrated pipette to recover survivors (allows clear definition of cidal end-point as 99.9% kill of initial inoculum).

Factors related to poor performance

---

1. Use of uncalibrated pipette/standard loop to recover survivors.
2. Use of inoculum of $<10^5$ cfu/ml (both make it impossible to reach or measure a 99.9% kill as end-point).

It is not now recommended that individual laboratories perform MBC or SBT determinations but rather refer strains to local or national laboratories with expertise in these tests.

6 Automated methods

Automated methods of antimicrobial susceptibility testing are not commonly used in the United Kingdom. They are likely to have an increasing role in the near future as departments grow larger, laboratory information management systems (LIMS) become more integrated to other health care IT, and 24 hour working becomes more frequent. Automated methods have been recently reviewed from a North American and British perspective (31, 32).

One of the most important developments is that of automated readers for disc susceptibility testing. These systems are of special use with standardized methods such as the BSAC disc susceptibility method. They employ the use of a camera or scanner to capture an image of the plate then use image-analysis software to measure zones and derive categorical sensitivity results. Such automated readers will usually be directly linked to LIMS to facilitate report formulation. Most work best on clear or semi-clear agars and are less good when reading zones on blood-based media. They all require the operator to check the plate images on screen prior to reading. A number of systems are presently available in the UK including Accuzone, Aura Image, BioMIC, BioVideobact, Mastascan Elite, Osiris, ProtoZONE, and SIRSCAN.

These systems have the advantages that they reduce transcription errors, reduce operator variability, allow for automatic interpretation, as well as links to 'expert' software and enhance the ability to provide resistance epidemiology at a local, national, or international level. In addition the software can be used to monitor IQA performance of the disc test method.

The second major area of application of automated systems are based on broth dilution techniques. Basically a broth microdilution tray, gallery, or strip containing dried antimicrobials or other reagent are rehydrated when inoculated with bacteria in a broth suspension. Such methods are usually used to provide an organism identification as well as a categorical susceptibility result or MIC. Some systems are highly developed including a robotic capacity. There are three main systems in widespread use, the Microscan Walk Away System, Sensititre ARIS (Automatic Reading and Incubation System), and the Vitek. In the UK the Vitek is the most commonly used automated system in use but market penetration is at present relatively modest.

The Microscan Walk Away System uses standard size microtitre trays in which the test organisms grow. Growth is detected photometrically (after overnight incubation) or fluorometrically if the short incubation methods are used. Preparation of plates for incubation is manual using a multipoint inoculator but computer algorithms manage the data produced. The Sensititre ARIS also uses standard size microtitre trays. After inoculation they are placed in the incubator of the system and monitored fluorometrically following hydrolysis of fluorogenic substrates. The system is usually run overnight. In contrast to the above two systems the Viteck uses a thin plastic card not microtitre trays. The card contains 30 wells linked by capillaries through which the bacterial test suspension passes to inoculate the wells and rehydrate reagents in the wells. Cards are available to perform isolate identifications as well as susceptibility testing. Growth is determined turbidometrically hourly for up to 15 hours and the MIC calculated. The system has three main components a filler/sealer, reader/incubator, and computer analysis module. The more automated Vitek 2 has a robotic element to allow for initial sample processing including inoculum preparation, bacterial inoculum density verification, and filling and sealing and finally card disposal.

These systems also all have the advantages of automated disc susceptibility zone readers in terms of data transfer, analysis storage, and use of 'expert' software. In the past systems such as Virtek had problems with the detectors of some β-lactamase mediated resistance in Gram-negative bacteria as well as low level glycopeptide resistance in enterococci and now staphylococci.

These systems also tend to be more expensive in terms of reagents as well as the initial cost of purchase, or ongoing cost related to lease or reagent rental. They are less flexible in the range of agents which can be tested when compared to manual methods and, as they cannot be used in all circumstances, an alternative must be available.

At a more basic level multipoint inoculation systems can be regarded as a primitive form of automation for identification and susceptibility testing using breakpoint methods. In addition, most broth microdilution tray or strip galleries, which contain dosed antimicrobials for rehydration, are linked to some sort of reader for use in recording visually derived end-points.

7 Expert systems

An 'expert system' is a knowledge-based computerized system which assists in making decisions. Most automated antimicrobial susceptibility testing instruments operate some form of expert system. The ATB Expression and the Vitek (bioMerieux) and the Phoenix (Becton Dickinson) all operate a rule-based expert system. They have the advantage that fixed (often large) batteries of anti-biotics are tested so bespoke rules may be used. Most commercial automated zone readers, e.g. the Osiris (Sanofi Pasteur); the Aura Image (Oxoid); the Mastas-canElite (Mast); the BioMIC (Giles) and the SIRSCAN (i2a) use rule-based expert systems and expert systems are included in instruments capable of reading agar-incorporation breakpoint plates (e.g. Mastascan). Expert systems may also be designed to run on a laboratory information system.

Expert systems can apply rules of different types.

(a) Recognition of new resistances of public health concern, e.g. penicillin-resistant β-haemolytic streptococci; meropenem-resistant Enterobacteri-aceae; metronidazole-resistant anaerobes, or linezolid-resistant Gram-positive organisms. These results should be checked, as the likeliest explanation is error in identification or in the susceptibility test. If results are confirmed, the isolate should be referred to a reference laboratory. The expert system must not be able to alter a resistant result to susceptible.

(b) Inherent resistance to antibiotics, e.g. ampicillin-resistant *Enterococcus faecalis* (probably *E. faecium*); ampicillin-susceptible *Klebsiella* spp.; nitrofurantoin-susceptible *Proteus mirabilis*; colistin-susceptible *Serratia marcescens*, or aztreonam-susceptible Gram-positive organisms. Incorrect identification is again the most likely cause of error. The system may, on the basis of these rules, alter a susceptible result to resistant.

(c) Inconsistent results, e.g. methicillin-resistant, penicillin-susceptible *S. aureus*.

(d) Addition of comments to isolates such as multi-resistant Gram-negative bacteria, MRSAs, glycopeptide intermediate *S. aureus*, vancomycin-resistant enterococci, or penicillin-resistant pneumococci; alert organisms such as *Streptococcus pyogenes*, or enteric isolates capable of faecal–oral spread. They may also advise against certain organism/antibiotic combinations particu-larly where resistance may emerge through high frequency mutation, e.g. fusidic acid resistance in staphylococci; clindamycin resistance in erythromycin-resistant staphylococci; some third-generation cephalosporins for Enterobacteriaceae.

(e) Use of indicator antibiotics to assist in interpretation, e.g. oxacillin to detect resistance to penicillinase-resistant penicillins in staphylococci and peni-cillin resistance in *Streptococcus pneumoniae*; cefaclor to detect non-β-lactamase resistance in *Haemophilus influenzae*; nalidixic acid to detect fluoroquinolone resistance in *Neisseria gonorrhoeae* and *H. influenzae*.

(f) At their most advanced, expert systems may carry out interpretative read-ing. Here, the resistance phenotype rather than results for individual antibiotics is used. The mechanism of resistance is derived from the phenotype and from the mechanism certain inferences can be made, such as expected results for agents not tested, suggestions for further agents to test, and agents most likely to be useful *in vivo*. Interpretative reading may also detect anomalous speciation or errors in antimicrobial susceptibility tests and permits study of the epidemiology of resistance determinants.

Beta-lactams are particularly suitable for interpretative reading since there is a wide range of resistance mechanisms giving different phenotypes. With glycopeptides, validation and differentiation of vanA, B, and C in enterococci is possible. For aminoglycosides, interpretative reading may be possible but there is a problem with isolates possessing multiple modifying enzymes. Interpretative reading is generally not applied to macrolide/lincosamide/streptogramin antibiotics although inducible and constitutive enzymes may be differentiated. Tetracycline analogues are hardly ever tested but interpretative reading is possible. Quinolone resistance is class related. No scheme can predict resistance mechanisms present in unidentified coliforms and interpretative reading requires that organisms are speciated. It is also necessary to include a wider range of agents than is commonly tested in the UK. It is also necessary to test agents with a high diagnostic value for interpretative reading. For a review of phenotypes to use in interpretative reading, see Livermore, Winstanley, and Shannon (33).

There are some limitations of expert systems:

(a) The continual need to update the system to cope with new resistance mechanisms.

(b) Organisms producing unexpectedly large or small amounts of enzyme may evade the system.

(c) There is a clear need to detect organisms that are resistant by means of impermeability or efflux.

(d) With certain genera, e.g. *Acinetobacter*, the relationship between resistance mechanism and phenotype is poorly defined.

(e) Other organisms with novel resistance mechanisms will not be detected if their phenotype is typical of an organism with a known mechanism.

(f) Probably the biggest limitation is that organisms commonly have multiple resistance determinants, e.g. multiple aminoglycoside modifying enzymes (34); multiple TEM and SHV enzymes (35) including multiple ESBLs (36); organisms with ESBLs may also contain *AmpC* genes on plasmids or be porin-deficient (37).

Despite their limitations, expert systems can improve quality and ensure consistency in result reporting. They can play an important role in local and national surveillance of antibiotic resistance and in education.

8 Clinical relevance and epidemiological outputs

Data from human studies guided by experimental animal and *in vitro* models support the concept that a parameter representing an integration of a measure of antibacterial potency and pharmacokinetics of a drug can be used to predict clinical or bacteriological outcomes (38). This process of combining a susceptibility measure, usually MIC, and pharmacokinetics to predict bacteriological or clinical outcomes is usually termed pharmacodynamics. In human studies pharmacodynamic parameters such as Cmax/MIC, AUC/MIC, and T > MIC have been shown to predict outcome: a Cmax/MIC of >10 for aminoglycosides is predictive of good clinical outcomes in patients with Gram-negative pneumonia (39); an AUC/MIC of >100 for fluoroquinolones is predictive of good clinical and bacteriological outcomes in patients with Gram-negative ICU pneumonia (40); in community-acquired pneumonia due to pneumococci a fluoroquinolone AUC/MIC of >35 has been related to bacteriological outcomes (41); and finally for linezolid a T > MIC of >85% plus an AUC/MIC of >100 predicts clinical outcomes in patients with severe Gram-positive infection (42).

Antibiotic concentrations in patients' sera may vary by up to two-fold, but MIC values often vary over a 1000-fold range hence much of the variability seen in pharmacodynamic parameters observed in patients is related to changes in pathogen MIC values. However, due to the many other factors which determine clinical outcome in human infection, it has taken a long time to show that MIC or categorical susceptibility results are related to cure. In the last 25 years much data have been collected which clearly point to the conclusion that susceptibility test results have a prognostic significance in a wide range of clinical situations. In a retrospective study Lorian and Burns (43) were able to show that 81% (219/271) of patients improved when treated with an antibiotic to which the infecting organism was susceptible by disc test while only 3% (1/27) improved when the isolates were resistant to the agent used.

Further studies of patients with bacteraemia and a range of underlying conditions, indicated that categorical sensitivity testing based on MIC and BSAC breakpoints showed that 17% died related to bacteraemia if the therapy was inappropriate compared to 9% who received appropriate antibiotics (44).

Inappropriate antibiotic use in the management of ICU-associated bacteraemia with MRSA, coagulase negative staphylococci and *P. aeruginosa*, and bacteraemia in immunocompromised patients has also been associated with poor outcomes when compared to appropriate use (45, 46). Similar data are also available for patients with ventilator-associated pneumonia (47) and there is also information to suggest poor outcomes related to specific resistance mechanisms, such as treatment of ESBL producing *K. pneumoniae* with cephalosporins (48). A large scale review conducted about fifteen years ago concluded that for both nosocomial and community-acquired infections the mortality, likelihood of hospitalization and length of stay were usually twice as great for patients infected with drug-resistant strains as those infected with drug susceptible (49). In a new and different therapeutic area a number of meta analyses have now established that resistance to either the macrolide or 5-nitroimidazole component of the drug regimen used to treat *Helicobacter pylori* is an important predictor of therapeutic failure (50).

Given the prognostic value of susceptibility testing it is not surprising that laboratory databases have been used to monitor resistance from the public health perspective. Despite the problems with this approach related to sampling bias, lack of differentiation of colonization and infection, non-standard isolation and susceptibility testing, and repeated isolation of the same pathogen from multiple specimens from the same patient, this approach is reasonably cost-effective and very large databases can be put together rapidly if data from a large number of laboratories are used.

References

1. Acar, J. F. and Goldstein F. W. (1996). In *Antibiotics in laboratory medicine*, 4th edn. (ed. V. Lorian), p. 1. Williams and Wilkins, Baltimore.

2. Brown, D. F. J. and Blowers, R. (1978). In *Laboratory methods in antimicrobial chemotherapy* (ed. D. S. Reeves, I. Phillips, J. D. Williams, and R. Wise), p. 8. Churchill Livingstone, Edinburgh.

3. Stokes, E. J., Ridgway, G. L., and Wren, M. W. D. (1993). In *Clinical bacteriology*, 7th edn, p. 237. Edward Arnold, London.

4. Andrews, J. M. (2001). *J. Antimicrob. Chemother.*, **48**, Suppl. S1, 43.

5. King, A. (2001). *J. Antimicrob. Chemother.*, **47**, Suppl. S1, 77.

6. National Committee for Clinical Laboratory Standards. (2000). *Performance standards for antimicrobial disc susceptibility tests—7th edn; Approved Standard M2-A7.* NCCLS, Wayne, PA, USA.

7. National Committee for Clinical Laboratory Standards. (2001). *Performance standards for antimicrobial susceptibility testing. Ninth Informational Supplement M100-S9.* NCCLS, Wayne, PA, USA.

8. Olsson-Liljequist, B., Larsson, P., Walder, M., and Miörner, H. (1997). *Scand. J. Infect. Dis.*, Suppl. **105**, 13.

9. Report of the Comité de l'Antibiogramme de la Société Française de Microbiologie. (1996). *Clin. Microbiol. Infect.*, **2**, Suppl. 1, 11.

10. Brown, D. F. J. (1994). *Rev. Med. Microbiol.*, **5**, 65.

11. Ericsson, H. and Sherris, J. C. (1971). *Acta Pathol. Microbiol. Scand.*, Section B, Suppl. 217.

12. Gosden, P. E., Andrews, J. M., Bowker, K. E., Holt, H. A., MacGowan, A. P., Reeves, D. S., *et al.* (1999). *J. Antimicrob. Chemother.*, **42**, 161.

13. Brown, D. F. J. (1990). *J. Antimicrob. Chemother.*, **25**, 307.

14. Brown, D. F. J. (2001). *J. Antimicrob. Chemother.*, **48**, Suppl. S1, 65.

15. Bignardi, G. E., Woodford, N., Chapman, A., Johnson, A. P., and Speller, D. C. E. (1996). *J. Antimicrob. Chemother.*, **37**, 53.

16. Van Griethuysen, A., Pouw, M., van Leeuwen, N., Heck, M., Willemse, P., Buiting, A., *et al.* (1999). *J. Clin. Microbiol.*, **37**, 2789.

17. Livermore, D. M. and Brown, D. F. J. (2001). *J. Antimicrob. Chemother.*, **48**, Suppl. S1, 59.

18. M'Zali, F. H., Chanawong, A., Kerr, K. G., Birkenhead, D., and Hawkey, P. M. (2000). *J. Antimicrob. Chemother.*, **45**, 881.

19. Carter, M. W., Oakton, K. J., Warner, M., and Livermore, D. M. (2000). *J. Clin. Microbiol.*, **38**, 4228.

20. Walsh, T. R., Bolmstrom, A., Qwarnstrom, A., *et al.* (2001). *J. Clin. Microbiol.*, **39**, 2439.

21. Wootton, M., Howe, R. A., Hillman, R., Walsh, T. R., Bennett, P. M., and MacGowan, A. P. (2001). *J. Antimicrob. Chemother.*, **47**, 399.

22. Waterworth, P. M. and del Piano, M. (1976). *J. Clin. Pathol.*, **29**, 179.

23. The British Society for Antimicrobial Chemotherapy. (1991). *J. Antimicrobial Chemother.*, **27**, Suppl D.

24. Hanberger, H., Nilsson, L. E., Maller, R., and Isakson, B. (1991). *Antimicrob. Agents Chemother.*, **35**, 1710.

25. Brown, D. F. J. and Yates, V. S. (1986). *Eur. J. Clin. Microbiol.*, **5**, 726.

26. Johnson, M. M., Hill, S. L., and Piddock, L. J. V. (1999). *Antimicrob. Agents Chemother.*, **43**, 1862.

27. Baker, C. N., Stocker, S. A., Culver, D. H., and Thornsberry, C. (1991). *J. Clin. Microbiol.*, **29**, 533.

28. Faiers, M., George, R., Jolly, J., and Wheat, P. (1991). *Multipoint methods in the clinical laboratory*. Public Health Laboratory Service, London, 14.

29. The British Society for Antimicrobial Chemotherapy. (1998). *Heart* **79**, 207-10.

30. MacGowan, A. P., McMullin, C. M., James, P., Reeves, D. S., and White, L. O. (1997). *J. Antimicrob. Chemother.*, **39**, 277.

31. Ferraro, M. J. and Jorgensen, J. H. (1999). In *Manual of clinical microbiology*, 7th edn. (ed. P. R. Murray), p. 1593-1600. A. S. M. Press, Washington.

32. Felmingham, D. and Brown, D. F. J. (2001). *J. Antimicrob. Chemother.*, **47**, S1, 81.

33. Livermore, D. M., Winstanley, T. G., and Shannon, K. P. (2001). *J. Antimicrob. Chemother.*, **48**, Suppl. S1, 87.

34. Shaw, K. J., Hare, R. S., Sabatelli, F. J., *et al.* (1991). *Antimicrob. Agents Chemother.*, **35**, 2253.

35. Essak, S. Y., Hall, L. M., Pillay, D. G., and Livermore, D. M. (2001). *Antimicrob. Agents Chemother.*, **45**, 88.

36. Bradford, P. A., Cherubin, C. E., Idemyor, V., Rasmussen, B. A., and Bush, K. (1994). *Antimicrob. Agents Chemother.*, **38**, 761.

37. Pangon, B., Bizet, C., Bure, A., *et al.* (1989). *J. Infect. Dis.*, **159**, 1005.

38. MacGowan, A. P. and Bowker, K. E. (1999). *J. Chemother.*, **9**, Suppl. 1, 77.

39. Kashuba, A. D. M., Nafziger, A. N., Drusano, G. L., and Bertino, J. S. (1999). *Antimicrob. Agents Chemother.*, **43**, 623.

40. Forrest, A., Nix, D. E., Ballow, C. H., Goss, T. F., Birmingham, M. C., and Schentag, J. J. (1993). *Antimicrob. Agents Chemother.*, **37**, 1073.

41. Ambrose, P. G., Grasela, D. M., Grasela, T. H., Passarell, J., Mayer, H. B., and Pierce, P. F. (2001). *Antimicrob. Agents Chemother.*, **45**, 2793.

42. Rayner, C. R., Forrest, A., Meagher, A. K., Birmingham, M. C., and Schentag, J. J. (2000). *40th Interscience Conference on Antimicrobial Agents and Chemotherapy*, Abstract 1390, p. 29. American Society for Microbiology.

43. Lorian, V. and Burns, L. (1990). *J. Antimicrob. Chemother.*, **25**, 826.

44. Phillips, I., King, A., Gransden, W. R., and Eykyn, S. J. (1990). *J. Antimicrob. Chemother.*, **25**, Suppl. 59.

45. Ibrahim, E. H., Sherman, G., Ward, S., Fraser, V. J., and Kollef, M. H. (2000). *Chest*, **118**, 146.

46. Behrendt, G., Schneider, S., Brodt, H. R., Just-Nubling, G., and Shah, P. M. (1999). *J. Chemother.*, **11**, 179.

47. Rello, J., Gallego, M., and Mariscal, D. (1997). *Am. J. Respir. Crit. Care Med.*, **156**, 196.

48. Paterson, D. L., Ko, W. C., von Gottberg, A., Mohapatra, S., Casellas, J. M., Mulazimoglu, L., *et al.* (1998). *36th Infectious Diseases Society of America*, Abstract 1885a, p. 188.

49. Holmberg, S. D., Solomon, S. L., and Blake, P. A. (1987). *Rev. Infect. Dis.*, **9**, 1065.

50. Jenks, P. J. (2002). *Br. Med. J.*, **325**, 3.

Chapter 8

Antimicrobial assays

David S. Reeves and Les O. White[a]

Department of Medical Microbiology, Southmead Hospital,
Bristol BS10 5NB, UK.

1 Introduction

An antibiotic was originally defined as a substance produced by a micro-organism which inhibited the growth of other micro-organisms. However many drugs loosely referred to as antibiotics are semi-synthetic derivatives of natural antibiotics (e.g. various penicillins and cephalosporins) or compounds produced solely by chemical means (e.g. sulfonamides, 4-quinolones). In addition there are true antibiotics which have useful anticancer rather than antimicrobial properties. For this reason it has become customary to refer to antimicrobial antibiotics and other antimicrobial drugs as antimicrobial agents, a term which is often reduced to antimicrobial. This terminology will be used in this chapter.

For many years after their introduction, antimicrobials were only infrequently assayed in samples from patients. The main reason for this is that antimicrobials usually have a large therapeutic index and are given in large doses without causing harm. Outside the clinical field however, assays have been extensively used in the development and control of antimicrobial drug production, but the methods used are suitable mainly for high concentrations in non-biological matrices (a matrix is the substance, such as plasma, serum, or water, in which the antimicrobial is prepared or presented), and have a level of accuracy and reproducibility in excess of that needed for clinical use.

The widespread use of gentamicin after its introduction in 1964 proved a powerful stimulus for using blood assays since its useful therapeutic range of concentrations (from therapeutic to toxic) is narrow and the toxic effects are frequently irreversible. Over the past 20 years there has been an increasing use of antimicrobial assays to monitor concentrations in samples from patients, mainly those receiving an aminoglycoside (streptomycin, gentamicin, netilmicin, tobramycin, amikacin), but also chloramphenicol, vancomycin, teicoplanin, some other antimicrobials including some antifungals and antivirals. A variety of techniques have been applied to assays. Initially, most were done by microbiological methods (Section 5) but non-microbiological techniques are now widely used.

---

[a] Dr White died during the preparation of this edition.

Some are immunoassays (Section 6), based on competition for specific antibody directed against the antimicrobial, the pre-eminent routine assay used for antimicrobials being fluorescence polarization immunoassay (FPIA). The other widely used technique is high performance liquid chromatography (HPLC), usually used for analytes for which immunoassays are not available (Section 7).

2 Clinical application of antimicrobial assays

2.1 General considerations

Not every patient receiving an antimicrobial requires the monitoring of its concentration in blood or other body fluids, and in many types of antimicrobial therapy monitoring would needlessly waste resources. Furthermore there should be a relationship, however weak, between concentration and toxicity or efficacy to justify measuring levels.

2.1.1 Relationship of concentrations to efficacy

Information on this is scanty. It is known, however, that certain doses of antimicrobials (presumably those recommended for normal use) regularly cure infection, and it is also known in general terms the concentrations that such doses produce in the blood. Information is lacking on whether treatment failure is accompanied by low concentrations, but this is not surprising since there are many other factors causing failure and, in any event, blood concentrations of most antimicrobials are well above those needed for therapy because of their low toxicity. Most information relating blood concentrations to efficacy concerns aminoglycosides and glycopeptides. This was reviewed by Reeves and White (1) and more recently by MacGowan et al. (2). Early studies on the efficacy of gentamicin given at a frequency of more than once a day showed that for most systemic infections, including bacteraemia, post-dose concentrations of >5 mg/litre were associated with a more favourable clinical outcome (3–8). For pneumonia caused by aerobic Gram-negative bacilli, higher concentrations were needed (>7–8 mg/litre). For once-daily dosing, now the most commonly employed modality of aminoglycoside therapy, there are no published data relating efficacy to post-dose levels in humans, although one is suggested by animal models (9, 10).

With vancomycin, Zimmermann et al. (11) in a retrospective review found that pre-dose concentrations of >10 mg/litre combined with post-dose levels >20 mg/litre were associated with fewer fever days and an improved rate of fall of WBC but not with mortality or reduced length of stay. Prospective studies (12, 13) did not find an association between clinical outcome and pre-dose concentration.

Retrospective reviews on the use of teicoplanin have been able to demonstrate an association between levels and clinical outcome. In infections with S. aureus such studies have shown that a pre-dose level of 20 mg/litre, or high pre-dose levels in general, were related to a better clinical outcome (14, 15), and higher concentrations may be needed in bone infections (16).

For other agents, reliance has to be made on the expected concentrations from published pharmacokinetic data; these have been reviewed by Wise (17) and, for injectable agents, by Reeves and Paton (18). When co-trimoxazole is used for the treatment of PCP efficacy appears to be related to maintained concentrations of 5 mg/litre of trimethoprim (19–21).

In a patient unexpectedly not responding to treatment with an antimicrobial to which the infecting pathogen is sensitive, a possible cause may be inadequate concentrations, perhaps due to abnormal pharmacokinetics in a very ill patient, or even the accidental administration of the wrong antimicrobial. Similarly, if the patient suffers an ill-effect which may possibly be an adverse reaction of the antimicrobial then a measurement of concentrations in the blood may show these to be excessively high. Only by measuring blood concentrations can the existence of concentration-dependent effects be established. Certainly when oral therapy is used to treat a serious infection, checks of concentration in blood may be useful because of the unreliability of absorption of many agents. Monitoring levels can also show up failures of compliance, or prescription or administration errors, both causes of otherwise unexplained failure of therapy.

2.1.2 Relationship of blood concentration to toxicity

There is rather more substantial evidence of this than with efficacy (1, 2). High pre-dose levels of aminoglycosides have been associated with ototoxicity: strepto-mycin >3 mg/litre (22); gentamicin 2 mg/litre (23, 24). High post-dose levels have been said to be associated with ototoxicity, but the recent increased use of once-daily therapy (in which post-dose levels are transiently very high) has not been followed by a rise in ototoxicity, and thus contradicts the previous impression. Mattie *et al.* (25) and MacGowan and Reeves (26) have reviewed the matter. It is clear that aminoglycosides are nephrotoxic but relating raised levels to toxicity is difficult since it is usually unclear as to whether they are the cause or effect of impaired renal function. While a number of authors, among them Matzke *et al.* (27) and Li *et al.* (28), have shown an association between raised pre-dose levels (>2 mg/litre for gentamicin) and renal toxicity, a causal relationship is unclear with any particular level.

Very high (>60 mg/litre) pre-dose levels of teicoplanin have been associated with neutropenia (29). There is no clear relationship between high levels of vancomycin and ototoxicity, but high pre-dose levels may be predictive of nephro-toxicity (30). It is thought that therapeutic drug monitoring of vancomycin may reduce the incidence of nephrotoxicity (31, 32).

High levels of chloramphenicol are associated with toxicity which can be fatal. The so-called 'grey baby syndrome' can occur in other age groups. It may be caused by accidental overdosage. Serum levels may be very high (>100 mg/litre), but toxicity can occur at lower levels (>40 mg/litre) (33).

During therapy with co-trimoxazole high levels of sulfamethoxazole or its metabolites may cause toxic or unwanted effects. Levels of >200 mg/litre have been associated with leucopenia (34). It is generally thought that levels should be kept below 100 mg/litre.

Benzylpenicillins have been thought to be the cause of convulsions when plasma (>100 mg/litre) or CSF (>10 mg/litre) levels are high (35).

Leucopenia has been related to high levels of flucytosine (>100 mg/litre).

2.2 Indications for monitoring

2.2.1 Aminoglycosides

In view of the frequency of litigation over aminoglycoside toxicity, it is advisable that all patients receiving aminoglycosides for more than 24 hours have their serum levels monitored. When this is impossible because of non-availability of assay services special efforts should be made to monitor concentrations in certain patients or consideration given to using an alternative antimicrobial.

2.2.2 Types of patients in whom monitoring of blood aminoglycoside concentration is essential

These include:

(a) Patients with impaired renal function, particularly if its degree is changing rapidly or unpredictably.

(b) Patients with life-threatening infections in whom it is essential to achieve adequate blood concentrations immediately.

(c) Patients receiving long courses (>7 days) of therapy, since previously stabilized levels may rise after this time.

(d) Patients with gross obesity, in whom levels tend to be high when dosed according to total body weight.

(e) Patients with pre-existing sensory loss (such as blindness) in whom deafness would provide a disastrous extra burden.

(f) Patients who have had previous courses of aminoglycosides, since they may already have some vestibular/cochlear damage.

(g) Patients receiving other drugs which can potentiate ototoxicity (such as frusemide) or renal toxicity (such as some of the older cephalosporins), or inactivate an aminoglycoside (such as carbenicillin).

2.2.3 Non-aminoglycoside antimicrobials; situations in which therapeutic monitoring may be advisable

These include:

(a) The use of a potentially toxic antimicrobial in a patient in whom excretion may be reduced. Examples include chloramphenicol in neonates, and benzylpenicillin, vancomycin, co-trimoxazole, or flucytosine in renal failure.

(b) When a patient with a life-threatening infection fails to respond to therapy with an antimicrobial active *in vitro* against the invading pathogen, having excluded other causes for the failure (such as an abscess), assays can provide confirmation that the expected concentrations are indeed present, for example teicoplanin (severe staphylococcal infections), rifampicin (tuber-culosis), fluoroquinolones.

(c) The giving of an antimicrobial by a route of uncertain absorption (such as orally) to treat a serious infection (for example, bacterial endocarditis).

(d) Checking the concentration in a body fluid, such as cerebrospinal fluid, where penetration is poor or uncertain.

3 Taking specimens for assays

Using standardized intervals at which blood samples are taken for assay in relation to dosing makes it easier to interpret the results and adjust dosage. Although multiple samples taken after a dose would provide more pharmacokin-etic information, it is us usually impracticable to take more than one post-dose sample and one immediately pre-dose. The former is often termed the 'peak' con-centration, although this is clearly a misnomer since the true peak concentration will occur immediately after an intravenous dose of an antimicrobial unless it is given as a hydrolysable pro-drug, such as chloramphenicol succinate (which hydrolyses in the blood to yield chloramphenicol). The pre-dose sample is taken immediately before a dose and is often called the 'trough' concentration. Follow-ing extravascular (intramuscular or oral) administration the blood concentration rises at a variable rate to a maximum and then falls. The interval between the dose and that maximum varies considerably, but is often about one hour with intra-muscular administration. For bolus intravenous administration a dose–sampling interval of 1 hour usually ensures that the distribution phase (during which blood concentration exceed, sometimes greatly, those in the tissues) has ended, and that concentrations are in the early elimination phase. This is recommended by the BNF for aminoglycosides. The recommended time is longer for vancomycin (two hours) since the distribution phase may continue for some time after the end of the infusion. Although accuracy of the timing of samples for assays should always be sought, in the circumstances of clinical activities it is recognized that sample may not be taken exactly on time. If this happens it is important to ensure that two conditions are met:

(a) It is better to take a post-dose specimen late rather than early so as to avoid it being during the distribution phase, when levels may be unrepresentatively and worryingly high.

(b) The exact time of the sample, and preferably that of the dose, should be recorded on the assay request form.

Pre-dose samples are less subject to interpretation errors if they are not taken on time because the plasma levels are changing slowly. They are therefore valu-able when monitoring therapy on a daily basis because any trend in changes would be of greater significance.

When the plasma half-life of an antimicrobial is very long, either as an inher-ent property or because there is reduced elimination, timing of samples is less critical, although it is still important to record the exact time and the dose–sample interval. Such samples are sometimes called 'random', although this is clearly a misnomer.

Samples should never be taken down an intravenous line which has been used for the administration of an antimicrobial. The very high concentration of drug in the fluid may well cause an error in the in observed putative plasma level even if the line has been flushed through with normal saline.

The important aspects of specimen collection are given in Protocol 1.

Protocol 1

Important points about collecting specimens for assays (when in doubt contact the laboratory for advice)

Equipment

- Plain tubes

Method

1 Unless otherwise specifically indicated, always take body fluid samples into plain tubes and separate the serum after clotting. Many assays are not validated for plasma.

2 Collect samples aseptically if possible, especially for microbiological assays. Samples should be refrigerated as much as possible.

3 Venous blood is preferable, but adequate samples from neonates can be obtained by heel pricks.

4 When in doubt, ask the laboratory about the type and minimum volume of sample.

5 Do not take peak samples earlier than 1 h post-dose (see Section 3). Very high transient concentrations may be found (during the so-called distribution phase) which have little relationship to efficacy or toxicity. Also a slight delay could result in a large change in the levels found.

6 (a) For most antimicrobials take the post-dose (peak) sample 1 h after a dose. Take the pre-dose (trough) sample just before the dose preceding the peak sample is given.

(b) It is recommended to take vancomycin post-dose samples 2 h after the end of the infusion.

(c) For antimicrobials taken intravenously as pro-drugs (erythromycin, chloramphenicol) take the peak sample 1.5–2 h post-dose to allow adequate time for hydrolysis of the pro-drug.

(d) For some oral antimicrobials (e.g. rifampicin) the time to peak concentration may be highly variable and it might be advisable to take more than one sample post-dose (e.g. 1 and 2 h or even 1, 2, and 3 h).

7 The most frequent cause of patently ridiculous results (those which seem pharma-cokinetically impossible) are:

   (a) Drawing a blood sample down the same intravenous cannula used for giving the antimicrobial.

   (b) Failure to give the dose.

   (c) Dose given at wrong time.

   (d) Giving an iv dose into an infusion tube through which the fluid is running very slowly. The dose will thus take a long time to enter the blood.

   (e) Giving the wrong drug.

8 When submitting the sample inform the laboratory about all antimicrobials the patient has received in the last 72 h.

9 If there is likely to be a delay in the laboratory receiving the sample, seek advice on the stability of the antimicrobial in question. Immediate separation of serum or plasma and storage at −20 °C may be advisable.

4 Methods of assay

Assay methods for antimicrobials fall into two main types: microbiological and non-microbiological.

(a) Microbiological methods are based upon response of a population of micro-organisms to differing concentrations of antimicrobial.

(b) Non-microbiological methods employ principles, such as immunological binding or chromatographic separation (both are described in more detail below).

4.1 Characteristics of assay methods: microbiological vs. non-microbiological

In considering whether to use any method, its characteristics should be examined in relation to its intended use. It is particularly important to remember that the needs of an assay for examining samples from normal volunteer studies may differ from those for blood samples from patients with, say, renal failure. The method should therefore always be validated in the circumstances of its use.

When considering the characteristics below it will become clear that, with regard to clinical samples and providing a clinical service, microbiological assays perform poorly in many respects compared with immunoassays or HPLC. In other situations, e.g. pharmacokinetic studies, many of its drawbacks are less important and microbiological assay compares more favourably as a rational method of choice.

4.1.1 Specificity

Poor specificity is a major problem with microbiological assays. The specificity of any assay may be affected by:

(a) Other antimicrobials, perhaps those co-administered with or given previously to the antimicrobial to be assayed.

(b) Metabolites with antimicrobial activity (for example, desacetyl cefotaxime).

(c) Inactive metabolites or degradation products. These will not interfere with microbiological assays but may adversely affect non-microbiological assays, including some immunoassays.

(d) Non-antimicrobial drugs, which may affect microbiological assays (anti-tumour agents) and non-microbiological assays, particularly HPLC.

In samples from patients, problems may arise because the requesting clinician fails to inform the laboratory of concomitant or recent prior antimicrobials. Prior antimicrobials are a particular problem when they have a naturally long elimination half-life in the blood or the patient has renal failure. No microbiological nor non-microbiological assay can be guaranteed to show complete specificity, although commercial immunoassays for aminoglycosides show very high specificity, and this is most likely to become apparent when dealing with complex problems in very sick patients. It is essential to keep this in mind when interpreting levels from patients.

4.1.2 Precision (reproducibility)

Because microbiological assays depend on a biological response their precision is inherently less good than that of non-microbiological methods. They are, however, capable of giving adequate precision for clinical and pharmacokinetic purposes provided sufficient replication is used, which usually entails running samples and calibrators in triplicate. This can give a precision of ±10–20% at the 95% confidence limits. Non-microbiological assay are inherently more reproducible. This, together with the often sophisticated instrumentation used, makes it easy to obtain a precision of better than ±5–10% at 95% confidence limits.

4.1.3 Sensitivity

This is the lowest concentration of antimicrobial which can be assayed at the required degree of precision. If this has not been determined experimentally for concentrations below that of the lowest (non-zero) calibrator (definition of calibrators: *one or more solutions of known drug concentration used to calibrate the assay*) then the concentration of that calibrator should be taken as the limit of sensitivity. Limit of sensitivity may vary with the matrix (e.g. serum, urine) in which the sample is presented and with presence of potentially interfering substances. Sensitivity is usually adequate for microbiological assays of clinical samples since one expects to find sufficient concentrations to inhibit sensitive bacteria. HPLC methods may not easily give sufficient sensitivity for assays in blood but on the other hand immunoassays can have such high sensitivity that they can be designed to require only a tiny sample volume.

4.1.4 Speed

In the clinical situation slow turn round is a major disadvantage of microbiological assays. The minimum time to produce a zone of sufficient readability to give adequate precision is at least five hours with a plate bioassay for gentamicin when using *Klebsiella* spp. as indicator organism. With slower-growing organisms incubation is usually 'overnight' (i.e. about 18 hours). For clinical purposes it is highly desirable that an assay result be available before the next dose of antimicrobial is due to be given so that dosage can be appropriately modified if necessary. Certainly the result should be available within two dose intervals. Non-microbiological assays are in general considerably quicker than microbiological assays, the result for a single sample being available within hours or even minutes.

4.1.5 Range of concentration

The calibration curve for inhibition zone size versus logarithm of concentrations for bioassays is non-linear if taken over a wide range of concentrations, and thus it is best only to use the middle part of it. The range of concentrations covered by this 'almost linear' part is about 16-fold. Samples within this range may be assayed directly, but higher concentrations require dilution. This can lead to an unacceptable delay in reporting when an out-of-range sample requires repeating. Some non-microbiological assays (e.g. HPLC) have a linear response over a wider range of concentrations, so that samples from patients can usually be assayed at the first attempt. Immunoassays are often so rapid that dilution and re-assay of high concentrations causes little delay or inconvenience.

4.1.6 Sample size

For many clinical applications, a sample of up to 1 ml of serum is usually available, but from neonates 100 μl or less is usual. Since microbiological plate assays need at least a triplicate application of sample to maintain their precision, and each application to the plate takes 50–100 μl, their use for neonatal samples is severely limited. Sample size is rarely a problem with immunoassays or HPLC.

4.1.7 Costs

Agar plate diffusion assays require only inexpensive consumables and equipment when done on the small number of samples sent for clinical purposes, although a computer is invaluable for recording the zone sizes and calculating the results. Automated equipment for measuring and recording zone diameters is invaluable when large numbers of assays need to be performed, as for example in pharmacokinetic research. Microbiological assays do however require skilled and experienced technical staff to give the best results.

Conversely, immunoassays usually come in commercial kit form to run on expensive dedicated analysers. Since both the consumables and equipment are expensive, a laboratory should consider carefully when investing in such instrumentation. Several types of commercial immunoassay systems are available for assay of gentamicin and not all necessarily perform equally well or are suited to all laboratories. The least expensive option may not necessarily be the best choice; many factors should be taken into consideration when making a choice including cost, ease of use, speed, adaptability, sample capacity, popularity, quality of performance, and customer service support. The degree of skill required by the operator of most sophisticated analysers is reduced but proper supervision is essential and senior staff trained in servicing and trouble-shooting must be available.

In the case of HPLC, equipment is expensive but consumables are less expensive than with immunoassays. Skilled, well-trained staff capable of setting up the equipment, dealing with servicing, and trouble-shooting issues are essential. Repair of HPLC equipment often takes longer than repair of dedicated analysers (which can often be repaired in <24 hours) and therefore back-up equipment is essential if an uninterrupted service is to be maintained.

5 Microbiological assays

Some 25 years ago there was a variety of microbiological assay techniques in common use. These included agar diffusion on a flat plate, agar diffusion in capillary tubes, broth dilution, turbidimetry using broth cultures and, in addition, rapid microbiological methods based on chemiluminescence, urease, or ATP production (36, 37). Over the years most of these techniques fell by the wayside virtually leaving the agar plate diffusion method as the only one in use. This use is now minimal and because of this the method will not be described here. The reader is referred to the previous edition of this book (38), where it is given in some detail, and a chapter by Andrews (39).

6 Immunoassays

6.1 General principles

The two essential reagents for an immunoassay are:

(a) Antibody reagent containing immunoglobulin with specific activity for the drug to be assayed. This immunoglobulin may be monoclonal or polyclonal. Its concentration must be limited, that is there should be insufficient to bind to all the tracer in the tracer reagent.

(b) Tracer reagent, comprising drug (or a close derivative of the drug) which has been chemically labelled with a tracer atom or molecule and which will compete with drug for the specific immunoglobulin binding sites in the antibody reagent. A tracer atom could be a radioactive isotope (in which case the assay is a radioimmunoassay). A tracer molecule could be an enzyme (enzyme immunoassay), a fluorescent dye (fluoroimmunoassay), or any other tagging molecule.

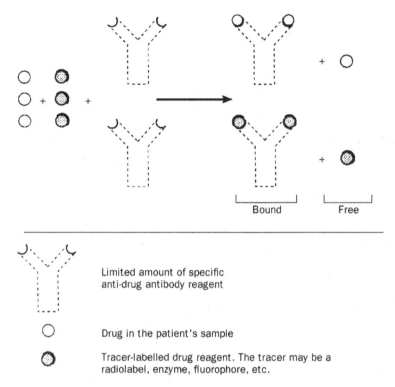

Figure 1 Principle of a competitive binding immunoassay.

Reagents (a) and (b) are mixed with sample and the tracer and any drug in the sample compete for the limited number of antibody binding sites (Figure 1) in such a way that measuring the proportion of bound or unbound tracer can be used (through the use of a calibration curve) to determine the concentration of drug in the sample. If the separation of bound from unbound tracer is required the assay is called a heterogeneous or separation immunoassay. Radioimmunoassays are separation immunoassays. If a separation step is not required then the assay is a homogeneous or non-separation immunoassay. Immunoassays are in general highly sensitive and highly specific. High sensitivity translates in the clinical situation into 'requires only small volumes of sample' making immunoassays ideal for all patients, including neonates. High specificity essentially eliminates the major drawback associated with the bioassay. Since the early 1980s commercial homogeneous immunoassays have become the methods of choice for clinical aminoglycoside assays. This is because they are not only highly specific and highly sensitive (like all immunoassays) but in addition do not use radioisotopes, are very quick, technically simple, easily automated, and highly reproducible. The first successful immunoassay for aminoglycosides was an enzyme immunoassay (EMIT) (see ref. 40) developed and marketed by Syva. It essentially caused the demise of bioassay for clinical aminoglycoside assays and by 1984 had become the most popular method in the UK. EMIT was subsequently overtaken by a type of fluoroimmunoassay (polarization fluoroimmunoassay or FPIA) and FPIA is now the method of choice for aminoglycoside assay used by the majority of clinical laboratories. The FPIA will be discussed in greater detail below. For more information on immunoassays the reader should consult White and Lovering (40) and Marks (41).

6.2 Reagent constitution and storage

Virtually all immunoassays for antimicrobials will be performed using commercial equipment and kits and other reagents will have batch numbers and expiry dates. No materials should be used after their expiry date and all must be stored according to manufacturers' instructions. Some reagents may require storage frozen or at a specific temperature. Thawing and re-freezing may or may not be permitted. If re-freezing is allowed a log should be maintained of dates of thawing and re-freezing. If reagents are freeze-dried and require constitution before use, necessary volumes of water to be added should be accurately measured with a pipette. The appropriate quality water must be used for reconstitution. If deionized water is specified that is what should be used. Inappropriate sources of water may contain interfering substances. Never reconstitute materials in tap-water.

6.3 Calibration

Most immunoassays in use today do not require calibration every time an assay or batch of assays is processed. A calibration curve for a particular assay is run, stored in the analyser if it passes certain statistical requirements, and is subsequently used to calculate the results for successive batches of assays. Calibrators supplied by the kit manufacturers will normally comprise a drug-free blank and up to five additional calibrators. Analysers are normally programmed to run calibrators in duplicate as a test of reproducibility. It may be possible to over-rule this setting and run single calibrators and although this appears to cut costs it is not recommended as it eliminates this check on the reproducibility of the instrument.

In an immunoassay the relationship between calibrator concentration and response (measure of bound or unbound tracer) is, as with bioassays, not linear. Most immunoassay calibration curves are sigmoid. The analyser will be programmed with appropriate mathematical functions for curve fitting and determining goodness of fit. Many analysers will only accept a calibration curve when it meets pre-programmed statistical criteria for acceptance. These criteria might include the following:

(a) Minimum acceptable reading.

(b) Minimum span between reading of highest and lowest calibrators.

(c) Maximum allowable divergence of duplicate readings.

(d) Goodness of curve fit.

Since calibration is performed infrequently then the accuracy of the results must be carefully monitored by the frequent use of internal control samples. Internal control results will act as a guide to when an assay needs recalibration (see Section 8.1).

6.4 Internal control

The performance of immunoassays must be monitored by the regular use of internal control samples (Section 8). These may be purchased from the kit supplier or a third party. Immunoassays should be controlled with three samples covering the low end, the mid range, and the top end of the calibration curve. For example, where the range of gentamicin calibrators is 0.5–10 mg/litre controls of around 1 mg/litre, 4 mg/litre, and 8 mg/litre are recommended.

Controls should be run every day that assays are performed and some laboratories choose to run at least one control in every batch of assays.

6.5 Fluorescence polarization immunoassay (FPIA)

Fluorescent compounds absorb light energy and then, after a very short period of time (approx. 10 nanoseconds), release some of that energy as light of a longer wavelength. Fluorescein absorbs light at 481–498 nm and fluoresces at 525–550 nm. If a solution of drug labelled with fluorescein is illuminated with plane polarized light then the fluorescence loses its polarization as a result of the random Brownian motion of the molecules between absorption and emission. If however this labelled drug is bound to a large molecule such as specific antibody then polarization is retained. There is therefore a relationship between degree of polarization and degree of antibody binding which can be used as the basis for an assay (Figure 2). Because the parameter being measured is a difference in polarization rather than a difference in intensity then potential sources of interference such as background fluorescence are minimized. The commercial success of FPIA was due to the design of a dedicated analyser (Abbott TDX) on which the assays were performed. The TDX can perform 20 gentamicin assays in less than 20 minutes and requires only 50 µl of sample. Calibration curves are very stable, lasting many weeks, and assays are very reproducible with relative standard deviations of better than 3–4%. The Abbott TDX has been followed by the Abbott TDX/FLX and Axsym analysers which perform similarly. Other FPIA kits are now available for other analysers and several manufacturers make kits designed to be run on the TDX/FLX. The following antimicrobial assays can be performed on the Abbott TDX: amikacin; gentamicin; netilmicin; teicoplanin; tobramycin; vancomycin. Abbott originally also marketed a kit for streptomycin assay but unfortunately this was withdrawn some years ago.

6.5.1 Assay of very high and very low aminoglycoside concentrations

The popularity of once-daily aminoglycoside therapy has substantially extended the normal therapeutic range. Trough gentamicin/tobramycin/netilmicin

279

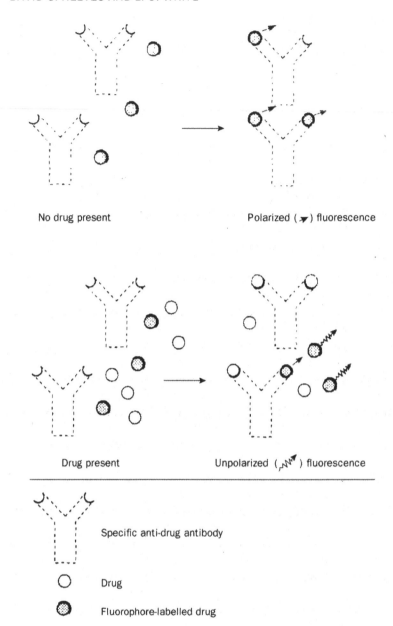

No drug present

Polarized (⟶) fluorescence

Drug present

Unpolarized (⟿) fluorescence

Specific anti-drug antibody

○ Drug

◉ Fluorophore-labelled drug

Figure 2 Principle of a fluorescence polarization immunoassay (FPIA).

concentrations of <0.5 mg/litre and peak concentrations of >10 mg/litre will be encountered routinely. The TDX/FLX analysers have a 'dilution protocol' which can be used to assay either high or low concentrations (42) with high precision and accuracy without the need for manual dilution. The variations of the protocol are described in Protocol 2.

Protocol 2

Dilution protocols for aminoglycoside assays on Abbott TDX/FLX analysers

Equipment and reagents

- Analyser
- Assay sample

A. Dilution protocol for high concentrations

1 Press ASSAY × (assay number) EDIT.

2 Press NEXT, SMPL VOL is displayed.

3 Edit the display to any fraction (usually a half) of the displayed value (minimum acceptable value 0.5).

4 Press STORE, STOP.

5 Run the assay. The analyser will pick up the reduced volume of sample and make the appropriate correction when printing out the result. The run printout will display the message DILUTION PROTOCOL and the volume setting.

6 The analyser will automatically reset to the normal mode for the next run.[a]

B. Reverse dilution protocol for low concentrations

1 Follow part A, steps 1 and 2.

2 Edit the display to a multiple of the displayed value (maximum acceptable value 5.0).

3 Press STORE, STOP.

4 Run the assay. The analyser will pick up the increased volume of sample and make the appropriate correction when printing out the result. The run printout will display the message DILUTION PROTOCOL and the volume setting.

5 The analyser will automatically reset to the normal mode for the next run.[a]

[a] System parameter 2.3 (RST SPL) must be set to 1 (default).

6.5.2 Potential pitfalls

Although FPIA assays are highly specific the following should be borne in mind when interpreting clinical assays. Certain aminoglycosides cross-react but not necessarily 100% (Table 1). It is therefore essential that the correct drug is specified on the request form. Although it seems unlikely problems can arise. In the last 20 years the following errors have been encountered:

(a) Newborn twins, one treated with gentamicin, one treated with netilmicin. Drugs transposed on the forms.

(b) A cystic fibrosis patient on Nebcin®. Nebcin® is tobramycin but person completing the request wrote it up as netilmicin.

Table 1 Possible cross-reactivity with aminoglycoside immunoassays

Assay for	May cross-react with
Gentamicin	Netilmicin
Netilmicin	Gentamicin
Tobramycin	Amikacin, kanamycin
Amikacin	Tobramycin, kanamycin

The TDX/FLX assay for vancomycin cross-reacts with its inactive degradation product CDP-I (43). This breakdown product can accumulate in renal patients dosed infrequently and trough levels measured on a TDX/FLX may be as much as a 100% overestimation of microbiologically active vancomycin. A new vancomycin assay formulation for the Abbott Axsym, and some other immunoassays for vancomycin, do not cross-react with CDP-I.

7 High performance liquid chromatography (HPLC)

HPLC is the abbreviation for both high performance and high pressure chromatography. The term high performance is preferred since this is the *raison d'être* of the test; high pressure is a secondary effect.

7.1 General principles and terms

A liquid mobile phase comprising one or more solvents with or without added solutes is pumped through a column packed with a solid stationary phase. A liquid sample containing the compounds to be separated is introduced into the mobile phase by means of a valve operated device called the injector. Separation of the various compounds in the sample occurs by differential retention on the stationary phase. After separation the eluant from the column phase passes through a detector where the separated compounds produce a response (such as absorption of UV, fluorescence, etc.). In any mobile phase/stationary phase combination flowing at a given rate individual eluting compounds can be presumptively identified by their retention time (time from point of injection to the apex of the response [usually referred to as a peak on a chromatogram] in the detector produced by the eluting compound). The compound is quantified by measurement of peak height or peak area of the chosen peak in the chromatogram with reference to a calibration curve derived from one or more calibrators of known concentration.

7.2 Characteristics

The run time required to analyse a single sample will be several minutes. A run time of 10 minutes means, however, that it will take 100 minutes to assay ten samples and 1000 minutes (>16 hours) to assay 100 samples. This low sample capacity compared with bioassay or immunoassay means that full automation is essential if large numbers of samples are to be assayed. Automation is no problem but the necessary equipment is expensive.

High reproducibility and high sensitivity are achievable but the former depends on the sample preparation procedure and quality of the injector. Sensitivity depends to a large extent on the detector used. Detection by UV absorption will, for many antimicrobials, give sufficient sensitivity for measurement of blood levels but an (unfortunate) exception are the aminoglycosides.

High specificity is possible and mixtures of antimicrobials do not usually present a problem. Indeed, very closely related compounds, such as the individual components of gentamicin, can be separated by HPLC, although this still, however, leaves the problem of how to quantitate them at the concentrations found in blood. It should, however, be remembered that whereas only co-administered antimicrobials may interfere with a bioassay any drug might interfere with an HPLC assay; therefore knowledge of all other drugs in the sample may be important. HPLC can also be used to assay inactive pro-drugs (for example, chloramphenicol succinate), metabolites (penicilloic acids), and breakdown products.

7.3 Principles of separation—reverse phase

For rapid efficient (see below) separation, modern analytical HPLC methods use microparticulate stationary phases. These have particle sizes from 3-5 μm and are usually packed in stainless steel analytical columns approx. 4 mm in internal diameter and 10-30 cm in length. Sometimes a short guard column containing similar stationary phase is placed in front of the analytical column to protect it and lengthen its useful life. The high performance (speed, efficiency) relies on these microparticulate packings. Correct packing of these analytical columns is essential and most laboratories will buy them off the shelf, packed and ready to use.

Although any type of chromatography may be performed as HPLC the most commonly used method in the clinical situation is reverse (or reversed) phase chromatography, so named because it is the reverse of traditional (or normal phase) chromatography. Traditional chromatography (normal phase) used a hydrophilic stationary phase (such as paper) and a hydrophobic mobile phase such as a mixture of organic solvents. In reverse phase the opposite is true, the stationary phase being hydrophobic and the mobile phase being hydrophilic. Hydrophilic mobile phase formulations will usually contain a proportion of water and be water miscible, meaning that watery samples such as plasma can be injected, and allowing for the possibility of relatively simple sample preparation procedures.

7.3.1 Reverse phase packings

Reverse phase packings are usually based on chemically modified silica. Reacting the surface hydroxyl groups of silica with an organochlorosilane is used to manufacture so-called C_3, C_8, or C_{18} packings depending on the length of the carbon chain of the organochlorosilane. C_{18} or octadecyl packings (often called ODS or C18 packings) have been used in numerous applications and very many commercial products with slightly differing separation properties are available. A published method or standard operating procedure (SOP) will usually state the make of packing material used. Commonly encountered C_{18} packings include Hypersil ODS, Spherisorb ODS, and Microbondapak C_{18}. More information can be found in Koenigsberger (44) or White and Lovering (40). In reverse phase chromatography the mobile phase is usually pH 2–6 since silica dissolves at higher pH values. In acid mobile phase the ionization of acidic compounds is suppressed and reverse phase separations can be devised. For the separation of basic compounds the mobile phase can be modified by the addition of an ion-pair reagent. In ion-pair chromatography the ion-pair reagent (for example heptane sulfonic acid or octane sulfonic acid) forms a dynamic ion-pair with any positively charged compounds and this ion-pair interacts with the stationary phase and is retained to a greater or lesser extent. Ion-pair chromatography can also use basic ion-pair reagents such as tetrabutylammonium hydroxide.

To achieve any given separation with a chosen stationary phase the mobile phase is formulated with water, organic solvent (such as methanol or acetonitrile), and modifier (such as buffer or ion-pair reagent) to produce the required separation in the shortest possible time.

7.3.2 Efficiency and selectivity

An HPLC method can be defined by two parameters, selectivity and efficiency.

Selectivity (often called alpha or α) is a measure of the ability to separate two compounds A, the compound of interest, and B, (say) anything else:

$$\alpha = (V_B - V_0)/(V_A - V_0)$$

where V_0, V_A, and V_B are the volumes of mobile phase pumped from the point of injection to the elution of the solvent front (unretained material), A and B.

Efficiency is a measure of peak broadening as the compound passes down the column. A commonly used formula for efficiency (N or number of theoretical plates) is:

$$N = 5.54(R_t/W_{hh})^2$$

where R_t is the retention time of the chosen peak and W_{hh} is the width of this peak at half-height measured in the same units (e.g. seconds) as R_t.

7.4 Equipment

A working HPLC set-up is sometimes called a chromatograph (not to be confused with the printout containing the peaks, the chromatogram). The essentials

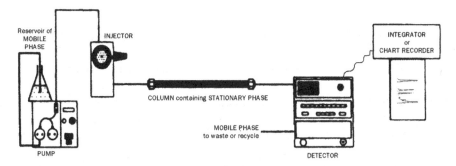

Figure 3 Typical HPLC equipment (manual injection).

for HPLC are pump, injector, detector, and data recording/manipulating device. A typical HPLC set-up is shown in Figure 3.

Mobile phase from a suitable reservoir is pumped through the column containing the stationary phase. Microparticulate stationary phase will cause a high pressure in the system and a good HPLC pump should be capable of delivering an accurate, reproducible, pulse-free flow of up to 3 ml/min or more against back pressures of up to 3–4000 psi (optimally the flow rate would be 1–2 ml/min and the back pressure would be <2000 psi).

The injector introduces the sample into the flowing mobile phase, must be capable of leak-free operation under normal back pressure, and must have good reproducibility. The most common type of injectors will allow 2–200 μl injections, and may be manual or fully automated.

HPLC detectors measure UV absorbance, fluorescence, electrochemical activity, or change in refractive index. UV absorbance detectors have the greatest applicability in the clinical field and may be either fixed (selectable) wavelength (usually 254 or 214 nm) or allow any wavelength (between 190 and 600 nm) to be selected by means of a monochromator. Detectors have analogue output suitable for either computing integrators (usually 1 volt full scale output) or a chart recorder (often 10 millivolts full scale output). More recent ones may also have direct digital output.

HPLC equipment should be regularly serviced; failure of one component will render the whole instrument unusable, unless spares are available.

7.5 Sample preparation

Unlike bioassay or immunoassay where untreated serum may be used as the sample most HPLC procedures will require some form of sample preparation before serum can be assayed. The simplest form of sample preparation is protein precipitation with an organic solvent (methanol, acetonitrile) or acid (7% perchloric acid). Some HPLC procedures may involve more complex and time-consuming steps such as solid phase extraction, solvent extraction, sample drying and reconstitution, etc. Urine samples may present less of a problem and may merely require diluting, since drug concentrations may be high and there will be little or no protein present.

7.6 Calibration

As with other assays, calibrators and calibration are required. Advice on their preparation is given in Protocol 3. However, since there is a simple linear relationship between peak height or area and concentration, single point calibration may be sufficiently accurate for clinical assays (this is determined during method validation). Calibrators may need to be made up in an appropriate matrix (such as serum). However, during method validation, recovery experiments comparing peak height from aqueous solutions with those from serum samples will be performed. If ~100% recovery is obtained then aqueous calibrators may be used. As with other assays, appropriate internal controls should be processed with every batch of samples.

Protocol 3

Advice on the preparation of accurate stock solutions for use in the preparation of working calibrators

Equipment and reagents

- Analytical balance
- Volumetric flask
- Antimicrobial powders
- Diluent

Method

1 Never use dosage formulation for preparing calibrators. The drug may be present as an inactive pro-drug (e.g. chloramphenicol succinate) or contain additional inert ingredients (especially tablets). The declared potency may be nominal and a slight excess of drug over that stated may be present.

2 Obtain powder for laboratory use or a laboratory reference powder with a declared potency. Manufacturers will often supply such material on request (often free of charge). Reference material can also be purchased. Note that international reference material will have potency declared in terms of International Units. It will be necessary to know the conversion factor for conversion to mg/litre.

3 Ensure that powders are stored and handled according to the suppliers information. Some powders may be hygroscopic and absorb atmospheric moisture rapidly. Damp powders will lose their potency rapidly. A bottle of powder stored in the cold should always be brought to ambient temperature before opening to avoid condensation. Aminoglycoside powders may have potency stated as 'as-is' or 'dry'. Aminoglycoside powders should be dried by heating at 110 °C if dry potency is given. Powders should be stored in a desiccator.

4 If kept dry most antimicrobial powders will remain stable for at least one year in an air-tight container at 4 °C. If in doubt about stability get advice from the supplier/manufacturer.

Protocol 3 continued

5 Use a properly maintained calibrated analytical balance capable of weighing to at least 0.1 mg. Use only scrupulously clean equipment.

6 Weigh an appropriate amount of powder to make a convenient stock solution of (say) 1000 mg/litre. Remember to take the potency into account. If sufficient material is available weigh at least 50 mg of powder with an accuracy of ±0.1 mg. If only a small amount of powder is available a microbalance capable of weighing accurately to 0.01 mg may be required.

7 Transfer all the powder to a volumetric flask by carefully washing with diluent. Make up to the volumetric mark with appropriate diluent.

Note: Some substances will not be readily soluble in water and a small volume of acid (e.g. lactic acid for trimethoprim), or alkali (e.g. 0.1 M sodium hydroxide for sulfonamides), or organic solvent (e.g. 2–3 ml of ethanol for 10–50 mg of rifampicin or chloramphenicol), or warming may be necessary to achieve solution. Suppliers/manufacturers should be able to supply appropriate information.

7.6.1 Internal standard

Some HPLC methods use an internal standard. This is quite different from a calibrator and is a chemical added to the samples and calibrators prior to sample preparation. The chosen internal standard is a compound which is chemically stable, chemically similar to the drug being assayed, at a concentration producing a 20–80% full scale response, baseline separated from the drug being assayed, and reproducibly recovered from any sample preparation procedure.

When an internal standard is used then quantitation is based on the peak height or area ratio to the internal standard height or area in the same chromatogram, rather than just on peak height or area alone.

An internal standard can improve assay reproducibility, especially if a complex sample preparation procedure and/or an injector with poor reproducibility is being used.

7.7 Methods for individual antimicrobials

Numerous HPLC methods have been published and the reader is advised to consult individual chapters in Reeves et al. (45) and Reeves and Ullmann (46). Methods for assay of benzylpenicillin, chloramphenicol, ciprofloxacin, or flucytosine in human serum, suitable for therapeutic monitoring, are summarized in Table 2. HPLC procedures should not be used for clinical assays until they have been fully validated in-house. Protocol 4 describes a method for the assay of benzylpenicillin in serum. It is an unpublished method used for therapeutic drug monitoring in the authors' laboratory.

Table 2 Summarized HPLC methods for therapeutic monitoring of antimicrobials

HPLC parameter	Benzylpenicillin	Chloramphenicol	Ciprofloxacin	Flucytosine
Column	Hypersil 5 ODS	Hypersil 5 ODS	Spherisorb ODS II at 50°C	Hypersil 5 C8
Mobile phase	Methanol/water/ phosphoric acid (35 : 64 : 1)	Methanol/water/ phosphoric acid (25 : 74 : 1)	Tetrabutyl ammonium phosphate plus acetonitrile (5%), pH 3	Aqueous octanesulfonic acid (5 g/litre)
Detection	UV absorbance 214 nm	UV absorbance 214 and 254 nm	Fluorescence: excitation 310 nm emission 445 nm	UV absorbance 214 nm
Sample preparation	Protein precipitation with acetonitrile	Protein precipitation with acetonitrile	Protein precipitation with methanol	Protein precipitation with perchloric acid
Internal standard	No	No	No	No

Protocol 4

HPLC method for the assay of benzylpenicillin in serum

Equipment and reagents

- Stationary phase: Hypersil 5 ODS 100 × 4 mm (HPLC Technology, Macclesfield, UK)
- Mobile phase: methanol/water/phosphoric acid (35 : 64 : 1, by vol.) pumped at 1 ml/min
- Detection: UV absorbance at 214 nm
- Acetonitrile

Method[a,b]

1 Mix the sample with an equal volume of acetonitrile.

2 Shake and sediment the precipitate by centrifugation.

3 Inject 20 μl of the clear supernatant.

[a] The assay does not use an internal standard. Single-point calibration is by the use of an aqueous solution of benzylpenicillin 50 mg/litre subjected to the same sample preparation.

[b] Performance expectations: the lower limit of detection depends on the quality of the detector but should be at least 1–2 mg/litre. Calibrators and controls should be freshly prepared each day.

8 Quality assurance

In the hospital laboratory Clinical Governance is about ensuring a consistently high quality of care for patients through the provision of timely, accurate, laboratory investigations and their interpretation, and accepting that it is the responsibility of the department in which we work, ourselves included, to provide this care. Quality assurance is a field in its own right (Chapter 10) (47). Quality assurance includes good laboratory practice, laboratory accreditation, use of SOPs, correct storage of reagents, process control, correct maintenance of equipment, appropriate training of staff, appropriate record keeping ensuring unbroken audit trails, regular audit and quality improvement programmes. It also includes the use of internal controls and, where available, external quality assessment (EQA).

8.1 Internal controls

Internal controls are samples processed alongside clinical samples to evaluate the quality (accuracy, reproducibility) of the results for the clinical samples. In the field of assays internal controls are samples of known concentration run on a day-to-day basis and have already been mentioned in Sections 6.3 and 7.6. Immunoassays require at least three concentrations (low, medium, high) covering the range of the calibration curve. With HPLC two or even one internal control will probably be adequate. Essentials for the correct use of internal controls are:

(a) Careful record keeping—daily control values should be recorded and/or plotted (day of month vs. concentration).

(b) Setting limits of result acceptability, with medical relevance taken into account. Plus or minus 10% (medium and high concentration) or ±15% (low concentration) are generally accepted as adequate for clinical antimicrobial assays.

(c) Following rules in the event of results being outside acceptable limits. These would determine whether or not to accept the clinical results, and the need for assay recalibration, equipment maintenance, etc.

8.2 External quality assessment (EQA)

EQA (sometimes called proficiency testing) is a means whereby the quality of the results from one laboratory is measured by comparing the results of a large number of laboratories processing identical samples. In the UK United Kingdom National External Quality Assessment Schemes (UK NEQAS) are pre-eminent in providing EQA programmes for clinical laboratories. Many disciplines and tests are covered (see the web site www.ukneqas.org.uk) and, in the antimicrobial assay field, assays for amikacin, chloramphenicol, flucytosine, gentamicin, netilmicin, tobramycin, and vancomycin are currently covered. Monthly samples for assay are circulated to circa 250 participating laboratories and quality of results is scored on the basis of a statistical formula taking both inaccuracy (bias) and irreproducibility into account. More details of the antibiotic assay scheme can be found on the web site (www.ukneqasaa.win-uk.net). In the UK participation in EQA is not mandatory, but accredited laboratories are required to participate in approved EQA programmes. There are procedures for dealing with any UK clinical laboratories which persistently perform poorly in any EQA programme. Laboratories with appropriate internal control procedures would normally be expected to perform acceptably in EQA programmes unless a gross error (e.g. processing the wrong sample, transposition error, clerical error) were made.

9 Clinical interpretation

The final step of any clinical antimicrobial assay is interpretation of the result with regard to the patient. The significance of the result should initially be assessed by a trained medical microbiologist who should then contact the relevant clinician to advise on appropriate action (if any). Many antimicrobial assay results have immediate and direct relevance to the management of the patient and should therefore be faxed, telephoned, or delivered electronically as soon as they are available (even if the levels are 'normal') and not merely delivered in the mail. The basis for the relevance of results has been discussed elsewhere (1, 2) and in this chapter (Sections 2.1.1 and 2.1.2).

So-called 'normal' ranges are usually applied to antimicrobials which are assayed routinely. Raised pre-dose (trough) concentrations indicate potentially toxic drug accumulation and low pre-dose concentrations may be below the MIC for the infecting organism. The significance of high post-dose (peak) levels in relation to toxicity is less clear but low peak levels of some antimicrobials usually suggest efficacy may be compromised. It is becoming a common practice to assay only trough concentrations. However, a trough streptomycin concentration of <1 can only be interpreted as normal if it matches a peak level of 15–45 mg/litre. A patient who had never received any streptomycin would have a trough of <1 mg/litre yet (assuming streptomycin was indicated) the dosage regimen could hardly be considered appropriate. Since many aminoglycosides are often now administered once-daily it is essential that the dosing regimen is known before interpretation can be made. For example a trough gentamicin level of 2 mg/litre will be 'normal' with traditional dosing but 'toxic' (meaning a dosage adjustment is indicated) with once-daily administration. With some antimicrobials (for example, teicoplanin or ciprofloxacin) it is necessary to know details of the pathogen before levels can be interpreted. Trough ciprofloxacin concentrations of 0.4 mg/litre might be adequate to treat an *Haemophilus* infection but not *Pneumococcus* or *Pseudomonas*. A trough teicoplanin level of 10 mg/litre might be considered inadequate for treatment of MRSA endocarditis. Interpretation of blood levels is a constantly changing area and the clinician needs to keep up to date with the current literature. Table 3 summarizes some 'normal' and 'toxic' concentrations.

Table 3 Antimicrobial concentrations in the blood

Antimicrobial	Normal (effective)[a] range (mg/litre)	Potentially toxic concentration[b] (mg/litre)
Gentamicin, netilmicin or tobramycin	*Traditional dosing* Infective endocarditis:[c] Pre < 1, Post 2–3 Other infections: Pre < 2, Post 5–8	*Traditional dosing* Pre > 2
	Once-daily dosing Pre < 1, Post > 10, or 8 hour post 1.5–6	*Once-daily dosing* Pre > 1, or 8 hour post-dose > 6
Streptomycin	Pre < 5, Post 15–45	Pre > 5
Amikacin	*Traditional dosing* Pre < 10, Post 15–25	*Traditional dosing* Pre > 10
	Once-daily dosing Pre < 5, Post > 40	*Once-daily dosing* Pre > 5
Vancomycin	Pre 5–10, 1 hour post 20–40, 2 hour post 18–26	Pre > 10, ??Post > 50
Teicoplanin	Severe staphylococcal infection: Pre > 20	All infections: Pre > 60
	Non-staphylococcal endocarditis: Pre 10–15, Post > 40	
	Other severe non-staphylococcal infection: Pre > 10	
Benzylpenicillin	Varies with the pathogen	> 100 (serum), > 10 (CSF)
Flucytosine	Pre 30–40, Post 70–80	> 100
Chloramphenicol	Pre < 10, Post 15–25	> 40

[a] Levels below the normal range may indicate that a dosage increase is indicated.

[b] A potentially toxic concentration is a concentration prompting a dosage reduction to avoid/minimize toxicity rather than a concentration likely to cause toxicity.

[c] When used in combination with a cell wall-active antimicrobial.

References

1. Reeves, D. S. and White, L. O. (1981). In *Therapeutic drug monitoring* (ed. A. Richens and V. Marks), p. 445. Churchill Livingstone, Edinburgh.

2. MacGowan, A. P., Reeves, D. S., and Wise, R. (1999). In *Clinical antimicrobial assays* (ed. D. S. Reeves, R. Wise, J. M. Andrews, and L. O. White), p. 1. Oxford University Press, Oxford.

3. Noone, P., Parsons, T. M. C., Pattison, J. R., Slack, R. C. B., *et al.* (1974). *Br. Med. J.*, **i**, 477.

4. Noone, P., Pattison, J. R., and Davies, G. G. (1974). *Postgrad. Med. J.*, **50**, Suppl. 7, 9.

5. Noone, P. and Rogers, B. T. (1976). *J. Clin. Pathol.*, **29**, 652.

6. Moore, R. D., Smith, C. R., and Lietman, P. S. (1984). *Am. J. Med.*, **77**, 657.

7. Moore, R. D., Smith, C. R., and Lietman, P. S. (1984). *J. Infect. Dis.*, **149**, 443.

8. Moore, R. D., Lietman, P. S., and Smith, C. R. (1987). *J. Infect. Dis.*, **155**, 93.

9. Freeman, C. D., Nicolau, D. P., Belliveau, P. P., and Nightingale, C. H. (1997). *J. Antimicrob. Chemother.*, **39**, 677.

10. Kashuba, A. D. M., Bertino, J. S., and Nafziger, A. N. (1998). *Antimicrob. Agents Chemother.*, **42**, 1842.

11. Zimmermann, A. E., Katona, B. G., and Plaisance, K. I. (1995). *Pharmacotherapy*, **15**, 85.

12. Ryback, M. J., Cappelletty, D. M., Kang, S. L., Levine, D. P., *et al.* (1996). *Abstracts of the 36th Interscience Conference on Antimicrobial Agents and Chemotherapy*, Abstract A-36. ASM, Washington DC.

13. Ryback, M. J., Cappelletty, D. M., Rulting, R. C., Mercier, R. C., Houlihan, H. H., Kepster, M. E., *et al.* (1997). *Abstracts of the 37th Interscience Conference on Antimicrobial Agents and Chemotherapy*, Abstract A-46. ASM, Washington DC.

14. Wilson, A. P. R., Gruneberg, R. N., and Neu, H. (1994). *Int. J. Antimicrob. Agents*, **4**, Suppl. 1, S1.

15. MacGowan, A. P., White, L. O., Reeves, D. S., Reed, V., *et al.* (1997). *Abstracts of the 37th Interscience Conference on Antimicrobial Agents and Chemotherapy*, Abstract A-45. ASM, Washington DC.

16. Greenberg, R. N. (1990). *Antimicrob. Agents Chemother.*, **35**, 2392.

17. Wise, R. (1999). In *Clinical antimicrobial assays* (ed. D. S. Reeves, R. Wise, J. M. Andrews, and L. O. White), p. 27. Oxford University Press, Oxford.

18. Reeves, D. S. and Paton, J. H. (1987). *Care of the Critically Ill*, **3**, 100.

19. Lau, W. K. and Young, L. S. (1976). *N. Engl. J. Med.*, **295**, 716.

20. Winston, D. J., Lau, W. K., Gale, R. P., and Young, L. S. (1980). *Ann. Intern. Med.*, **92**, 762.

21. Sattler, F. R., Cowan, R., Nielsen, D. M., and Ruskin, J. (1998). *Ann. Intern. Med.*, **109**, 280.

22. Line, D. H., Poole, G. W., and Waterworth, P. M. (1970). *Tubercle*, **51**, 76.

23. Nordstrom, L., Banck, G., Belfrage, S., Juhlin, I., *et al.* (1973). *Acta Pathol. Microbiol. Immunol. Scand. Sect. B*, Suppl. **241**, 58.

24. Mawer, G. E., Ahmad, R., Dobbs, S. M., McGough, J. G., *et al.* (1974). *Br. J. Clin. Pharmacol.*, **1**, 45.

25. Mattie, H., Craig, W. A., and Pechere, J. C. (1989). *J. Antimicrob. Chemother.*, **24**, 281.

26. MacGowan, A. P. and Reeves, D. S. (1994). *J. Antimicrob. Chemother.*, **34**, 829.

27. Matzke, G. R., Lucarotti, R. L., and Shapiro, H. S. (1983). *Am. J. Nephrol.*, **3**, 11.

28. Li, S. C., Ioannides-Demos, L. L., Spicer, W. J., Berbatis, C., Spelman, D. W., *et al.* (1989). *Med. J. Aust.*, **151**, 224.

29. Wilson, A. P. R. and Grüneberg, R. N. (1997). In *Teicoplanin, the first decade*, pp. 137–44. The Medicine Group, Abingdon.

30. Farber, B. F. and Moellering, R. C. (1983). *Antimicrob. Agents Chemother.*, **23**, 138.

31. Welty, T. E. and Copa, A. K. (1994). *Ann. Pharmacother.*, **28**, 1335.

32. Fernandez de Gatta, M. D., Calvo, M. V., Hernandez, J. M., Caballero, D., *et al.* (1996). *Clin. Pharmacol. Ther.*, **60**, 332.

33. Glazer, J. P., Danish, M. A., Plotkin, S. A., and Yaffe, S. J. (1980). *Pediatrics*, **66**, 573.

34. Fong, I. W. (1998). *Abstracts of the 38th Interscience Conference on Antimicrobial Agents and Chemotherapy*, Abstract 1226. ASM, Washington DC.

35. Lerner, P. I., Smith, H., and Weinstein, L. (1967). *Ann. N. Y. Acad. Sci.*, **145**, 310.

36. Reeves, D. S. and Bywater, M. J. (1976). In *Selected topics in clinical bacteriology* (ed. J. De Louvois), p. 21. Bailliere Tindall, London.

37. White, L. O. and Reeves, D. S. (1981). In *Therapeutic drug monitoring* (ed. A. Richens and V. Marks), p. 456. Churchill Livingstone, Edinburgh.

38. Reeves, D. S. (1989). In *Medical bacteriology: a practical approach*, 1st edn. (ed. P. M. Hawkey and D. A. Lewis), p. 195. IRL Press, Oxford.

39. Andrews, J. M. (1999). In *Clinical antimicrobial assays* (ed. D. S. Reeves, R. Wise, J. M. Andrews, and L. O. White), p. 35. Oxford University Press, Oxford.

40. White, L. O. and Lovering, A. M. (1999). In *Clinical antimicrobial assays* (ed. D. S. Reeves, R. Wise, J. M. Andrews, and L. O. White), p. 45. Oxford University Press, Oxford.

41. Marks, V. (1981). In *Therapeutic drug monitoring* (ed. A. Richens and V. Marks), p. 155. Churchill Livingstone, Edinburgh.

42. White, L. O., MacGowan, A. P., Lovering, A. M., Holt, H. A., *et al.* (1994). *J. Antimicrob. Chemother.*, **33**, 1068.

43. White, L. O., Edwards, R., Holt, H. A., Lovering, A. M., *et al.* (1988). *J. Antimicrob. Chemother.*, **22**, 739.

44. Koenigsberger, R. (1981). In *Therapeutic drug monitoring* (ed. A. Richens and V. Marks), p. 131. Churchill Livingstone, Edinburgh.

45. Reeves, D. S., Wise, R., Andrews, J. M., and White, L. O. (ed.) (1999). *Clinical antimicrobial assays*. Oxford University Press, Oxford (ISBN 0 19 922325 4).

46. Reeves, D. S. and Ullmann, U. (ed.) (1986). *High performance liquid chromatography in medical microbiology*. Fischer, Stuttgart (ISBN 3 437 10983 9).

47. Snell, J. J. S., Brown, D. F. J., and Roberts, C. (ed.) (1999). *Quality assurance principles and practice in the microbiology laboratory*. Public Health Laboratory Service, London (ISBN 0 901144 45 2).

Chapter 9
Laboratory computing in medical microbiology

Andrew M. Lovering

Department of Medical Microbiology, Southmead Hospital, Bristol
B10 5NB, UK.

1 Introduction

There can be few, if any, clinical microbiology laboratories in the UK that are
without some form of computer system. Indeed, many laboratories will be running their second, or even, third generation of system and most will be acutely
aware of the relative advantages and disadvantages of a laboratory computer system. Consequently this chapter will not address the basic principles and methods
of operation of microbiology laboratory computer systems, as these will be familiar to most readers, but highlight some of the developing issues in Information
Technology (IT) that are impacting on microbiology laboratories. For those readers unfamiliar with such basic principals the chapter by MacGowan et al. (1) and
the paper by Kenny (2) are strongly recommended.

All too often computer, or IT, systems used in pathology laboratories are viewed
in isolation to either the developments that are occurring within the organization
to which that laboratory belongs or to those within the health community as a
whole. Awareness of how IT systems within microbiology interact in the wider
information structure of health care provision and how planned developments
are likely to impact on the operation of these IT systems is of value in a number
of areas. From the junior staff trying to make sense of the apparent redundancy
in the information that must be entered into the system to the senior managers
who must assess whether their system continues to meet current operational
requirements, understanding of these broader issues is important.

2 Laboratory computers in microbiology

2.1 Stand-alone systems (Laboratory Information Management Systems—LIMS)

Laboratory computer systems have been used in medical microbiology for over
twenty years. The first systems were home-grown systems, largely tailored to the

laboratory requirements and owing more to the enthusiasm of a few members of staff within the department than any strategic direction in IT. Such systems were largely autonomous, free-standing units and have served many laboratories well over the years. Their popularity resulting more from an absence of commercial systems at the time of development than a laboratory's preference for a home-grown system. They are, however, difficult to maintain as the systems knowledge base is invested in a limited number of individuals and have proved poorly responsive to the changing IT needs of the health community. In many cases, the systems are running on outdated hardware with obsolete software and have little or no capability for upgrading, frequently being termed legacy systems.

2.2 Systems integrated with other hospital systems (Hospital Information Systems—HIS)

Since the mid 1980s there has been a move towards integration of the health care computer systems within an organization under a central IT strategy. This approach has varied between the integration of a number of stand-alone systems onto a common hardware platform through to the development of fully integrated health care systems. Although integration of stand-alone systems onto a common hardware platform has facilitated ward, and general practice, access to enquiry functions, these systems remain largely autonomous with little in the way of shared data. In contrast, integrated health care systems address most aspects of a hospital's activity within a single computer system, all be it with individual department modules. This approach allows the use of a relational database with one master record per patient, common coding structures and maintenance functions and, in theory, the ability to conduct data enquiries across the system. Unfortunately, although popular with ward- and community-based users, such systems have proved expensive to install, maintain, and upgrade, somewhat cumbersome in use, and have committed organizations to a single software product rather than 'cherry picking' of the best systems. As a consequence they have not proved popular with hospitals and with the move towards an electronic patient record (EPR) their value has been largely superseded.

2.3 Feeder systems to electronic patient records (Integrated Laboratory Information Management Systems—ILIMS)

Traditionally with laboratory computer systems the findings of an investigation are communicated back to the requester as a paper report, sometimes with results additionally available on ward-based VDU enquiry. However, over the last decade general practices have increasingly used computers, rather than paper, to store patient records and thus issuing of paper reports by laboratories does not meet the modern requirements of many general practitioners. In many practices, clerks must enter pathology reports onto the practice computer from the paper reports received from the laboratories and for them it is highly desirable to receive electronic copies of the report which can be directly integrated into the patient's records. More recently similar developments have been occurring within secondary care provision and with the implementation of electronic patient records within hospitals by 2005 a key requirement of the White Paper 'Information for Health; 1999' (3) the way that pathology laboratories communicate results to users is set to change.

With an electronic patient record, data are stored in a patient-based system, which has its own database and enquiry functions, and which serves as a gather system to collate information from various sources. These items of information may be entered manually; such as when recording medical histories, or captured electronically from other computer systems, such as the pathology system. However, the way that results are displayed is governed by the team that supply the EPR rather than by the departments that supply the data. In theory, a user could receive microbiology results from two different laboratories and have them integrated into a patient's notes without being aware of the independent sourcing of the requests. Although pressures from health care providers will continue to dominate the choice of laboratory computer systems, provided data can be exported in a format recognized by the EPR, the particular system in operation within the laboratory is of lesser importance to the provider. Consequently, laboratories should be afforded greater freedom to choose the system that best fits their departmental requirements than has been seen over the past few years.

3 Core elements of a microbiology computer system

When considering laboratory computer systems it is easy to be distracted by the additional functionality present in the system and ignore the core functionality. It can not be stressed enough that if the core functions of a computer system do not work efficiently, no amount of secondary functionality will make it a good system. The following functions are generally considered as core elements of a laboratory IT system.

3.1 Requesting

3.1.1 Data entry

For each request made of the laboratory there is a need to record basic information identifying the patient, the person making the request, the sample type, time and method of collection, and the investigation required. These data have been entered traditionally by hand from a request form and it goes without saying that it should be possible to enter these data with a minimum of key strokes, or by using automated methods such as bar code readers, entering common requests in a shorthand form, and cloning patient details across when multiple specimens are received. With the wider introduction of EPR it is not unreasonable to expect that as well as receiving results electronically users should be able to make requests electronically; which, in theory, alleviates some of the data entry requirements and potential errors. Electronically requested specimens may, or may not, arrive with a request form but on entering the sample identity number these details should be available, pre-filled, on the requesting screens. For laboratories that operate using the request form as a worksheet rather than recording details directly onto the computer system (paper versus paperless working) (3) there will also be a requirement to print worksheets.

Although electronic requesting of investigations is a simple concept it generates difficult issues relating to integration of the different coding schemes that are used to identify the same information. This is commonly addressed by creation of a mapping routine. Within a single organization it is relatively easy to implement a mapping whereby when a user of the hospital EPR submits a sputum sample using a code of SP this information is correctly transmitted to the microbiology system where the code of SPU is used. This process is not so easy to implement when dealing with general practice EPRs from multiple suppliers and the adoption of national electronic data interchange standards (currently EDIFACT—see Section 3.4.2) are essential. In the same way, although clinical diagnosis and details can be transmitted as free text, primary care users would expect to use the Read Coding scheme which is in use within their system and laboratory systems should be able to recognize this and any other accepted thesaurus of coded clinical terms (3).

3.1.2 Linkage into patient administration systems

In general microbiology computer systems fall into two categories; those that have linkage into the main patient administration computer system (PAS) and those that do not, with the systems linked to PAS being further divided on whether the linkage is bi- or uni-directional. In a bi-directional link, when a patient's details are entered in the microbiology system a search is made on the PAS system for a patient with the corresponding details and, if found, the patient number and details from the PAS system are used for the microbiology request. If no patient record is found on the PAS system with the relevant details a new patient record is set up on the PAS system. For a uni-directional system this recording of a new patient details on PAS is missing and the patient 'exists' only within the microbiology system. The problem with a uni-directional system occurs if that patient is subsequently admitted to hospital and a PAS record created. Unless specific routines to identify duplicate patients are in place, such as using the New NHS Number, a second record for the same patient will be created in the microbiology system and that patient's microbiological history will be fragmented. This may cause problems for ward-based staff trying to look up microbiology results using the hospital accession number of the patient and it will certainly cause problems when trying to implement an EPR within the hospital. If possible, with the requirement for EPR in the near future it would appear logical for laboratories implementing a new computer system to consider these issues and how they can be resolved.

3.1.3 Risk categorization for samples and patients

Despite all the arguments about the use of universal precautions there remains the requirement for accurate knowledge about the potential risks posed to staff by a specimen. Although such information is sometimes supplied as part of the clinical details this is a notoriously unreliable process and there should be a way to assign risk status within the laboratory IT system. This risk flag may either be attached to the patient where the risk remains for some time, or to a particular sample, or group of samples, where only certain sample types constitute a risk. Ideally there should be the capability for risk status to be either attached for life or a finite period and it is desirable if risk categorization, once entered, can be transmitted to other disciplines within pathology or for example to nursing modules where the patient is infected with say MRSA.

3.2 Result entry

3.2.1 Text- or test-based systems

Although some early microbiology computer systems were text based, whereby a report was simply entered as free text, most systems in use today are based upon tests and results. Within an investigation each discrete unit is identified as a test to which a result can be attached, such as red blood cells in a urine microscopy. These tests can be either the tests that are reported back to requesters, as in the case of the red blood cells, or intermediate tests that are used as part of a pathway to a final result, such as DNase. Although adoption of a test-based system allows use of shorthand codes the important benefit it brings is to permit the implementation of automatic validation and authorization routines. Free text entries are normally excluded from any validation rules and are usually restricted to comments attached to the report by the person clinically reviewing or authorizing the report.

3.2.2 Single and batch result entry

For most microbiological investigations results are entered for each of the elements, or tests, in the investigation on a single specimen basis, and most readers who have seen a microbiology computer system will be familiar with this. However, in some areas of the microbiology laboratory, such as virology and serology, where samples are batched it is useful to be able to enter the same result or result profile against a series of specimens without calling each one up individually.

3.2.3 Linkage to automated equipment

Although there are very few analysers used in a clinical microbiology laboratory it is often desirable for these to be linked into the main microbiology computer system. Typical systems that would warrant linkage would be blood culture analysers and, with the adoption of standardized sensitivity testing methods, automated readers. The linkage can be either uni- or bi-directional. In an uni-directional interface the user enters a link laboratory number on the automated equipment and the findings are then sent using this number to the main computer system. In a bi-directional interface, having entered the laboratory number the automated equipment requests patient demographic and investigation detail from the main computer, before returning the findings of the investigation. In terms of the final computer report there is little difference between the two approaches, but as many of the analysers have their own software to allow them to run as stand-alone units, use of the bi-directional interface allows use of the functionality present in the automated equipment—such as statistical or epidemiological analysis. Occasionally linkage of blood culture analysers to laboratory systems may cause unnecessary problems and thought will need to be given to the process by which data are transmitted. For example, with the current generation of blood culture analysers which have continuous monitoring it may be unhelpful for a patient record to be updated in the early hours of the morning to the effect that the blood culture is positive, without laboratory staff having the opportunity to confirm the finding. In this case a buffering system on either the blood culture system or laboratory system may be needed.

3.2.4 Electronic input of results from reference centres

Very few microbiology laboratories process all of the samples they receive, with most referring certain types of request on to specialist centres. Although the workload generated by these referred samples is relatively modest, such as specialist serology, in certain cases, such as routine virology, it can be substantial. Most laboratories will receive the reports from the specialist centre, manually enter them onto the laboratory computer, and then issue reports to the original requesters. This is frequently a time-consuming process and can lead to errors in data entry. With the introduction of the X400 NHSnet, linking health care providers with a secure communications pathway, receiving reports directly back into the requesting laboratory's computer system is an interesting possibility. The theory of this is only marginally more complex than for receiving results from a blood culture analyser and relies more on co-operation between the requesting and reference centres than technological advances.

3.2.5 Split site working

Allied to the problems of receiving results from reference centres has been the trend for amalgamation of laboratories and centralization of services. While clearly a single computer system on the various sites that make up a centralized pathology service will be the best solution to IT requirements, electronic data transfer between the IT systems on the individual sites may adequately address the issue in the short-term. This may be particularly the case when the organization, or organizations, served by the laboratories have implemented an electronic paper record. However, issues of common working practices and staff interchange between the laboratories are clearly influenced by the commonality of the IT systems on the various sites, but are not insurmountable.

3.2.6 Near patient testing

At present, unlike in some of the other pathology disciplines, near patient testing is uncommon in microbiology; being restricted mainly to dipstick testing of urine. Under the guidance for CPA Accreditation responsibility for training, and by inference quality assurance, in near patient testing remains with the pathology department rather than the unit undertaking the testing. As it is rare for the results of near patient testing to be recorded, other than in the patient notes, it is difficult to see how audit of the performance of near patient testing can be undertaken. With access to the pathology computer systems normally possible at the site of testing, and required under the guidance for Clinical Governance (4–6), there should be no reason why near patient testing results should not be entered onto pathology computer systems. This would simply require setting up access facilities to the system for the ward-based staff undertaking the near patient testing.

3.3 Validation, system actions, and authorization

These three functions, in various roles, make up the operational core of a modern laboratory information management system. Validation routines determine whether a piece of data entered into the computer is a possible response, system actions govern what happens as a consequence of entering that item of data, and authorization routines assess the potential significance of the data item entered. The three items have a high degree of overlap and are collectively termed a rules base. While it is unlikely to encounter a current commercial product that is without a rules base, there are large differences in the operational functionality of the rules base in different systems. Consequently, purchase, or operation, of a system with only a very rudimentary rules base may lead to many hours a day manually approving reports which could have been automatically approved in a system with a more comprehensive rules base.

3.3.1 Validation

This is the process that ensures that the data entered into the computer system is a possible finding. This can vary from disallowing entry of sample collection dates in the future to preventing a user from recording that a strict anaerobe grew aerobically. Clearly there will be instances where a possible but rare event occurs, in these cases a warning may be given to the user but the data accepted.

3.3.2 System actions

Having entered a valid piece of data, system actions are used to determine any further action that needs to be taken and are sometimes called cascade requesting. Typical examples would include booking a pre-set work schedule for a particular specimen type, ordering the appropriate sensitivity tests when a particular organism is isolated, or suppressing one of the sensitivity tests if the organism is resistant. System actions can be effectively used to support standard operating procedures within a laboratory as they prompt users to follow work protocols.

3.3.3 Authorization

This is the process of determining whether the potential significance of the data item entered requires approval by a technical or medical reviewer before being released back to the requester. It goes without saying that the objective of authorization routines should be to deal automatically with the bulk of the routine and negative findings from the laboratory and only send the significant findings for authorization by a reviewer, flagging any unusual results.

3.3.4 Logic rules, decision trees, knowledge bases, and expert systems

Although in the earlier examples use has been made of single tests, in microbiology, more so than haematology and chemistry, it is the totality of the report, in association with patient and specimen factors, which govern its clinical relevance. Consequently, for the most efficient and satisfactory use of a rules base it is desirable to be able to link or chain together the individual elements of an investigation to form logic rules and decision trees that describe common circumstances (1). These are likely to include elements such as patient age, sex, type, specimen type, and the findings of the individual tests that made up the investigation rules. This would then allow a midstream urine sample from a female general practice patient aged 16–60y, which had a raised white cell count in the microscopy and grew a pure growth of coliforms, sensitive to the primary agents tested, to be classed as an event not necessarily needing to be authorized by a medical reviewer. Unfortunately, the more flexibility that is introduced into the rules base the more complex the system is to set up and maintain, but ultimately a more satisfactory system is achieved.

During the 1990s great advances were made in the theory of systems design in relation to the way in which knowledge is stored and can be applied in IT. This lead to the hope that expert systems would enter into pathology IT. These would have the potential to improve overall quality by making even non-routine laboratory services error-free and more predictable, and have essentially no human involvement. To date this has not happened and other than a few publications describing such systems, introduction of these would appear unlikely within the near future (7, 8).

3.4 Returning results to requesters

Traditionally returning the results of an investigation to the original requester has involved issuing of a paper report and, at the time of writing, this remains the primary data source for legal purposes. The printed report being augmented by the availability of results on VDU enquiry and direct telephoning of results. For the foreseeable future paper reporting will remain an essential feature of laboratory computer systems but with electronic data interchange becoming the major way in which reports are returned to requesters it may be necessary in the future only to print out reports for certain requesters or locations.

3.4.1 Paper reports and direct VDU enquiry

The importance of good report design and screen displays for VDU access should not be underestimated. These should indicate whether the report is provisional, interim, final, supplementary, or a copy report. Additionally they should indicate who authorized the report and whether the report has been printed or sent electronically. It is essential that there should be flexibility with regard to the production of reports in different formats for different investigations and according to the department's present and future needs. Although few microbiology investigations are suited to graphical display, there should be the potential for the production of summary reports which contain information combined from individual investigations; such as pre- and post-dose antibiotic assays, or sick and convalescent serology samples.

3.4.2 Electronic reporting to primary care

Issuing of electronic reports to general practice has been increasing since the mid 1990s and its wider implementation is seen as a priority issue within primary care. Early messaging systems utilized locally derived protocols for the transmission of reports but with the adoption of the United Nations Directories for Electronic Data Interchange for Administration, Commerce and Transport (EDIFACT) as the NHS standard for electronic data interchange, all laboratory systems should be moving to this standard (9). Although the Pathology EDIFACT message defined the transmission protocols for electronic data interchange (EDI) between hospitals and general practice, microbiology was largely outside of the scope of the original NHS-funded project. As a consequence, although for Clinical Chemistry and Haematology individual tests are mapped to Read Codes (9) and sent as single entities, for microbiology the whole report is sent as a single text element. The significance of this is that within primary care it will not be possible to conduct analysis of the content of the returned reports, for epidemiological or antibiotic audit purposes. Furthermore differences will remain between the way in which reports from different microbiology laboratories are displayed leading to a greater requirement for validation of the quality of returned reports than in Clinical Chemistry or Haematology (see Section 3.4.4).

3.4.3 Electronic reporting to secondary care

Although standards exist for EDI between pathology laboratories and primary care providers, few exist for EDI between pathology laboratories and secondary care providers. As a consequence most organizations implementing an electronic patient record have developed their own protocols for data exchange, frequently based around commercial data exchange and mapping software packages. Although initially the easiest option, this approach largely locks the laboratory and the secondary care provider together, making it difficult for the laboratory to replace its computer system or the secondary care provider to source its pathology services from an alternative centre without a lengthy, and expensive, interfacing exercise. It would appear much more logical to move towards a national standard on EDI between pathology laboratories and secondary care providers and so avoid many of these problems.

3.4.4 Issues of data quality and ownership in EDI

In purchasing and implementing IT systems laboratories spend considerable time and effort in ensuring that the printed reports and VDU enquiry screens present data in a logical and unambiguous way. With the increasing use in both primary and secondary care of EDI for reporting some interesting issues relating to data ownership and quality assurance have arisen. With EDI a laboratory transmits an electronic copy of the report back to the requester's computer system which then displays the report using its own display functions. Consequently, although the report sent electronically mirrors the data held in the laboratory IT system, there is no guarantee that this will be displayed in an acceptable format on the requester's computer system. So although it is widely considered that the responsibility of the laboratory ends with assuring that the EDI message is accurate, it would appear prudent for laboratories entering into EDI arrangements to review how reports will be presented to the end user. This is particularly important, as despite the fact that the paper report is the primary information source, it is clear that many requesters are using EDI as their primary data source without reference to the paper reports. Specific issues that should be addressed when reviewing the display of EDI data include assuring that critical information is easily identified and that adequate procedures are in place for multiple reports, to ensure that only the most current information is displayed.

4 Secondary functions

4.1 Access, security, and audit

The goal of any IT system is to provide information at the point of use, to those who need it, when they need it. Against this must be balanced the technical difficulties of doing so, the costs involved and, increasingly, issues of patient confidentiality. Traditionally laboratory IT systems have had poor functionality in these areas: for instance, some still do not have ward and primary care-based access to enquiry functions, many operate using generic passwords which rapidly become common knowledge, and most have only rudimentary audit capabilities. These aspects of a laboratory IT system are increasingly becoming of importance, with access to information at the point of use a feature of Clinical Governance (4) and issues of patient confidentiality addressed in the Caldicott Report and other secondary publications (10, 11). Although users of laboratory IT systems are health care professionals and do so, in the vast majority of cases, with regard to the sensitivity of the data stored within the system, attention still needs to be given to restriction of data availability, hopefully without impairing the ability of an individual to perform their job. This needs to be backed-up by an effective audit system; not just to police the system but to allow the reasons for an error to be identified and help prevent that error occurring again. In early IT systems comprehensive audit capability was limited by data storage capacity but with the advances in computer technology this is no longer an issue. Some of the key features of security within a laboratory IT system would include:

(a) Individual user logon with regular password changes.

(b) Access only to routines that the user requires.

(c) Preventing of 'browsing' within the system.

(d) The ability to restrict the records for prominent patients.

(e) The ability to restrict knowledge that certain investigations have been undertaken to authorized individuals (e.g. HIV testing).

(f) The ability to restrict knowledge to authorized individuals that investigations on patients have been requested from certain locations (e.g. GUM clinics and certain Child Health Clinics).

(g) The ability to audit trail both data entry and enquiry functions.

4.2 Laboratory management functions

Although these have frequently featured prominently in both the description of laboratory IT systems and statements of need when procuring systems, in practice they have tended to be of only marginal value. A number of reasons may be identified for this which include; poorly developed software, widely differing needs and requirements between laboratories, better tools outside of the laboratory IT system, the resources needed to operate the management functions. However, probably the main reason relates to the relative infrequency with which such information is actually useful for managerial purposes. Clearly the added value that such functions provide will differ between laboratories and typical functions that are included in current IT systems include (12):

(a) Workflow tracking and contract monitoring.

(b) Monitoring laboratory and individuals performance for work throughput and accuracy.

(c) Audit of compliance and enforcement of standard operating procedures.

(d) Stock control systems.

(e) Pricing and costings modules.

(f) Quality control monitoring.

4.3 Data extraction

All laboratory IT systems will have the capability to provide analysis of the data stored within them, with most operating a bespoke enquiry and report generator. With such data enquiry systems the user enters a series of criteria and the system returns the records which satisfy those criteria, usually in the form of a print or table. Although this approach may be satisfactory for many of the departmental information requirements, in practice such enquiry packages are difficult to use and, in general, functionality falls far short of even the most basic PC-based package. A much more satisfactory approach is to provide a data extraction routine within the laboratory IT system which will allow export of data into third party software for subsequent analysis. This can be achieved either by physical export and import of data or by providing links for the third party software into the reference files of the laboratory IT system.

Information requests from pathology IT systems were a major feature of the contract driven approach to health care provision in the 1990s and most laboratories will be familiar with requests for workload data. Of interest during this time was the infrequency of requests directly related to the way in which patients were managed. Even with the introduction of Clinical Audit (6), the publication of the House of Lords report detailing the importance of surveillance, Clinical Governance (4), and the difficulties in infection control caused by MRSA, information requests relating to patient management remain rare. This is difficult to understand as the importance of epidemiological data is well established and infection control is closely associated with microbiology services. However, with the increasing importance of infection control within trusts and the introduction of specific infection control packages, this situation is likely to change and information to support infection control is likely to become an increasing feature of laboratory IT systems.

5 System maintenance and development

When introducing a computer system, departments should expect the system to be flexible enough to meet the changing requirements of the department or respond to national initiatives, such as the introduction of the New NHS Number. Although for most microbiology laboratories changes will largely be restricted to the work patterns undertaken within the laboratory, which can be addressed through system maintenance, there will remain the need for regular, substantive, developments to the system (12, 13). These may be to address the level of functionality within the system or simply to fix known problems. However, such developments are costly if funded on an individual site basis and are, consequently, best addressed as part of the support contract rather than as bespoke developments.

6 Procurement of a new system

Even with continuing development there will come a time when the IT system will need replacement. This may be due to under-investment during the life of the system such that it is uneconomic to bring it up to the required level of functionality, an obsolete operating system or hardware platform with excessive maintenance costs, or simply that the product no longer fits into the departmental or organization's approach to computing. However, with the increasing drive towards EDI, providing data can be produced by EDI, pressures for change resulting from the requirements of the organization to which the laboratory belongs may diminish, along with the will to pay for such changes.

The process of selection of a pathology IT system has become an increasingly complex and lengthy process subject to various articles of legislation regulating public sector procurement, such that laboratories are unlikely to engage in such a process without specialist assistance. Since 1993, all substantial public IM&T investment has needed a properly structured business case which is based on good investment appraisal, a clear plan for benefits realization, sufficient skilled and experienced staff to complete the installation, commitment from all levels of the purchaser and proper project control, with structured training and post-implementation evaluation. Currently within the UK such purchases are made through an agreed process; Procurement of Information Systems Effectively (POISE) (14). Although such a process is beyond the scope of this chapter, the key points are summarized in Table 1, and the reader is directed to the excellent articles by Feltham (15), Moritz *et al.* (16), and Kenny (2) detailing the process and giving advice on the preparation of statements of need.

References

1. MacGowan, A. P., McCulloch, S. Y., and Lovering, A. M. (1996). In *Practical medical microbiology* (ed. J. G. Collee, A. G. Fraser, B. P. Marmion, and A. Simmons). Churchill Livingstone, London, UK.
2. Kenny, D. (1993). *Clin. Chim. Acta*, **222**, 147.
3. Information for Health. (1999). HMSO, London, UK.
4. HSC 1999/065 (1999). Clinical governance in the new NHS. Department of Health, London.

Table 1 The key stages in the Procurement of Information Systems Effectively (POISE) process

Stage 1: Planning
1. Verify and understand the business goals, expected benefits and lifetime costs, strategy, and funding.
2. Research and understand the current market, confirm that there are potential solutions.
3. Agree to scope and content of the procurement, understand purchaser's organization; agree on the approach to be taken in the procurement.
4. Document objectives, budget constraints, resources, and overall timetable.
5. Establish a project board.

Stage 2: Preparation
1. Define the business problem as the Detailed Statement of Need (DSON).
2. Produce and approve the Summary of Need (SON).
3. Produce a project advertisement that reflects the purchaser's needs and meets legal obligations of European Community.
4. Produce the contract framework including relevant terms and conditions.

Stage 3: Purchase
1. Issue advertisement and select capable vendors.
2. Issue SON to selected vendors and receive responses for evaluation.
3. Select vendors capable of providing solutions that meet all mandatory requirements in SON.
4. Review and evaluate selected vendors to product manageable shortlist.
5. Issue contract framework and negotiate draft contracts with each shortlisted vendor.
6. Invite tenders and receive best offers for final evaluation.
7. Evaluate offers and award contract to most economically advantageous solution.
8. Publish award notice and debrief unsuccessful vendors.

Stage 4: Performance
1. Implementation of the contract, acceptance of the information system, and payment to vendor.
2. Post-implementation activities to complete the Benefits Realization Programme.
3. Monitor and review the project against the original business goals.

5. HSC 1999/123 (1999). Governance in the new NHS controls assurance statements 1999/2000 risk management and organisational controls. Department of Health, London.

6. A First Class Service—Quality in the new NHS. (1998). HMSO, London, UK.

7. Peters, M. and Broughton, P. M. G. (1993). *Ann. Clin. Biochem.*, **30**, 52.

8. Blick, K. E. (1997). *Clin. Chem.*, **43**, 908.

9. Executive Letter EL (92) 34 (1992). Adoption of UN/EDIFACT as the NHS standard for Electronic Data Interchange of structured messages.

10. The Caldicott Committee. (1997). Report on the review of patient—identifiable information. Department of Health, London.

11. HSC 1999/053 (1999). For the record managing records in NHS Trusts and health authorities. Department of Health, London.

12. Brown, D. F. J. and Amphlett, M. (1999). In *Quality assurance—principles and practice* (ed. J. Snell, D. Brown, and C. Roberts). Public Health Laboratory Service, London, UK.

13. Bund, C., Heinemann, G. W., Jager, B. *et al.* (1998). *Pharm. Acta Helv.*, **72**, 349.

14. HSC 1999/143 (1999). Review of NHS procurement implementing the recommendations. Department of Health, London.

15. Feltham, R. K. A. (1995). *Medinfo*, **8**, 549.

16. Moritz, V. A., McMaster, R., Dillon, T., and Mayall, B. (1995). *Pathology*, **27**, 260.

Chapter 10

Quality control and quality assurance

W. A. Hyde

Independent Consultant, 2 Calder Avenue, Hindley Green,
Wigan WN2 4TR, UK.

P. K. Curley

Department of Microbiology, Leeds General Infirmary,
Gt George Street, Leeds LS1 3EX, UK.

1 Introduction

The late European Committee for Clinical Laboratory Standards produced a
document on quality control for microbiology, which stated (1):

> "Internal quality control is the set of procedures undertaken by the staff
> of a laboratory for the continual evaluation of laboratory work and the
> emergent results, in order to decide whether they are reliable enough to
> be released to clinicians or epidemiologists.
>
> External quality assessment which is a term that should be used in pre-
> ference to external quality control (since it is not a system for exerting
> control), refers to an objective system of retrospectively comparing results
> from different laboratories by means of an external agency."

A definition of assurance in the Collins dictionary (2) is given as 'freedom from
doubt'.

A more comprehensive definition of quality control would be the method by
which an organization ensures that the product or information which it provides,
is as near perfection as possible given the constraints of time, budget, and ability
of the staff employed.

Good quality control in the pathology laboratory begins with the recruitment
policies and ends with report validation.

The influence of Clinical Pathology Accreditation (CPA) (UK) Ltd. (3) and similar
schemes in other countries together with the introduction of Good Laboratory Practice with the use of Standard Operating Procedures (SOPs) into clinical

laboratories has led to greater understanding of the steps necessary to achieve the aims set out in the above definitions.

2 Personnel

2.1 Recruitment policies and staffing structures

Quality control should encompass all aspects of the organization and management of the department. This starts with a good recruitment policy to ensure that quality staff are placed in roles where they can effectively fulfil the requirements of the role and thus contribute to team and organizational objectives.

Quality people = Quality service = Quality organization

Whenever someone leaves, there is an opportunity to reassess the situation and ascertain whether or not the post needs to be filled in the same way. The staffing structure of the department should be constantly reviewed. When a post becomes vacant it may be better filled by a different grade or the same grade but with enhancement points. In either case a working pattern with more flexible hours could well improve the quality of service provided.

For reasons of quality and safety there is a limit to the number of unqualified staff such as the Medical Laboratory Assistant (MLA) grade who should be employed. The ratio of unqualified to qualified staff will vary according to the needs of different laboratories (4).

It is inevitable that existing staff may have to adapt to changing working practices in the quest for providing the best service. However when a more gradual change is possible new staff can be employed and given clear job descriptions including any unsociable hours, thus assisting in a smooth transition.

Having determined what is required, in addition to a Job Description (now obligatory for CPA) a Personnel Specification should be prepared. This sets out the characteristics required of a particular post, for example the qualifications, experience, and individual skills. Alternatively a Role Profile may be developed which sets out these requirements on one form.

Interviews should be properly constructed and carried out by appropriately trained staff using properly validated selection techniques. Applicants for technical posts should provide evidence of their degree and State Registration. For other grades, appropriate tests such as typing tests can be used in addition to the interview to ensure a sufficiently high standard of accuracy can be achieved.

2.2 Training and organization

All new starters need an Induction course, which may be on several levels: first, an overview of the organization and its structure followed by an induction into the specific department of employment. Induction at this second level can also be partly job/grade specific and should be broadened to include returnees after maternity leave or extended sick leave, and those whose roles may have changed.

Good training is essential to maintain quality and should be comprehensive and structured. The use of an in-house logbook for trainee Biomedical Scientists has long been an invaluable addition to the official Council for Professions Supplementary to Medicine (CPSM) logbook and is now a requirement for a CPSM accredited laboratory in the UK. This form of record keeping can be used when training all new staff in the laboratory or office, regardless of grade and, in an abbreviated form, for returnees to work.

Once induction and training are complete staff should be best utilized according to the predetermined structure. It would be counterproductive to have highly trained Biomedical Scientists pouring plates except in an emergency, and dangerous for Medical Laboratory Assistants to read Gram films. The Institute of Biomedical Sciences (IBMS) has guidelines for duties which are not appropriate for MLA grade staff (4) and these should be adhered to for reasons of quality and safety.

Training of established staff should continue by regular rotation through sections, updates by attendance at courses and symposia, lunchtime lectures, and participation in Continuing Professional Development (CPD) schemes.

More senior staff should be encouraged to pursue management qualifications and attend any relevant in-house courses on topics such as recruitment, appraisals, and quality issues.

The organization of a department has clear implications for the quality of results produced. The responsibilities of all senior members of staff must be understood. A departmental senior team must meet regularly to discuss all organizational and methodological changes before they can be implemented. Full departmental meetings should also be held at which changes and problems can be discussed openly. All staff should be encouraged to give their points of view.

This type of team building leads to good staff relations, smooth organizational changes and, inevitably, better results.

2.3 Standard operating procedures

Over the last few years, an increasing number of laboratories have become CPA accredited, SOPs have become a way of life in clinical laboratories. Although probably the most time-consuming task in preparation for accreditation they are an invaluable adjunct to Quality Assurance.

Prior to this system, quality could be as variable as the staff: methods could be changed or modified according to whoever was performing them. However, a clear concise written instruction for a procedure in which all staff must be trained should be agreed and authorized as departmental policy. If all staff adhere to the agreed procedure the quality of the service is, therefore, enhanced.

In the UK there is no definitive SOP, but only guidelines, an example of which was published in the IBMS Gazette: August 1992 (5). This provides a very useful basis to work from and may be modified according to the procedure. These guidelines showed that SOPs may have a series of standard headings, some of which are not required for administrative SOPs. In other SOPs, headings such as

Area of Application could be used at the start of a section, to cover all procedures in that section. The heading Quality Control underlines the need to have some form of QC in place for every procedure. The principle of the procedure can be very brief, or, in the case of laboratory tests as explicit as possible for training purposes. Indeed, a well written SOP with explanations and diagrams in addition to a concise, easy to follow method page provides a useful aid to completing an in-house log book with its requirement for personal notes. If a kit test is being used there is no need to write an SOP under the usual headings. A copy of the kit insert can be used, provided all the manufacturer's instructions are adhered to. If there is any deviation from these instructions they must be justified, documented, and attached to the kit instructions to ensure quality is maintained and in case of litigation.

Standard Operating Procedures for all equipment in the laboratory are also required. These are sometimes referred to as Equipment Operating Procedures (EOPs), which can be included in and cross-referenced with the SOPs. EOPs are needed for every piece of equipment and should include location, service schedule, decontamination procedure, safe use, and electrical testing. SOPs and EOPs should cross-reference with Control of Substances Hazardous to Health assessments (COSHH) (6) and Risk Assessments and vice versa.

All such documentation should be updated as necessary and reviewed annually, which means that any system used must have facilities for updating. A type of eight digit index code may be useful in this respect consisting of a prefix for the section, followed by a code for the test, followed by a two figure number which can easily be changed each time there is an alteration or new version. This facilitates up to 99 versions, e.g. SRTDxG01 means: SR = serology section, TDxG = gentamicin assays using TDx, 01 = the version.

All SOPs which are no longer current should be clearly stamped 'Superseded' and the date on which they were superseded should coincide with the implementation date of the replacement SOP.

A format such as this ensures conformity in writing SOPs thus maintaining quality.

2.4 Logistics and organization

The organization of the department should be decentralized, with responsibilities for such areas as supply and equipment monitoring devolved to section level and responsibility for budgeting and ordering remaining with the appropriate senior member of staff.

This type of decentralization has three advantages:

(a) It gives the responsibility for keeping up stocks to the users.

(b) It ensures that users know the costs involved, thus preventing wastage.

(c) It should free the more senior staff to monitor the technical work of the department.

2.5 Specimen collection and transport

The training of medical and nursing staff in the requirements of specimen collection and transport is vital; it cannot be assumed that they are aware of the different transport and storage requirements for each type of sample. It is particularly vital for important samples such as CSF, blood cultures, viral and chlamydia samples. Theatre staff must be made aware that if pus is found a large sample rather than a swab must be sent to the laboratory. A simple sheet showing the various types of swabs and their use can easily be prepared and sent to wards and departments. A more detailed information document for staff using laboratory services should be available, and form an integral part of training and induction of medical and nursing staff. This does not substitute for a close working relationship between laboratory and departments such as ICU, Theatre, and SCBU.

If swabs are used it is important that the correct type is chosen as there is huge variation between survival times of bacteria on different types of swab and in transport media. Stuart (7) introduced his formulation in 1949 and there have been many variations on this theme since then. There is little doubt that the introduction of charcoal by Amies in 1967 (8) extended the survival times of bacteria and proved its superiority over Stuart's and Amies' without charcoal. The Wadsworth Institute (9) recommend the use of Cary–Blair for anaerobes and this is still the best clear transport medium for all organisms. A recent paper from Roelofsen *et al.* (10) showed that survival of bacteria on dry foam swabs could be as good as in transport media. These swabs may be more acceptable to those laboratories who don't like charcoal swabs.

Many workers have shown that survival of bacteria on swabs is far better at 4 °C than at room temperature or 37 °C (11).

2.6 Specimen handling and report validation

2.6.1 Specimen handling

All specimens handled by the laboratory should be correctly labelled with the patient's name, date of birth, and hospital number (or NHS number). Request forms should also be completed to an agreed standard. It is the responsibility of the requesting clinician to ensure that this is done. Laboratory staff should not process any specimens if there is insufficient information to guarantee the result being reported on the correct patient. If there is any doubt, medical advice should be sought.

Training given on induction should emphasize the need to check specimen details against request form information.

Most laboratories now have fully computerized booking and reporting systems, and some use a barcode numbering system. The laboratory number on the specimen must, of course, be identical to that on the request form. If computers are connected to hospital patient identification systems, they can be used to check patient details on request forms against patient records.

As information systems become more sophisticated and paper requests are replaced by electronic requesting, full sample labelling must continue even if barcodes are used. It is essential whenever new systems are introduced that the SOPs are amended and staff are trained in order to safeguard the standards of the laboratory.

Clerical errors are responsible for many more serious mistakes than are technical errors!

2.6.2 Report validation

The main purpose of report validation is to make sure that the report reflects the test results obtained and is consistent with previous reports. Computers can help when cumulative records are available. An unexpected test result can highlight the possibility of an incorrectly labelled sample or request form and should immediately be investigated.

All reporting staff should be aware of possible anomalies which could affect the result, e.g. peculiar antibiotic susceptibility patterns. Many checks can now be built into computer systems to prevent erroneous results from being reported. Anomalous results should not be edited without investigation for new bacterial variants, misidentification, media, or antibiotic disc failure.

However, a perfectly feasible result, but on the wrong patient, can only be avoided by staff diligence in double-checking patient identification. It is good practice whenever a significant result is found which has serious diagnostic implications that it is checked and confirmed by a senior member of staff as soon as is practicable.

3 Culture media quality issues

3.1 Storage conditions

These reagents are sensitive to heat, light, and especially moisture. Provision of adequate and appropriate storage is essential as much of the material used is of a sensitive nature and may be expensive to replace if incorrectly stored. The influence of incorrect storage on the final result is shown in Table 1, where the failure to tighten the cap of a pot of media results in the failure to isolate salmonella.

Dry media stored under optimum conditions will keep for two to three years unopened. After first opening it should keep for up to six months, but as is shown

Table 1 Deterioration of SS agar stored under various conditions for six months

Storage conditions	Moisture gain (%)	Salmonella recovery (%)
Unopened bottle, cool, dark, dry	0.0	100
Loose cap in light on bench	1.1	47
Loose cap in autoclave room	4.4	22

in Table 1 this depends entirely on proper handling. It is good practice to repeat quality control on media which has been stored for two years or more before opening. Media which has visibly deteriorated, e.g. lumpy or discoloured should not be used.

3.2 Preparation of culture media

3.2.1 Commercial source

Manufacturer instructions should be followed wherever possible, but it should be understood that these instructions refer to production of 1 litre volumes using an autoclave. It is impossible for manufacturers to produce protocols for every variation of volume or method in current use. Preparators must be used for volumes greater than 2 litres. The amount of heat input into larger volumes of media using hot plates or gas rings will inevitably lead to some destruction of the nutrient quality of the medium, and when bile or bile salts are in the formulation they may precipitate.

Media manufacturers would prefer to use F.O. units (12) which indicate total heat input rather than relying on the traditional '121 °C for 15 minutes' which is difficult to define and almost impossible to monitor.

The ultimate control of this process must be by using bacteriological performance criteria defined in the quality control procedures.

3.2.2 'In-house' produced media

Great care must be taken when producing media from raw materials using formulae taken from commercial catalogues. These formulations do not show definitive weights of components. All manufacturers give a disclaimer either on the label or in the catalogue which states that: 'these formulations may be adjusted to ensure that performance criteria are met'. Nutrient sources are variable, and for example, agar-agar can have a wide range of gel strengths. Chemicals and dyes, even pure grades, do not have a bacteriological specification and each must be individually quality controlled by substitution and comparison with components of known performance characteristics. It follows that all new raw materials used in 'in-house' formulations must be subjected to this type of testing.

3.2.3 HACCP (Hazard Analysis and Critical Control Point) (13)

This system of control was instituted into the US space programme to eliminate the possibility of accidents due to either systems or mechanical failure. The system has now been adopted throughout industry and can be applied to virtually any process of manufacture, production, or even R&D. Formal HACCP systems may be introduced with benefit into many of the procedures carried out in clinical laboratories, from blood cultures to producing culture media, which are presently controlled using informal fragmented HACCP type procedures.

A **Hazard** as defined in the food industry is a source of danger, unacceptable contamination, growth of bacteria, or survival of bacteria. In a clinical microbiology laboratory, it could be defined as 'any weakness in the system which can adversely influence the production of an accurate report on the material taken from the patient and sent for analysis'. This could embrace everything from the decision to take a sample to the appreciation and correct interpretation of the report, involving communication, training, logistics, budgets, staffing, and infrastructure.

A **Risk** is the likely occurrence of a hazard.

A **Critical Control Point** (CCP) is the location or step in the procedure at which control can be exerted over a hazard so that it can either be prevented or eliminated, or controlled to acceptable levels.

A typical HACCP programme is as follows:

1. Hazard analysis.

2. Identification of critical control points.

3. Establishment of CCP criteria.

4. Monitoring procedures for CCPs.

5. Protocols for deviation of the CCP.

6. Record keeping.

7. Verification.

Bolton (14) proposed a similar system for Quality Assurance in Food Microbiology laboratories described as 'all those planned and systematic actions necessary to provide adequate confidence that a product or service will satisfy given requirements for quality'. He used a modified HACCP system to control the flow of the sample from acceptance to reporting using the term 'Quality Assessment Point' instead of Critical Control Point to describe the points at which the result could be influenced.

A modified HACCP scheme is outlined in Table 2 showing the steps taken in culture media preparation and the possible points where problems can occur, the steps to be taken to control these problems, and the verification that these steps were effective in controlling the problems.

Evaluations of large batches of media which are to be used over a period require comprehensive quality assessment.

Media purchase decisions should never be made on administrative or budgetary criteria alone. Frequently used culture media such as Columbia agar or CLED should be purchased on an annual basis after first requesting a sample from a manufacturer of a large enough batch, and testing it extensively in comparison with the current batch. This needs to be done quickly but carefully, as manufacturers cannot hold large stocks which cannot be sold. This approach gives the user confidence to cut the amount of daily quality control to that necessary to show that the production method has been carried out correctly, and should lead to better control and savings.

Reference must be made to European Standard EN 12322:1999 (15). This gives details of the definitions and the methods for storage, selection, and correct use

Table 2 HACCP applied to culture media preparation

Control point	Hazard/critical limits	Records, control, verification, corrective action
Ordering	Too little/too much.	Regulated delivery taking account of seasonal variation of use.
Unopened storage	Out of date media.	Stock rotation system.
Opened storage	Moisture gain.	Tighten caps; store in cool, dry atmosphere.
Weighing	Balance accuracy; ±0.1 g.	Check daily; both ends of scale.
	Dust.	Wear mask; use hood.
Water	Out of specification >10 μS.	Check deionizer or still; must be less than 10 μS.
Mixing and soaking	Undissolved lumps.	Mix well; allow time to soak.
Sterilization by boiling	Explosive boiling/boiling over.	Mix constantly; wear glasses and gloves.
Sterilization by autoclaving	Failure to sterilize 121 °C ± 2 °C 15 min.	Check temperature and pressure records; use biological controls; external check on controls and instruments.
Preparators	Failure to sterilize/ overheat/out of control (manufacturers spec).	Check controls with external monitors.
Cooling	Too hot/too cold 47 °C ± 2 °C.	Use water-bath or incubator to control cooling; check temperatures.
Supplements	Wrong/outdated/poor quality/badly stored/wrong diluent. (Check spec.)	Rotate and check stock; check appearance; final bacteriological QC.
Pouring plates	Volume incorrect ±1%.	Check pump set-up.
	Contaminated plates >5%.	Check tubing; sterilize, and dry immediately.
	Lumpy media.	Check cooling temperatures, if large volume of supplement warm to 47 °C before adding.
	None or limited growth/<90% recovery target for organisms.	Use separate tubing for each selective medium especially those with dyes or antibiotics.

Table 2 (*Continued*)

Control point	Hazard/critical limits	Records, control, verification, corrective action
Cooling and setting	Uneven depth.	Set on flat surface; check with spirit level.
	Bubbles.	Check tubing for leaks.
Drying	Too dry/wet plates.	Check times and temperature of drying cabinet; preferably dry overnight under laminar flow.
Quality control	Not sterile >5% contamination.	Autoclave or preparator checks. Note type of bacteria, if spores check autoclave, if vegetative check supplements, pump tubing, drying system.
	Wrong colour.	Check supplement, pH, and correct media.
	Failure to grow target organisms.	Check correct media; check pump tubing;
	<90% recovery.	check water.

of culture strains, though the method it gives for the preparation of working cultures is inaccurate and incomplete; not showing a recovery step into a good nutrient broth before using cultures taken from storage. It is vital that such a recovery step is introduced before inoculating bacteria onto selective media. Failure to do this will result in unpredictable and varying results which may be blamed on the media. This type of error is the most common mistake encountered when investigating complaints from clinical laboratories to media suppliers.

A useful reference for laboratories involved in large-scale manufacture and supply of ready prepared media is that produced in the United States of America by the NCCLS. This organization produces guidelines and standards for many aspects of clinical microbiology (16).

If a thorough evaluation of the annual batch purchase has been carried out a simple quality control can be used to ensure that there has been no breakdown in the HACCP controls, using an organism intended to grow and others to show the supplements have been added (see Tables 3 and 4).

This type of QC can be easily done using Mossell's ecometric technique (17), which is described in full in the 1st edition of *Medical bacteriology: a practical approach*.

3.3 User problems

3.3.1 Water quality

Tap-water should never be used; pH measurement of water is useless unless a special low ion electrode is used, or potassium chloride is added to the water.

Table 3 Culture collection strains for quality control

QC organisms	ATCC	NCTC
Acinetobacter calcoaceticus	15309	5866
Bacteroides fragilis	25285	9343
Campylobacter jejuni	—	11168
Candida albicans	18804	—
Closttridium perfringens	13132	11229
Corynebacterium diphtheriae	19409	3984
Enterobacter cloacae	13047	10005
Escherichia coli O : 111	—	9111
Haemophilus influenzae	—	10479/11931
Neisseria gonorrhoeae	19424	8375
Proteus mirabilis	25933	—
Pseudomonas aeruginosa	27853	10662
Salmonella senftenberg	—	10384
Serratia marcescens	13880	10211
Staphylococcus aureus	25923	657
Staphylococcus epidermidis	14990	11047
Streptococcus faecalis		775
Streptococcus pneumoniae	—	10319
Streptococcus pyogenes	—	8198
Vibrio fluvialis	—	11218

Conductivity is the best method to detect impurities; the water for culture media must read <10 microsiemens.

3.3.2 Balances

Balances for commercial media should be accurate to 0.1 g and the preparation of in-house media 0.1 mg. They must be checked daily at each end of the weighing scale, using standard weights.

3.3.3 Mixing

Water must be measured separately from the powder, i.e. one-third of the volume is added and allowed to soak for 10 minutes, and mixed well before adding the remainder.

3.3.4 Heating

Use the least heat for the least time; if sporing bacteria will not grow on a medium it does not need autoclaving.

3.3.5 Pouring

Agar media must be cooled to 47 °C before pouring to prevent evaporation and subsequent loss of volume and concentration of selective agents. Plastic tubing

319

Table 4 Suggested quality control organisms for daily control of media

Medium	Incubation conditions[a]	Test organism	Expected result
Blood agar bases	37 °C in O_2	Str. pyogenes	Good growth, β-haemolysis
		Str. pneumoniae	Good growth
CLED (Sandy's or Bevis)	37 °C in O_2	Staph. aureus	Good growth and distinction
		Str. faecalis	
		E. coli	Typical colony lactose +ve
		Pr. mirabilis	No swarming. Blue
Hoyles medium	37 °C in O_2	C. diphtheriae (non-toxinogenic)	Typical colonies
		Staph. aureus	No growth
MacConkey agar No. 2	37 °C in O_2	E. coli	Typical pink colonies
		Pr. mirabilis	Pale colonies, no swarming
		Staph. aureus	Pink colonies, good growth
		Str. faecalis	Deep red colonies, good growth
Mannitol salt	37 °C in O_2	Staph. aureus	Good growth, yellow colonies
		E. coli	No growth
Sabouraud agars[b]	37 °C in O_2	Cand. albicans	Good growth
		E. coli	Poor growth
TCBS	37 °C in O_2	Vibrio Group F	Typical yellow colonies
		Pr. mirabilis	No growth
Sensitivity test agar	37 °C in O_2	Staph. aureus	Sensitive to: trimethoprim, sulfonamide,
		NCTC 6571	tetracycline, nitrofurantoin, gentamicin.
		Ps. aeruginosa	Sensitive to: gentamicin, colistin,
		NCTC 10662	ceftazidime.
		E. coli	Sensitive to: trimethoprim, sulfonamide,
		NCTC 10418	ampicillin, nitrofurantoin, cephalexin. Look for good growth and adequate and reproducible zone sizes which should be recorded.
Selective media for Neisseria gonorrhoeae	37 °C in CO_2	Cand. albicans	No growth
		Staph. aureus	No growth
		Proteus spp. (trimethoprim-sensitive)	No growth
		Ps. aeruginosa	No growth
		N. gonorrhoeae	Good growth, small colonies
Chocolate agar	37 °C in 10% CO_2	H. influenzae	Good growth
DNase agar[c]	30 °C in O_2	Staph. epidermidis	Negative after adding N HCl
		Staph. aureus	Positive after adding N HCl

Table 4 (*Continued*)

Medium	Incubation conditions[a]	Test organism	Expected result
Campylobacter medium	44 °C in 6% O_2 (Skirrow) 37 °C in 6% O_2 (blood-free)	*C. jejuni* *Staph. aureus* *E. coli*	Good growth No growth No growth
Gentamicin or neomycin blood agar	37 °C, no O_2 10% CO_2	*B. fragilis* *E. coli*	Good growth No growth
Nalidixic acid		*Staph. aureus*	Good growth
Tween blood agar			

[a] All media are incubated for 18 h at 37 °C.

[b] Medium should not be dark; gel must be firm. Chloramphenicol should be added to make it more selective.

[c] Very few false positive results are found following incubation at 30 °C.

used for pouring selective media should be identified with coloured tape. This is particularly essential with media containing antibiotics, which will be absorbed into the tube and will leach out into the next batch of media.

3.3.6 Drying

Plates should be dried by leaving inverted overnight in a laminar flow cabinet protected from direct sunlight.

3.3.7 Poured plates

Plates should be stored at 4 °C ± 2 °C. If they are purchased commercially the manufacturer should give an indication of use-by date. If poured in-house most non-selective plates will keep for up to 10 days, though some culture plates which are being produced semi-commercially by the Public Health Laboratory Service have been given a shelf-life of up to six months! This type of extension of shelf-life is only permissible after trials showing that there has been no deterioration of performance.

4 Maintenance and storage of control organisms

The two conflicting requirements of a storage system are:

(a) The long-term preservation of organisms in conditions which will maintain their characteristics.

(b) Ready access to the organisms for day-to-day use.

4.1 Long-term storage

Freeze-drying is perhaps still the best, though the most tedious, technique for long-term storage.

321

This technique has been described in detail many times elsewhere (19). The most common technique in use is the bead technique which can be purchased as a kit from Technical Service Consultants Ltd. Storage is best carried out at $-76\,^{\circ}$C to ensure the survival of most bacteria. A lower temperature can be used, but certain bacteria may not survive including *N. meningitidis*, *N. gonnorhoeae*, *H. influenzae*, and *Campylobacter* spp.

Other approaches include the gelatin disc method of Stamp (19), the paper strip method of Hawkey *et al.* (20) and the bead system of Feltham *et al.* (21). These methods all require the purchase of expensive equipment such as $-70\,^{\circ}$C freezers or freeze-dryers, or are tedious (gelatin disc).

4.2 Short-term storage for ready access

For day-to-day use for QC of media and as controls for diagnostic tests and susceptibility testing organisms need to be in a readily accessible form such as in broth, or on agar plates, or slopes. To prevent strains from losing their characteristics fresh subcultures should be taken from long-term storage at $-76\,^{\circ}$C (e.g. on beads) on a bi-monthly basis. They can then be subcultured on a weekly basis onto plates or slopes kept on the bench at room temperature (14). Prior to use their performance should be checked. Pneumococci, particularly, are known to lose sensitivity to optochin.

It has been suggested that polystyrene beads may be better for some species such as *Legionella* which can be kept at $4\,^{\circ}$C and subcultured on a weekly basis. Anaerobes and *Campylobacter* spp. can be maintained for a short time in cooked meat broths if kept at $37\,^{\circ}$C. *Neisseria* spp. and *Haemophilus* spp. need to be kept on chocolate agar in an atmosphere of 5% CO_2.

5 Equipment monitoring

The monitoring of equipment is part of the HACCP system in industry as part of ISO 9000. An EOP would be produced and each member of staff using the equipment would be required to keep a training record for it. Similar systems are in use in clinical laboratories in compliance with CPA standards. Equipment in use in clinical microbiology laboratories, such as automatic machinery for carrying out antibiotic estimations, must be monitored according to manufacturers' instructions, but one essential, common to all equipment is the need for cleanliness and a knowledge of decontamination techniques. This is particularly important when analysing blood products with the ever present danger of contamination with blood-borne viruses.

5.1 Temperature control

All temperature-controlled equipment should have a separate means of temperature reading in addition to that supplied by manufacturers. Instruments such as maximum and minimum thermometers can be screwed into or stuck with Araldite® on to the inside of refrigerators or incubators by the user. Uniformity of temperature within an incubator should also be monitored. Multiple temperature monitoring can be carried out using thermocouples connected to an electronic thermometer via a switching mechanism and the results recorded on a chart recorder (Comark Electronics). Comark also supplies data loggers which can hold information or download it to a central computer which can highlight variations from the acceptable. Another useful method is to use an infrared thermometer (Fisher Scientific) which can be used for measuring the temperature of sterilized agars before adding blood or antibiotics.

As with any aspect of quality control, monitoring is useless unless someone reads the instruments, records the results, understands all the implications, and takes action accordingly. A Senior or Chief Biomedical Scientist should have clear responsibility for supervising this duty. It should be instilled into staff that thermometers are to be read automatically every time they open the door of the incubator or fridge.

5.2 Control of anaerobic cabinets

Testing for the presence of oxygen in the chamber can be carried out using indicator strips, these should be changed every day as described in the Wadsworth Manual (9). A cheaper method is to open in the cabinet a tube of thioglycollate broth which contains resazurin indicator and cover it loosely with foil; if it goes pink oxygen is present. Biological indicators can also be used, but they only give retrospective indication that a problem has occurred. A suitable organism is *C. haemolyticum*. *Ps. aeruginosa* will grow on blood media in very low levels of oxygen; CLED would be a better medium to use with this organism as an anaerobic control. Desiccants and catalysts should be regenerated regularly, the frequency varying with the type of cabinet. In some cabinets the catalyst needs to be changed only after 12 months (Russkin) which gives a considerable saving of time and money. When necessary cabinets should be decontaminated with a disinfectant such as Virkon which does not affect the acrylic surfaces. Catalysts may have to be removed before decontaminating cabinets. If in doubt consult the manufacturer.

5.3 pH meter electrodes

The best electrodes for use in microbiology are those such as the Ross Orion 8155SC, which are embedded in resin or, for agar plates, flat-ended like Orion type 450C/B (Fisher Scientific). The flat-end type seem often to give results at variance with those obtained by insertion of the bulb type into the agar. Culture media companies use the results obtained with the bulb type. Between use electrodes should be washed in distilled water and kept in a pH 4 buffer during the day, and in saturated KCl solution overnight, to prevent the growth of contaminants. The pH meter needs to be checked *every time it is used*, using two buffers, pH 7 and pH 4. Colour-coded buffers work well and contain a preservative (BDH Ltd.). If a setting of pH 4 cannot be attained the electrode should be immersed in a solution of pepsin overnight (approx. 2 mg pepsin in 20 ml of 1 M HCl), then washed well in distilled water before recalibration. The meter should also be fitted with a thermistor to compensate automatically for temperature variation within the electrode. However, this does not compensate for the variation in pH which occurs due to heating. The medium must be cooled to room temperature before taking the reading. Reading the pH before autoclaving or sterilizing is pointless as the value will drop unpredictably after heating. It should be noted that pH values shown on media formulations for all manufacturers are the pH values at 20 °C.

5.4 Autoclaves and preparators

Laboratory autoclaves have undergone considerable changes from the original simple downward displacement machines with inlet valve and exhaust valve, and no electronics to go wrong! The best autoclaves now in use are extremely complex machines often incorporating pulsed evacuation, air ballasting, condensate containment, and fully automatic cycles. They cost little more than standard machines, rarely block, and should conform to possible future legislation and new working practices, including those in maintenance departments regarding 'permission to work certificates'. This is important in view of the report that older autoclave exhausts can become contaminated with organisms from the chamber, making these regulations difficult to comply with (22). However, these new autoclaves require considerable maintenance and quality control.

Commissioning new machines in the laboratory with the manufacturers present should be part of the task of the microbiologist. The types of loads and vessels the department will use in day-to-day working should be used in the commissioning tests. The tests should not be based on another laboratory's experience of how they run their autoclaves. In this way, automatic cycles, especially the culture media cycles, can be set for loads relevant to the laboratory. They must be controlled using a 'floating' thermocouple placed inside a flask or bottle containing the same material as the rest of the load, in the centre of the load, and not in a 'standard' bottle as found in many pharmacy autoclaves. The slow heating of agar-containing media makes this precaution imperative if good results are to be obtained.

Autoclaves have been superseded by agar preparators for the production of agar plates. Most media manufacturers would recommend that volumes of not more than 1–2 litres are sterilized by autoclaving; larger volumes being prepared in preparators. Routine QC of the finished media should check the performance of these instruments. If problems of sterility occur the tubing used to pump out the media should be investigated first as it is difficult to sterilize and easy to contaminate. After sterilization it may come out of the autoclave wet and, if not dried immediately, could start to grow any bacteria which have found their way into the packaging. If the tube is kept above 56 °C in an incubator or drying cabinet most bacteria will not grow.

Laboratories involved with the United Kingdom Assessment Scheme (UKAS) must have the temperature and pressure controls checked on an annual basis.

5.5 Pipettes

Automatic pipettes in the media room and throughout the laboratory should be checked monthly. This can most easily be done by weighing replicate amounts on a balance accurate to three decimal places. If there is any deviation from the original specification of the pipette it should be stripped, lubricated, and re-checked.

6 Quality control of laboratory tests and reagents

6.1 Chemicals and dyes

It cannot be assumed that the quality of commercially produced chemicals used in 'in-house' formulations is adequate for use in microbiological procedures. They do not have microbiological specifications. Chemicals and dyes are used in vast quantities in industry whereas their use in microbiology is comparatively small. Although a chemical is 99.9% pure it may contain enough inhibitory substance to eliminate all bacteria. Examples of this have included a batch of A.R. glucose which inhibited all staphylococci and one of sodium citrate which inhibited all salmonellae. Both chemicals met 'manufacturing specification'. The only chemicals which can be used with confidence are those labelled 'bacteriology tested' or as in the Sigma catalogue, 'used in cell culture'. If a new dye or chemical is to be used in any procedure it must be tested by substitution in a formula against a chemical of known characteristics.

Dyes have many synonyms and are sold by suppliers as OEM products; i.e. not produced by them but labelled by them which has led to mislabelling (23).

6.2 Staining techniques

Staining techniques can give misleading results either when the stains do not give correct reactions, or if the stains themselves become contaminated with organisms. Gram stains, especially crystal violet, can become contaminated with *Pseudomonas* spp., which will adhere to films, such as smears of CSF or blood, causing false results to be reported (24). The source of these organisms is often the deionized water used to make up the stains. These problems may be avoided by making small batches from concentrated stains and by ensuring that deionized water is used while fresh and is not allowed to stand around in large containers for long periods. Similar problems have occurred with contamination of water by saprophytic mycobacteria and false results have been reported in Ziehl–Neelson stains (25).

6.3 Kits and identification systems

It is expensive and unnecessary to quality control most identification systems on a regular basis. Sometimes, however, either on receipt of a new batch, or if there is some doubt about results, a suitable set of organisms needs to be used. Some companies such as API System S.A. give details of suitable quality control organisms as part of their instructions for use. These organisms can be valuable for other quality control work. It must be borne in mind, however, that certain manufacturers use different enzyme substrates to test for the same enzyme, and this can lead to problems of interpretation (26).

All kits and reagents must be stored according to manufacturers' instructions and used by the expiry date. A record should be kept of the date when each batch/lot number is opened so that an audit trail will always be able to trace a particular reagent used on a particular patient sample.

6.4 United Kingdom National External Quality Assessment Scheme (UKNEQAS)

This scheme, organized by the PHLS Division of Microbiological Reagents and Quality Control (DMRQC), is an exercise not so much in quality control but in comparing the results obtained from various laboratories in the UK and now in many parts of the world. This type of assessment is likely to be effective only if the QC sample is investigated in precisely the same way as any other clinical sample. In many laboratories, however, the investigation is carried out by the most senior Biomedical Scientist and bears little relation to routine procedures. A major advantage of the scheme as a training exercise lies in its supply of rare pathogens or bacteria which are notoriously difficult to grow or identify. DMRQC has a unique opportunity to compare the results of different methods. Laboratories which consistently perform badly are offered help confidentially.

As almost all laboratories in the UK participate it is now a requirement for CPA accreditation. Similar schemes exist in the USA, such as the Quality Assurance Service of the College of American Pathologists.

6.5 Internal quality control

Standard operating procedures should include procedures for both external quality assessment through NEQAS and internal assessment.

These internal measures can include simulated specimens (similar to NEQAS) from previously frozen clinical isolates that have proved difficult in order to monitor improvements in performance. They can also be used when training staff. Other measures can include duplication of patient samples processed by different staff members, and duplicate reading of Gram films and urine microscopies. Potential new methods should also be thoroughly tested in duplicate with the existing ones before their introduction, to ensure that quality is maintained.

Daily quality control should be a part of all routine diagnostic procedures. Identification tests such as DNase, coagulase, should incorporate positive and negative control strains. Antibiotic susceptibility testing should follow recommended guidelines using control strains of known minimum inhibitory concentration. The control organisms used for laboratory tests will in many cases be different from those used to test media.

Serological tests and immunoassays should always incorporate internal QC samples on every run. The results of these can be evaluated using a Shewhart plot (27, 28) to show any values outside the accepted standard deviation. Westgard rules (29), which define specific performance limits, can then be applied to detect both random and systematic errors.

A recent publication from the Public Health Laboratory Service on Quality Assurance gives extensive information on most of the issues discussed above (30).

7 Near patient testing

Near patient testing (NPT) is the term for any analytical process performed for, or by, a patient outside the traditional clinical laboratory. Advances in technology have led to the development of instruments and kits designed for use in this role and which are able to provide an increasing range of tests including those previously confined to a microbiology laboratory.

The IBMS has issued guidelines on NPT to supplement those issued by the Joint Working Group on Quality Assurance (31) which CPA (UK) Ltd. endorses and requires for accreditation. Even in NPT it is clear that the laboratory has a crucial role to play.

8 Audit and error logging

Quality assurance evaluation includes continuing audit of the service provided. CPA accredited laboratories are required to check regularly that they meet quality performance targets and that these audit activities are documented.

For any specimen an audit trail should be able to establish its turn around time, internal quality control testing, batch and lot numbers of media and reagents used, personnel involved in processing and authorization, and consumer satisfaction.

Linked in with audit are risk management and error logging. Risk management is an essential part of good practice in clinical laboratories. Improvements are always possible.

It is important to establish a 'no blame' culture in which staff are encouraged to report incidents which have led to, or could have led to an incorrect result being reported. In this way changes can often be made to a system to minimize human errors and prevent them from recurring. Once a change has been made, the process can be re-audited to monitor improvement. Any such changes, if permanently adopted, will require the updating of relevant SOPs, staff training, and possibly informing the users.

9 Conclusions

The importance of quality control and assurance is seen in every aspect of the work of the clinical laboratory. It is perhaps even more important in the microbiology department because of the subjective nature of the observations which form the basis of the result.

It is even more important in this situation to apply control wherever possible to ensure consistency of the methods. Results have been shown to be influenced by many factors from the recruitment of staff to the validation of the report. All laboratories are under pressure, but this should not be an excuse for cutting corners. The use of HACCP systems within the SOPs can give a great deal of control over the work of the laboratory and the quality of the results.

Acknowledgement

We would like to thank Dr I. Crawford for reviewing the text of this chapter.

References

1. European Committee for Clinical Laboratory Standards. (1985). Part 2: *Internal quality control in microbiology*, Vol. 2, No. 4. ECCLS, Lund.
2. Collins English Dictionary. (1991). 3rd edn. Harper Collins, Glasgow.
3. Clinical Pathology Accreditation (UK) Ltd. Version 7.0 July 1999.
4. Institute of Biomedical Sciences. IBMS Guidelines.
5. Fox, M., Ward, K., and Kirby, J. (1992). *Gazette of the institute of biomedical sciences*, p. 412. August.
6. Control of Substances Hazardous to Health Regulations. (1997). Biological Agents ACOP. HMSO Stationery Office, Norwich.
7. Stuart, R. D. (1959). *Public Health Rep.*, **74**, 431.
8. Amies, C. R. (1967). *Can. J. Public Health*, **58**, 296.
9. Summanen, P. *et al.* (ed.) (1993). *Wadsworth anaerobic bacteriology manual*. Star Publishing, California.
10. Roelofsen, E., van Leeuwen, M., Meijer-Severs, G. J., Wilkinson, M. H. F., *et al.* (1999). *Clin. Microbiol.*, **37**, 3041.
11. Hill, G. (1978). *J. Clin. Microbiol.*, **6**, 680.
12. Stumbo, C. R. (1973). *Thermobacteriology in food processing*, 2nd edn. Academic Press, New York.
13. Mortimore, S. and Wallace, C. (ed.) (1998). *HACCP A practical approach*. Aspen Publications.
14. Bolton, F. J. (1998). *Int. J. Food Microbiol.*, **45**, 11.
15. (1999). *In vitro medical devices, culture media for microbiology. Performance criteria for culture media*. BS EN 12322.
16. www.nccls.org (1996). *Quality assurance of prepared microbiological culture media*, 2nd edn. Approved Standard.
17. Mossel, D. A. A., Van Rossem, F., Koopmans, M., Hendriks, M., *et al.* (1980). *J. Appl. Bacteriol.*, **49**, 439.
18. Kirsop, B. E. and Doyle, A. (ed.) (1991). *Maintenance of microorganisms and cultured cells*. Academic Press.
19. Stamp, Lord. (1947). *J. Gen. Microbiol.*, **1**, 251.
20. Hawkey, P. M., Bennett, P. M., and Hawkey, C. A. (1984). *J. Med. Microbiol.*, **18**, 277.
21. Feltham, R. K. A., Power, A. K., Pell, P. A., and Sneath, P. H. A. (1978). *J. Appl. Bacteriol.*, **44**, 313.
22. Scruton, M. W. (1986). *Hosp. Eng.*, **40**, 24.
23. Gadsdon, D. R. (1986). *Med. Lab. Sci.*, **43**, Suppl. 1, S77.
24. Walsh, D. M. and Eberiel, D. T. (1986). *J. Clin. Microbiol.*, **23**, 962.
25. Collins, C. H. and Yates, M. D. (1979). *Inst. Med. Lab. Sci. Gaz.*, 578.
26. Heltberg, O., Busk, H. E., Bremmelgaard, A., Kristiansen, J. E., *et al.* (1984). *Eur. J. Clin. Microbiol.*, **3**, 241.
27. Levey, S. and Jennings, E. R. (1950). *Am. J. Clin. Pathol.*, **20**, 1059.

28. Westgard, J. O., Barry, P. L., Hunt, M. R., and Groth, T. A. (1981). *Clin. Chem.*, **27**, 493.
29. Westgard, J. O., Groth, T. O., Aronsson, T., Falk, H., *et al.* (1977). *Clin. Chem.*, **23**, 1857.
30. Snell, J. J. S., Brown, D. F. J., and Roberts, C. (ed.) (1999). *Quality assurance: principles and practice in the microbiology laboratory.* Public Health Laboratory Service, London.
31. Joint Working Group on Quality Assurance. (1992). *Guideline on the control of NPT and procedures performed on patients by non-pathology staff.* JWGQA, Diagnostic Services Ltd. Mast House, Derby Road, Liverpool L20 1EA.

Chapter 11

Laboratory investigation of health care-associated infection

Peter M. Hawkey

Public Health Laboratory, Birmingham Heartlands Hospital,
Birmingham B9 5SS, UK.

Kevin G. Kerr

Department of Microbiology, University of Leeds,
Leeds LS2 9JT, UK.

1 Introduction

Whilst most hospital microbiology laboratories are very busy processing the large numbers of specimens detailed in the previous chapters, they will also be required periodically to investigate and direct the control of episodes of cross-infection. Although this chapter will concentrate on hospital-acquired infection (nosocomial infection), it is increasingly recognized that the infections previously regarded as typically nosocomial in origin, such as those caused by methicillin-resistant *Staphylococcus aureus*, may emerge, and be transmitted, in the community. Indeed the UK Department of Health Report *Getting ahead of the curve* (1) suggests that terms such as nosocomial infection are misleading and that 'health care-associated' infection is a more appropriate term.

In future, it is likely that hospital laboratories in the UK will become more involved with community cross-infection problems with the demise of the Public Health Laboratory Service in its present form.

Most of the techniques described here will be suitable for use in community outbreaks but some may require different application and interpretation. The techniques for the isolation and identification of organisms responsible for diseases which predominantly cause problems in the community are dealt with under the appropriate sections elsewhere in this book (bacterial meningitis, Chapter 2, Section 3; diphtheria, Chapter 3, Section 2.3; food poisoning, Chapter 6; cholera, Chapter 6, Section 5.3). Although the microbiology of food and water is of little interest to laboratories dealing exclusively with specimens from hospital patients, it may on occasions be necessary for those laboratories to examine such specimens. This chapter will not give specific methods but rather refer the reader to specialist publications on water (2) and food (3). At present in the UK, Public Health Laboratories can also offer assistance and advice, but with the establishment of the Health Protection Agency (http://www.hpa.org.uk/), these arrangements are set to change.

The investigation of suspected nosocomial infection must be undertaken in a logical and unbiased fashion, not by hasty assumptions of the nature of sources and routes of transmission. Details of an approach to the investigation of a suspected outbreak which will allow sound epidemiological and statistical analysis are given elsewhere (Chapter 12, Section 5). In the end it is the aim of every investigation to identify the source(s), the mode(s) of transmission, and the portal of entry into the patient.

1.1 Administration

No description of the role of the laboratory in the investigation of nosocomial infection would be complete without a system for the administration of the control of nosocomial infection. In the UK official guidelines for the management and control of hospital infection have been updated (4). Administrative arrangements in the USA differ slightly from the UK, mainly as a result of the lack of an equivalent to the clinical microbiologist, that role being taken by a hospital epidemiologist in the USA. In the US, the Joint Commission on the Accreditation of Healthcare Organizations (JCAHO: www.jcaho.org), as part of its hospital accreditation standards gives guidance on the key elements of infection control programmes, but allows hospitals some leeway in designing their own programs. In both countries the major decision making body is the Infection Control Committee (ICC), and practical support is provided by the Infection Control Practitioner (nurse) (ICN), both of whom have direct equivalents in the UK system.

In the UK the Infection Control Doctor (ICD) is an important member of the Infection Control Team (ICT), who provides leadership for the team. The post should be held by the Consultant Microbiologist who will be in a position to command respect from clinical colleagues and therefore be able to advise and lead the ICT and advise the Health Authority and Hospital and Primary Care Trusts in the control of hospital infection. The ICD will ensure that the policy made by the Control of Infection Committee is put into action. In some hospitals the ICN will be a Biomedical Scientist, in which case that individual will need to be sensitive to the needs and problems of the nursing staff.

The ICT will therefore consist of the ICD, ICN, Consultant Microbiologist (if not already the ICD), and a representative of management, who need not liaise on a day-to-day basis. Should an episode of cross-infection be identified, then the ICT may decide to deal with it themselves or, if it is a major problem, expand the ICT to an action group (AG). The AG is the ICT plus relevant clinicians, a senior nurse, and a Consultant in Communicable Disease Control. The AG will ensure that all steps to control the outbreak are taken, communicate with all affected groups, prepare a report for the ICC (ideally within 48 hours), review progress, and finally analyse the outbreak, making recommendations for prevention of future occurrences.

The Infection Control Committee will consist of the ICD, ICN, the Trust Chief Executive (or deputy), Consultant in Communicable Disease Control, and representatives from Clinical Governance and Clinical Risk Management Committees, as well as representatives of senior medical and nursing staff, including occupational health. The ICC may also co-opt or invite representatives from any other section of the hospital administration particularly from hotel services, pharmacy, engineering services, and operating theatres, as well as outside parties such as a senior Environmental Health Officer. It should meet at least four times annually to advise the Trust and formulate policies and programmes including audits

2 Sample collection

2.1 Surveillance

Surveillance as applied to nosocomial infection is an ill-defined term which implies some degree of effectiveness in the control of nosocomial infection. There is very little evidence to suggest that extensive ward-based surveillance programmes reduce significantly nosocomial infection rates. Haley (5) coined the term 'surveillance by objective' in which ICTs select high priority nosocomial infection problems and target these using specific surveillance strategies.

Laboratory-based surveillance is a valuable complement to these formal surveillance programmes. This is achieved by a visit from the ICN to the microbiology laboratory every morning to identify isolates of bacteria likely to be of importance in causing nosocomial infection. This work can be reduced if the laboratory uses a computer-based reporting system as infection control programs are often available (Chapter 9). If this surveillance is backed-up by frequent visits to the wards and discussion with ward staff, existing and undiscovered episodes of nosocomial infection will be brought to light for the ICT to consider.

It may be appropriate sometimes to carry out limited surveys of the prevalence of particular nosocomial infections, but these should always have a purpose, such as the discovery of an occult source.

A marked increase in the isolation rate of a bacterium usually indicates a problem of cross-infection, although obviously an increase in the prevalence in the community may lead to increased admissions to hospital. It must also be remembered that pseudo-outbreaks of infection occur from time to time. Pseudo-outbreaks are often suggested by an upsurge in recovery of unusual environmental Gram-negative bacteria or atypical mycobacteria from patient specimens. They may arise from contaminated anticoagulants being introduced into blood cultures via splashes (see Chapter 2). Others may result from contamination of irrigation or disinfectant solutions or because of poor cleaning of endoscopes (6) or unusual methods of specimen collection, such as a pseudo-outbreak of *Pseudomonas aeruginosa* infection on a haematology unit (7). On investigation, it was discovered that some personnel were retrieving stool specimens for surveillance cultures from lavatory pans.

Routine monitoring of the environment by culture is *not* indicated, except during the investigation of an outbreak. Evidence collected in the USA suggests that, although many fewer unnecessary environmental cultures are now taken, there is still room for further reduction (8).

2.2 Sampling protocols

2.2.1 Patients and staff

With the possible exception of patients on high-risk wards, such as neonatal and adult intensive-care units, there is no value in performing routine surveillance cultures on patients. Some laboratories may wish to survey patients on intensive-care units for the carriage of gentamicin-resistant coliforms, *P. aeruginosa*, *S. aureus* (including MRSA where it is thought to be a problem on adjoining wards). Coliforms and *P. aeruginosa* are best detected using rectal swabs, staphylococci by nasal swabs and/or perineal swabs plated on to appropriate selective media, see Table 1. Suggested guidelines for the prevention of MRSA infection in hospitals, including screening protocols, in the UK have been published (9). It should be borne in mind that the information gained from these cultures is unlikely to benefit the individual patient, so it should be regarded as a measure of the level of cross-infection in that unit.

Sampling of patients during outbreaks will be determined by the bacterium involved. Screening of patients on a regular basis (at least on admission and one or two times per week) at the most likely carriage site(s) will identify asymptomatic carriers and give an accurate picture of the spread of the organism which will assist in epidemiological investigations.

Screening of staff for nosocomial bacteria is an emotive subject and should not be undertaken unless there are likely to be tangible benefits to the patients and the action to be taken with those members of staff that are colonized is clear. It is, however, sometimes valuable to take hand-impression plates whilst investigating an outbreak of nosocomial infection. Two purposes will be served; first, a common potential route of cross-infection for many nosocomial bacteria will be identified, and secondly, the nursing and medical staff will be reminded of the importance of hand-washing (10).

2.2.2 Therapeutic substances

The microbiologist investigating an episode of nosocomial infection where the suspected mode of transmission of the bacteria is *via* a therapeutic substance is usually presented with a bewildering array of possibilities. The degree of sterility deemed appropriate for each type of substance ranges from the absolute in intravenous fluids to the relative in liquidized enteral feeds.

Whilst it is a cardinal rule that the sterility of no substance should be assumed, it is often appropriate to examine the non-sterile or easily contaminated sterile

Table 1 Suggested selective and differential media for the isolation of commonly occurring nosocomial bacteria

Bacterium	Medium	Commercial supplier[a]	Components and principle
Staphylococcus aureus	Mannitol salt agar (MSA)	B, D, G, L, O	7.5% NaCl inhibits bacteria other than most staphylococci, *S. aureus* usually ferments mannitol (yellow colonies), sometimes after 48 h. May not grow all strains of *S. aureus*. Coagulase tests performed directly from medium may give erroneous results. 'Third-generation' coagulase tests such *Staphytec Dry Spot Plus* (Oxoid) give better results.
S. aureus (methicillin resistant, MRSA)	MSA + 4 mg/litre methicillin[b] Blood agar + 4 mg/litre methicillin[b] Salt, phenolphthalein, methicillin agar (SPMA)[b,c] (17)		May not support growth of all MRSA strains. MRSA may be overgrown but all strains will grow. 5% salt, less inhibitory than MSA, not all *S. aureus* phosphatase positive (sodium phenolphthalein diphosphate split to give free phenolphthalein detected by exposure to NH$_3$, pink colour). There are also a range of commercially available media including ORSAB (Oxoid) and CHROMagar (M-Tech).
S. aureus (glycopeptide intermediately susceptible, GISA)			At present there is no selective differential agar for VISA, however, the presence of VISA may be suggested by subculturing suspect colonies to blood heart infusion agar plates supplemented with 6 mg/litre vancomycin, with a heavy inoculum and incubation for 24 h.
Streptococcus spp. and *Staphylococcus* spp.	Azide blood agar	B, D, G, O	5% NaCl and 0.2% NaN$_3$ inhibit most organisms except *Streptococcus* spp. and *Staphylococcus* spp. (although not all strains of the latter may grow). *Proteus* spp. are less susceptible to azide than other Gram-negatives and breakthrough growth may occur, although swarming is inhibited.
Streptococcus spp., including Lancefield gp A	Colistin, oxolinic acid, blood agar (COBA) (18)	L, O	Colistin 10 mg/litre and oxolinic acid 3 mg/litre provide good selection for streptococci, blood adds nutrients and provides indication of haemolysis.

Table 1 (Continued)

Bacterium	Medium	Commercial supplier[a]	Components and principle
Lancefield gp B streptococci	Granada medium[d] (19)		Trimethoprim is not only a selective agent but also stimulates production of red pigmentation. This is a property of folate inhibitors (some commercial preparations have included methotrexate). Pigment production may also be enhanced by placing a disc of a sulfonamide directly onto the plate where growth is expected to be reasonably heavy. Pigment production is also maximized by incubating anaerobically. A few strains of group B streptococci do not produce pigment and anaerobic atmosphere ensures red pigment production.
Enterococci	Kanamycin, aesculin, azide agar (20)	O	Developed for foods, but useful if enterococci thought to be causing nosocomial infection. Kanamycin and azide selective agents, enterococci hydrolyse aesculin causing black precipitate around colonies.
Vancomycin-resistant enterococci	Modified Lewisham medium (21)		Horse blood agar with vancomycin, aztreonam, and amphotericin B as selective agents. There is still no consensus on the best medium for the isolation of GRE from contaminated material, indeed there is no agreement on the optimum vancomycin concentration. Some authors report that recovery rates are increased by using an enrichment culture before plating to solid media (22). Commercially-prepared media are also available. Some contain meropenem as a selective agent—this may inhibit strains of *E. faecalis*.
Clostridium difficile	Cycloserine-cefoxitin agar[d] (23)	D, G, O	Characteristically green/yellow fluorescent colonies seen under long wave (360 nm) UV light, smelling of *p*-cresol. Gram stain morphology may be atypical if performed on colonies from this medium. Alcohol treatment of specimen before plating increases recovery. Lysozyme and taurocholate may also encourage spore germination. A commercially available medium (Oxoid) containing norfloxacin, moxalactam, and cysteine hydrochloride may be more selective than CCA and may increase recovery of *C. difficile*.

Organism	Media	Notes
Listeria monocytogenes	Oxford agar (24)	There are a large number of media for *Listeria* spp., mainly designed for isolation of these bacteria from foodstuffs. Several have been used in clinical microbiology. The selective components in Oxford agar are lithium chloride, cycloheximide, or amphotericin B, acriflavine, colistin, cefotetan, and fosfomycin. Aesculin and ferric ammonium citrate are differential agents with *Listeria* species growing as colonies with black halo. Recovery of low numbers of bacteria is enhanced by enrichment broth media. Enterococci also grow on this medium and hydrolyse aesculin. Diffusion of black aesculetin pigment into surrounding medium can be overcome by substituting cyclohexenoesculetin-β-d-glucoside/ferrous gluconate for aesculin/ferric ammonium citrate.
Klebsiella spp.	MacConkey, inositol, carbenicillin[c] agar (MICA) (25) with pre-enrichment in Koser's citrate broth	Few species of the Enterobacteriaceae ferment inositol, *Klebsiellae* do so and appear as pink colonies, 10 mg/litre Koser's citrate broth will increase recovery of small numbers.
Serratia marcescens	Deoxyribonuclease, toluidine blue,[c] cefalothin agar (DTBCA) (26)	Most Gram-negative bacilli are DNase negative, *Serratia* is usually positive and is routinely resistant to cefalothin (cefradine or cefazolin may be substituted). Toluidine blue is a metachromatic dye which is pink in the presence free nucleotides and blue with intact DNA.
Enterobacter spp.	Deoxycholate citrate, cystal violet, cefazolin, rhamnose[c] agar (DCCR) (27)	Not all Enterobacteriaceae ferment rhamnose, all species of *Enterobacter*, except a few strain of *E. agglomerans*, do. Cefazolin, crystal violet, and DCA are selective agents.
Proteus spp., *Providencia* spp., and *Morganella* spp.	*Proteeae* identification[c] medium (PIM)(28)	Medium contains tryptophan which *Proteeae* degrade to a brown melanin-like pigment, they also degrade the fine crystals of tyrosine in the medium producing clear zones around brown colonies. Clindamycin 5 mg/litre of colistin inhibit most Gram-negative bacteria. (N.B. 10% of *Proteeae* also inhibited.)

Table 1 (*Continued*)

Bacterium	Medium	Commercial supplier[a]	Components and principle
Pseudomonas aeruginosa	Nalidixic acid, cetrimide agar[c] (29) (various commercial formulations)	B, D, G, L, O	Cetrimide 300 mg/litre in original formulation supports the growth of many bacteria, however the addition of nalidixic acid (15 mg/litre after sterilization) and 200 mg/litre cetrimide provides a more selective agar. *P. aeruginosa* produces a blue/green pigmentation (pyocyanin), yellow fluorescence under UV light (fluorescein), and rarely pink/maroon pigment (pyorubin). Further tests needed to confirm identity.
	Phenanthroline, C-390[c] agar (PCA) (30)		Columbia blood agar supplemented with phenanthroline and C-390 (see Appendix II) is highly selective for *P. aeruginosa*, no other Gram +ve or −ve bacteria growing on the medium (30).
Pseudomonas spp. (other than *aeruginosa*)	Pseudomonas C-F-C agar[b] (31)	L, O	Very low concentration of cetrimide 10 mg/litre allows *Pseudomonas* other than *P. aeruginosa* to grow, selection increased with cefaloridine 25 mg/litre and fusidic acid 5 mg/litre.
Acinetobacter spp.	Leeds Acinetobacter medium (LAM)[c] (32)		Contains fructose, mannitol, sucrose, and phenol red and supplemented with cefsulodin, cefradine, and vancomycin. *Acinetobacter* spp. appear as pink colonies against a mauve background. *Stenotrophomonas maltophilia* and *Burkholderia cepacia* (oxidase positive) give colonies of the same colour, but the former produce opaque, flat colonies with a crenated edge, whereas *Acinetobacter* colonies are circular convex and smooth.
Stenotrophomonas maltophilia	Vancomycin, imipenem, amphotericin B agar (VIA)[c] (33)		Selective agar which also contains mannitol and bromothymol blue. *S. maltophilia* does not produce acid from mannitol and colonies are blue/green.
Burkholderia cepacia	BCSA medium (34)		Selective agents are crystal violet polymyxin B, gentamicin, and vancomycin; differential agents are sucrose, lactose, and phenol red. *B. cepacia* colonies appear greenish/brown with a yellow halo. There are a number of other media which are also commercially available, but BCSA is more selective and the bacterium grows faster on the latter.

[a] Commercial suppliers: B, BBL Microbiology Systems; D, Difco; G, Gibco; L, Lab M; O, Oxoid.

[b] Incubate for 48 h at 30 °C in air.

[c] These media are described in detail in Appendix II.

[d] Incubate for 20 h at 37 °C in anaerobic conditions.

products first. In the case of chronic, episodic cases of nosocomial infection, careful use of survey techniques such as case-control and cohort studies will be vital (Chapter 2). The routine sampling of commercially prepared substances labelled as sterile, and the in-use testing of disinfectants and antiseptics is inappropriate.

Solids can be emulsified in a quantity of nutrient broth using a vibrating mixer and then either plated directly or enriched by incubating overnight, followed by plating on a suitable selective and non-selective medium. Cream and oil-based products samples can be vortex mixed in modified Letheen broth (Oxoid) supplemented with 10% (v/v) Tween 80. Subcultures from the enrichment broth can be made to Letheen agar as well as other selective/differential media.

Heavily contaminated fluids can be plated directly on to solid selective media, but it is always useful to have a quantitative count for lightly contaminated fluids to help distinguish chance contamination. Traditionally this was achieved by preparing 10-fold dilutions of the fluid in sterile saline and then dropping duplicate 20 μl drops on to solid media and counting the colony-forming units. This is a time-consuming process; the alternative is vacuum filtration of a known volume of the fluid through a sterile 0.45 μm cellulose ester filter held in a suitable holder, such as the Sterifil Aseptic System (Millipore UK Ltd.). The filter is placed on the surface of a suitable selective agar medium and incubated for 18 hours at 37 °C. This method will allow large numbers of fluids to be processed in a very short time.

2.2.3 Equipment

The method of sampling equipment will be determined by the nature of the equipment. Most sites on equipment can be sampled with a cotton swab soaked in saline or nutrient broth. Containers and the lumens of tubes can be sampled as follows.

(a) Place 10–15 ml of nutrient broth in the article to be examined.

(b) Close by whatever means are available and vigorously agitate for 30 sec.

(c) Pour the nutrient broth out into a sterile container and either filter the whole volume or count an aliquot of the broth using 10-fold dilutions (see Section 2.3.2).

2.2.4 Environment

It is not necessary to routinely sample the environment unless an episode of environmentally derived cross-infection is suspected to have occurred. Quantitative or semi-quantitative sampling of the environment is essential, as comparisons between results can then be made.

The airborne spread of nosocomial bacteria is a comparatively rare event, so routine sampling of air will achieve little. However, if cross-infection is suspected to have occurred, then sampling with settle plates or a more sophisticated mechanical air sampler will be required. Although settle plates are an inexpensive way of enumerating airborne organisms, air turbulence will greatly affect

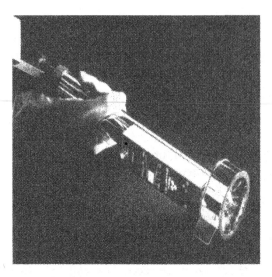

Figure 1 Hand-held Reuter centrifugal air sampler (Biotest RCS, Biotest UK Ltd.). The flexible agar medium strip is contained in the circular housing surrounding the impeller blades from different sites.

sampling. Also, in conditions of low humidity, particles <3 μm will remain suspended and not therefore be collected on a settle plate. Withstanding these limitations, a 9 cm Petri dish exposed for 15 minutes in still air will sample particles from approximately 1 cubic foot (11). Should a more rapid sampling technique, which can also sample from specific points, be required, then the hand-held Reuter centrifugal sampler (Biotest RCS, Biotest UK Ltd.) will fulfil that role (Figure 1). It is a hand-held instrument with a battery-operated electric motor that drives a multi-bladed impeller. Air is captured between the impeller blades and particles deposited by centrifugal force onto a flexible plastic strip containing wells of agar medium around the periphery of the impeller blades. The device performs poorly when sampling particles with a diameter of approximately 1 mm, unlike the cumbersome, noisy Casella slit sampler. The manufacturers' stated sampling rate of 40 litres/min is also an underestimate, 100 litres/min being a more accurate assessment (12). As most airborne bacteria-bearing particles found in hospitals are 4–20 μm in size, the Reuter instrument is the most practical one for routine hospital infection control procedures (13). Although standards for the level of microbial contamination of air have been suggested, they have not been widely adopted because agreement on the correlation of infections with levels of airborne contamination cannot be agreed (14). The best use of air sampling would seem to be during commissioning and servicing of clean areas and the investigation of specific episodes of nosocomial infection.

Whilst floors and other surfaces such as work tops and refrigerator doors are easy to sample, the value of such data is questionable, particularly when undertaken routinely. Smooth surfaces can be sampled using a moistened cotton swab; a sterilized card mask will enable a predetermined area to be sampled, take care to rub in a direction at right angles to the first used. A more precise quantitation of contamination may be obtained using Rodac (*Replicate Organism Direct Agar Contact*) plates, which are small Petri dishes filled with 16.5 ml of a non-selective medium, thus providing a meniscus of medium which protrudes from the dish. The plate is pressed against the dry surface to be sampled and the colonies counted after incubation.

Most water supplies within the hospital will be chlorinated, although it is worth remembering that hot water will lose all if not most of the chlorine present in it before heating. Water (and melted ice) can either be examined for evidence of faecal contamination (2), or, more usefully, in the hospital environment for the presence of nosocomial bacteria. This is most readily achieved by filtering 100 ml of water (less if heavily contaminated) through a 0.45 μm cellulose acetate filter using the technique described in Section 2.3.2 of this chapter. Bacteria, notably *P. aeruginosa*, will sometimes be found growing around tap outlets and in sink water traps. Whilst those in the latter situation are unlikely to be associated with nosocomial infection, tap nozzles can be sampled with a cotton swab. Organisms can be eluted by vortex mixing if a semi-quantitative result is required, otherwise plate the swab directly on to a suitable selective medium.

3 Specimen processing

3.1 Criteria for organism identification

The extent to which isolates of bacteria in a clinical laboratory are identified is always a matter for debate. Whilst a report of 'coliform' is perfectly adequate in an uncomplicated urinary tract infection, patently it is not appropriate for a blood culture isolate. Obviously problems can arise from differences in the level of identification when organism identities are used to collect surveillance data. Failure to sufficiently subdivide isolates may obscure cross-infection caused by a species. In addition, failures in procedures may cause 'pseudo-outbreaks'; if for instance an error occurs in the reading of coagulase tests, then coagulase negative staphylococci will be misreported as *S. aureus* (15). Similarly, pseudo-outbreaks can happen if antimicrobial resistance markers are used to identify clusters of nosocomial infection (16).

In general terms, if an episode of nosocomial infection is suspected, then isolates related to the causes should be as fully identified as possible. If a number of isolates belong to the same species, then some form of further subdivision must be used, such as typing.

3.2 Use of selective and differential media

Once the bacterium suspected of causing nosocomial infection has been identified, it will be necessary to delineate accurately the occurrence of that bacterium. The use of appropriate selective media will ensure that even small numbers of the cross-infecting bacterium will be identified, ensuring that all sources, routes of transmission, and portals of entry are known. It may also identify individuals who may be asymptomatically colonized by an outbreak strain, such as faecal carriers of an epidemic clone of glycopeptide-resistant enterococci. If the suspected epidemic strain is resistant to an antimicrobial to which the species is generally susceptible, then the compound can be incorporated into a suitable medium. It will be necessary to determine the MIC for the strain in question and check that it will grow on media containing the chosen concentration of antimicrobial. Using phenotypic characteristics of the bacterium under investigation, differential media can also be used to enhance its recovery in the laboratory, particularly in specimens which are likely to be heavily contaminated with other bacteria.

If an individual microbiologist has not had direct experience of investigating a particular nosocomial bacterium, then he or she may be uncertain as to the best selective medium. Table 1 gives details of a range of selective and/or differential media of value in the investigation of important nosocomial pathogens. It is particularly important to perform quality control on batches of unfamiliar media before they are used to determine whether they grow the bacterium under investigation.

4 Bacterial typing systems

4.1 Principles and use of bacterial typing systems

Most nosocomial infections are caused by a relatively limited number of bacterial species. This means that identification of bacterial isolates to species level will not allow the detection of cross-infecting strains and hence recognition of their source and route of transmission. Obviously the isolation of two or more epidemiologically related isolates of an unusual serovar such as *Salmonella cubana* strongly suggests cross-infection or a single source; the same cannot be said for two isolates of *Pseudomonas aeruginosa*.

Over the years a large number of different methods of subdividing species of bacteria (typing) have been developed and applied to many different species. No single typing system is perfect, and it is important to appreciate the strengths and weaknesses of the method that is used. An 'ideal' typing system for a bacterial species should perform well when judged by the following criteria.

(a) *Typing ability*. A method should be able to distinguish bacteria which are biologically or genetically similar but not identical, so that an additional method is unnecessary. If a method for example only types 50% of the strains encountered then it is a poor method.

(b) *Discrimination*. A typing method which exhibits a high degree of typability may well only divide the bacteria examined into a very small number of strains. The method would then be regarded as having poor discrimination or sensitivity. A method which exhibits good discrimination should recognize a reasonable number of types which correlate well with other methods and with epidemiological findings.

(c) *Reproducibility*. This is an important characteristic, as a method will be used over a long period of time and in different centres. However, the good performance of a method such as bacteriophage typing in other areas may outweigh a lack of stability. The technical complexity of a method will have a bearing on reproducibility as well as biological variations.

(d) *Applicability*. It is possible to develop a typing system using a laboratory collection of bacteria which has no value when used on clinical isolates of the same bacterial species. A typing method should therefore always be tested in field trials. The method should not be too complicated or expensive, as it will not be used by microbiologists. Centralization in reference laboratories will help improve availability of occasionally used methods.

Judgement should be exercised when deciding whether to type a group of isolates. Some laboratories may choose to type all isolates of bacteria commonly causing nosocomial infection, e.g. *Staphylococcus aureus* and *Pseudomonas aeruginosa*, particularly as methods may be used which can be automated to a certain extent. Smaller laboratories will rely on reference laboratories to carry out their typing so they may choose to be more selective. Good surveillance methods linked to epidemiological studies by infection control personnel would reduce the amount of typing done (see Section 2.1, this chapter).

A brief description of the various typing methods follows. Many of the methods are appropriate to the reference or research laboratory and are therefore not described in detail. The availability of methods for individual species will vary greatly from country to country. The typing methods described in detail here are those that might reasonably be attempted by a moderately large clinical microbiology laboratory.

When typing isolates from sites (such as environmental sources) where a range of subtypes can be expected it will be necessary to type more than one colony of the bacterial species to identify the epidemic strain. Obviously very large numbers of colonies cannot be typed, due to limitations on time and materials. However it should be remembered that if five colonies are typed then there is a 90% probability of detecting two equifrequent types. The probability falls rapidly if more than two types are present (35).

Phenotypic typing techniques.

4.2 Biotyping

Most laboratories now use a disposable, commercially-prepared gallery of biochemical tests to identify important bacterial isolates, such as the API 20E which utilizes 20 different biochemical tests. The use of this method will, therefore, provide a biochemical profile, in which different biotypes may be noticed such as urease positive *Providencia stuartii* or indole negative *Escherichia coli*. However, variations in the inoculum and duration of incubation can affect the results, so methods should be carefully standardized (36). The characters used in biotyping isolates are not always stable and can often be encoded on plasmids which are transferable and sometimes lost from strains, such as urease posi-tive *P. stuartii* (37). Biotyping schemes, specific to individual genera have been developed, e.g. *Acinetobacter* (38) and, although these may be more discriminative than commercially available identification systems, they often require prepa-ration of specialized media, are time-consuming to perform, and may not be suitable if large numbers of isolates are to be examined. Furthermore, biotyp-ing may not be useful, if bacterial species can be divided into only a very small number of types, e.g. *Staphylococcus epidermidis*, which cannot divided into any epidemiologically useful subgroups.

4.3 Antibiogram and resistogram typing

The determination of the pattern of susceptibility of a bacterium to a range of antimicrobial agents has been used many times to type organisms. It has advant-ages, as most laboratories will generate the new data as a by-product of the reporting of routine antimicrobial sensitivities to clinicians. When this informa-tion is handled in a computer (if MICs are used then sensitivity will be improved), then infection control software can 'flag' recurring patterns. Antibiogram typ-ing has no value in comparative studies, as stability (particularly if plasmids are involved) is a problem and because only a small number of agents are likely to give differing results, discrimination may be poor. This is especially true of sev-eral nosocomial pathogens such as enterococci which manifest little variation in antimicrobial susceptibility patterns. Nevertheless, antibiogram typing is simple to perform, is inexpensive, can be applied to most medically important bacteria, and it may be used to generate preliminary data which may indicate the need for more discriminative techniques.

Resistograms utilize the sensitivity of strains to different chemicals, thus building up a similar pattern to antibiograms. The same limitations apply as for antibiograms, and because of the small number of species for which systems have been developed; it is not worthwhile for a diagnostic laboratory to set it up as a routine procedure.

4.4 Serotyping

This is one of the oldest typing methods and is still used today. The Enterobacteria-ceae is the group of bacteria most commonly typed in this way, and schemes have been produced for almost all the genera and species. Serotyping to ident-ify O and H antigens is the basis of salmonella identification according to the Kauffman–White scheme (see Chapter 6). Serotyping schemes for Enterobacteria-ceae associated with nosocomial infection are described in detail elsewhere (39). Serotyping can be applied to many other bacteria including *P. aeruginosa*, *Legionella pneumophila*, and pneumococci. With other bacteria, such as *Listeria monocytogenes*, most isolates can be serotyped, but the majority of clinical isolates belong to a single serotype, 4b, which severely limits serotyping as an epidemiological tool in the investigation of clustes of listeriosis. Although there are problems with standardization of methods and production of antisera, serotype appears to be one of the most stable phenotypic markers in bacteria. For this reason serotyping is still widely used, but not normally in the clinical laboratory, isolates being referred to specialized reference laboratories that maintain standard panels of antisera. As the availability of such schemes will vary greatly from country to country, the problem should be discussed with the national reference laboratory.

4.5 Bacteriophage typing

Bacteriophages are viruses capable of replication within the bacterial cell, leading, in some cases, to lysis and release of infective bacteriophage particles. Typing schemes are developed by isolating a range of bacteriophages active against the bacterial species concerned (often from filtered sewage). The bacteriophage is purified and its activity against a large number of bacterial strains determined, and a set of bacteriophages is then selected to provide the maximum sensitivity for differentiating strains of bacteria. It is also a highly sensitive method, but suffers from being complex technically (environmental conditions can affect the sensitivity of bacteria to infection by bacteriophages) with many variables to be controlled. There is also a need to maintain the bacteriophage typing set in a viable state by serial passage. For these reasons, bacteriophage typing has largely remained in the province of the reference laboratory. It is particularly useful for further subdividing serotypes of *P. aeruginosa* and salmonellae and it remains a major typing method for *S. aureus*. A few larger hospital laboratories undertake bacteriophage typing of *S. aureus* as they have sufficient isolates to make the investment in materials and labour worthwhile. A method for bacteriophage typing *S. aureus* is given in the first edition of this book.

4.6 Bacteriocin typing

Bacteriocins are antibiotic-like, bactericidal substances which inhibit different strains of bacteria (40). The strain producing the bacteriocin is usually resistant to its action but, rarely, may be sensitive. By selecting suitable producer strains, isolates can be typed according to their sensitivity to a particular bacteriocin. Strains may also be typed by their ability to produce bacteriocins. Sensitivity to many bacteriocins is encoded on transferable plasmids, so stability of the method may sometimes be suspect. Bacteriocin typing has also been applied to *Shigella* spp., *E. coli*, and *Enterobacter* spp., amongst others, but the technique is rather labour-intensive and of limited typability and discriminative power and has now been superseded by other techniques. A method of pyocin typing of *P. aeruginosa* is described in the first edition of this book. A variant of bacteriocin typing, peculiar to swarming *Proteus* spp., relies on the Dienes phenomenon. It relies on both the sensitivity of a strain to a specific bacteriocin and that strain's ability to produce a bacteriocin (41). When differing strains of *Proteus* spp. swarm towards each other and meet, a 'ditch' is produced between the two strains into which neither strain will swarm. It is a simple method which can easily be applied in the smallest laboratory and can be used as a preliminary to more investigation using more discriminative techniques such as molecular methods (see below). A method is given in Protocol 1.

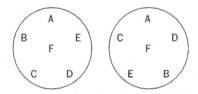

Figure 2 Positions of inocula for testing the Dienes compatibility of six strains of *Proteus* spp. in all combinations.

Protocol 1

Dienes typing method for *Proteus mirabilis* and *P. vulgaris*

Method

1 Inoculate the strains to be tested on to two blood agar plates in the positions indicated in Figure 2 (six strains A–F are shown in Figure 2). The inoculum can either be a small amount of a colony or a loopful of broth culture. Always include a strain from a different source to act as a positive control.

2 Incubate for 18 h at 30 °C: slow-spreading strains may require a longer incubation time.

3 Examine the plates under reflected light for lines of incompatibility. If the recommended pattern is used, all strains will be exposed to each other. Some strains may not swarm and become overrun by a neighbouring strain. Observing the origin of the contours of swarming growth will help recognize this problem.

4.7 Molecular typing methods

Dissatisfaction with phenotypic typing methods which often have poor discriminatory power and limited typeability and reproducibility has led to the widespread adoption of molecular methods many of which address the shortcomings inherent of more traditional techniques. There is now a bewildering array of choice with respect to molecular methods which has led to a feeling bordering on cynicism at the introduction of YATM (*Yet Another Typing Method*) which in turn is followed by more TBCA (*Totally Boring Clonal Analysis*) (42). Nevertheless, many of these techniques have emerged as extremely powerful epidemiological tools—for a review see ref. 43. Pulsed-field gel electrophoresis is generally regarded as the most discriminative molecular typing system for many nosocomial pathogens, however it requires equipment not widely available in most diagnostic laboratories. It is also expensive and time-consuming to perform. Accordingly, two methods, plasmid analysis and random amplification of polymorphic DNA (RAPD), are described here. These are relatively inexpensive and can be performed within one working day using equipment which is more widely available than that used for PFGE. Moreover, both methods do not require any a priori knowledge of the genetic structure of the bacteria under investigation. Furthermore, commercially produced kits can be used to further simplify these techniques for both plasmid extraction (e.g. Qiagen UK Ltd., Crawley) and RAPD-PCR (Amersham Pharmacia Biotoech, Little Chalfont, UK).

4.7.1 Plasmid analysis

A variety of rapid plasmid isolation methods have been described. The method given in Protocol 2 (44) is reliable and has the advantage that the plasmid DNA prepared can be digested with restriction endonucleases (Protocol 3).

Protocol 2

A rapid method for the isolation of bacterial plasmid DNA

Reagents

• See Table 2

Method

1 Inoculate 5–10 ml of Nutrient broth No. 2 (Oxoid) or similar medium in sterile 20 ml universal containers with the bacteria to be typed by plasmid profile.

2 Incubate with shaking at an appropriate temperature overnight (usually 37 °C).

3 Harvest the bacteria by centrifuging 1.5 ml at maximum speed in a microcentrifuge (MicroCentaur, MSE Scientific Instruments Ltd.) for 4 min using a 1.8 ml polypropylene Eppendorf-type tube. A pellet at least the size of a rice grain should be obtained. With some bacteria, such as coagulase negative staphylococci, it will be necessary to decant the supernatant, refill with fresh culture, and re-centrifuge until a large enough cell pellet is built up.

4 After decanting the supernatant, resuspend the pellet in 100 μl of reagent 1 to which 1 mg/ml of lysozyme (Sigma Chemical Co. Ltd.) has been added just before use. Lysozyme should be used when examining Gram-negative bacteria. For Gram-positive bacteria 1 mg/ml of lysostaphin (Sigma Chemical Co. Ltd.) is added instead, also just before use.

5 Incubate at room temperature for 15 min (Gram-negative bacteria) or 20 min at 37 °C (Gram-positive bacteria).

6 Add 200 μl of reagent 2 to achieve complete lysis of the cells, mix by gently inverting the tube two or three times. At this stage the solution will become clear and viscous.

Protocol 2 continued

7   After a period of 5 min at room temperature add 150 μl of reagent 3 and mix by inversion. The chromosomal DNA has now been precipitated. This is removed by centrifugation at 12 800 g[a] for 5 min.

8   Using a pipette, carefully remove 400 μl of the clear supernatant to a clean Eppendorf tube, taking care not to remove any chromosomal DNA.

9   Add 1 ml of ethanol and mix by inverting several times. Place the Eppendorf tube in liquid N_2 for 20–30 sec until a white condensate *just* starts to appear. An alternative method is to hold at –20 °C for 1 h. Centrifuge for 2 min. It is important to ensure that the hinges of the tubes are on the outside of the rotor so that the position of the feathery pellet can be predicted, thus avoiding damage to it.

10   Decant the ethanol, taking care not to disturb the pellet and resuspend in 400 μl of reagent 4.

11   Add 400 μl of the phenol reagent and mix briefly using a vortex mixer. Centrifuge for 2 min and carefully remove the *upper* phase into a clean tube, taking care not to take any phenol over.

12   Precipitate the DNA using ethanol as in steps 9 and 10, but do not resuspend the pellet.

13   Gently add 200 μl of diethyl ether to wash the pellet and centrifuge for 15 sec. Decant the ether and leave the tube inverted to allow any residual ether to evaporate.

14   Dissolve the DNA pellet in 20 μl of sterile distilled water and mix with 10 μl of loading buffer. The DNA can then be subjected to electrophoresis in either a vertical or slab agarose gel electrophoresis system. Many workers use TEB buffer to both make the gel (0.8%, w/v) and fill the apparatus. Stain the gel for about 20 min with TEB buffer or water containing a small amount of ethidium bromide (1 mg/ml).

15   Examine the gel on a UV transilluminator (302 nm, UV Products Ltd.). Bands may be recorded on a Polaroid camera for convenience using an orange filter or an imaging system.

[a] All centrifugation is carried out at approx. 12 800 g which represents maximum speed on an MSE MicroCentaur centrifuge.

Plasmid analysis can be applied to any bacterial species provided that they have plasmids which are stable. It is a valuable method for typing coagulase negative staphylococci. The routine laboratory will also find the method useful for sub-dividing serovars of food poisoning salmonellae; the gel in Figure 3 is taken from the investigation of such an outbreak.

4.7.2 RAPD-PCR

Random amplification of polymorphic DNA (RAPD), also known as arbitrary-primed PCR (AP-PCR) and multiple arbitrary amplicon profiling (MAAP) has been

Table 2 Reagents used in the rapid plasmid DNA isolation method

Reagent 1	50 mM glucose, 10 mM EDTA, 25 mM Tris HCl, pH 8.0	Glucose	901 mg
		Tris HCl[a]	222 mg
		Tris-Base[a]	133 mg
		Na$_4$EDTA	372 mg
		Distilled water to 100 ml	
Reagent 2[b]	1% SDS on 0.2 M NaOH	NaOH	0.8 g
		SDS	1.0 g
		Distilled water to 100 ml	
Reagent 3	3 M sodium acetate pH 4.8	Dissolve 24.6 g sodium acetate in 50 ml distilled water, add glacial acetic acid until pH 4.8, add water up to 100 ml	
Reagent 4	50 mM Tris HCl, 100 mM sodium acetate	Tris-HCl[a]	0.44 g
		Tris-Base[a]	0.265 g
		Sodium acetate	0.82 g
		Distilled water to 100 ml	
Phenol reagent	Add 40 ml of distilled water, 6 ml of 1 M Tris HCl[a] buffer at pH 8.0 and 5 ml of 2 M NaOH to 100 g of crystalline phenol ('Analar' grade), leave until phenol has dissolved		
TEB buffer	40 mM Tris HCl[a], 1 mM EDTA, 50 mM Boric acid pH 8.2	Make × 10 and then dilute for use. To make 1 litre of × 10:	
		Tris-Base[a]	60.5 g
		Na$_4$EDTA	3.7 g
		Boric acid	31.0 g
		Distilled water to 1 l	
		Check pH 8.2	
Loading buffer	40% w/v sucrose, 0.5 M Na$_4$EDTA, 0.5% w/v bromophenol blue	Na$_4$EDTA	16.5 g
		Sucrose	40 g
		Bromophenol blue	0.5 g
		Distilled water to 100 ml	

[a] Weights of Tris-Base and Tris-HCl refer to Trizma® compound supplied by Sigma Chemical Co Ltd.
[b] This reagent should be freshly prepared every 4 weeks.

used extensively to type bacteria of importance in health care-associated infection. In this technique, a short primer, typically around 10 bp in length, of a sequence which is not directed against a known complementary sequence hybridizes randomly at several points in the bacterial chromosome at very low annealing temperatures. If hybridization sites on the chromosome are in proximity, then the intervening sequences are amplified in the PCR and the resulting multiple products can be resolved on gel electrophoresis. A method suitable for use in the diagnostic laboratory is given Protocol 4.

Protocol 3

Procedure for digestion of plasmid DNA with restriction endonucleases

Method

1 Add to the ether-washed pellet from Protocol 2, step 13, 2 µl RNase solution (10 mg/ml—boiled to destroy nuclease activity), 1 µl of core buffer (varies according to restriction endonuclease used, manufacturers often supply buffer with the enzyme preparation), and 7 µl of sterile distilled water.

2 Spin for 15 sec in a microcentrifuge to mix.

3 Add restriction endonuclease in manufacturer's recommended amounts (5–10 units will usually give a complete digestion) and incubate for 2 h at the recommended temperature.

4 Load a suitable aliquot (5–10 µl) with loading buffer (5–10 µl) and electrophorese as in Protocol 2.

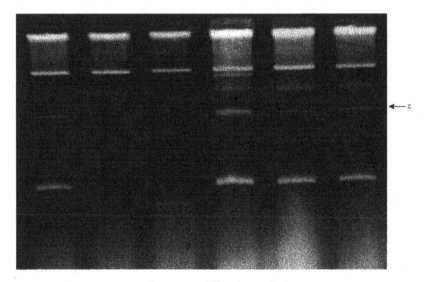

Figure 3 Plasmid profiles from isolates of *Salmonella typhimurium* made during an outbreak of food poisoning. Lanes 1, 5, and 6 show identical profiles of two plasmids and were all from faecal isolates from cases eating pork pies. Lane 4 is the blood isolate from the patient whose faecal isolate is in lane 5, it shows a slightly smaller deletion derivative of the larger plasmid. The isolates in lanes 2 and 3 were from cases not eating pork pies and show different profiles to the pork pie-associated strain (they were phage type 204 and 49 respectively; the isolates in lanes 1, 4, 5, and 6 were all phage type 12). The band attributable to chromosomal DNA is indicated (C). The faint band below the chromosomal DNA in lane 4 is the open circle form of the small plasmid, the majority of which is present in the covalently closed form.

Protocol 4

A method for RAPD-PCR

Method

1 DNA extraction. There are a number of commercially available kits for the rapid extraction of DNA from both Gram-positive and Gram-negative bacteria. If a 'quick and dirty' answer is required when examining a limited number of strains, genomic DNA used for RAPD-PCR can be prepared using simple extraction techniques. With some species, however, it may be necessary to use a commercial kit or a conventional procedure which results in more purified DNA. Pick colonies from a non-selective medium and suspend them in 200 µl of lysis buffer and boil for 5–10 min in a microcentrifuge tube in a water-bath.

2 Centrifuge for 2 min at 10 000 g. Aliquots of the supernatant can be used immediately for RAPD-PCR reaction, otherwise the DNA preparation may frozen at −20 °C until use.

3 Prepare a PCR mix (50 µl for each isolate to be tested), by adding:
   • 5 µl of 10 × PCR buffer
   • 5 µl of dNTPs
   • 2 µl of primer
   • 1 µl of *Taq* polymerase (5.0 U)
   • 35 µl sterile distilled water
   • 2 µl of template (as prepared in steps 1 and 2)
   There are many RAPD primers for individual bacterial genera and species which can be readily identified following a literature search.

4 Mix and overlay with 50 µl of mineral oil (if using a PCR cycler without a heated lid).

5 Programme the thermal cycler for one pre-denaturation cycle of 94 °C of 4 min followed by 35 cycles of 1 min at 94 °C (denaturation), 1 min at 35 °C (annealing), and 2 min at 72 °C (extension).

6 In a clean Eppendorf tube mix 20 µl of PCR product with 5 µl of loading buffer. Load the mixture into slots in a 1.5% agarose gel prepared with TAE buffer along with a 100 bp DNA ladder.

7 Electrophorese gels in TAE buffer at typically 5–10 V/cm gel length until the bromophenol blue tracking dye has reached three-quarters of the length of the gel. Stain gels by immersing in a plastic container with TAE buffer containing 0.5 µg/ml of ethidium bromide. (Caution! Ethidium bromide is carcinogenic—wear gloves.)

8 Photograph under UV light. If bands are unclear, it may be necessary to destain by further re-immersion in TAE buffer for 10–15 min.

The results of RAPD-PCR, in terms of typeability, and more importantly reproducibility, can be influenced by a large number of factors. These include purity

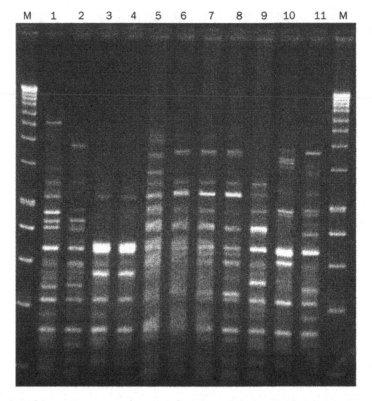

Figure 4 RAPD typing patterns of genomic DNA from potential metallo β-lactamase (MBL)-producing *P. aeruginosa* from Guangzhou, China. Lane M, 1 kb DNA ladder; strain 1, 2, 3, 4, 5, 6–9, 10–11 were the isolates from seven different hospitals, among them, strains 3, 4, 6–8 were proved to be MBL-producers by Etest screening using MBL strips. Strains 6–8 showed the same RAPD pattern and were isolated from the same hospital. Strains 3, 4 were also clonal but were isolated from different hospitals. (Courtesy of Dr J-H Xiong, University of Birmingham.)

of template DNA, length and sequence of primer, source of *Taq* polymerase, concentration of Mg^{2+} in the reaction buffer, and times/temperatures in the phases of the reaction. Trial and error, by varying each parameter in turn, may be required to achieve optimum results. An example of some isolates of *P. aeruginosa* typed by RAPD is shown in Figure 4.

References

1. Department of Health. (2002). *Getting ahead of the curve*. Download http://www.doh.gov.uk/cmo/idstrategy/idstrategy2002.pdf.
2. Environment Agency. (2002). *The microbiology of drinking water—methods for the examination of waters and associated materials*. Download: http://www.dwi.gov.uk/regs/pdf/micro.htm.
3. International Commission on Microbiological Specifications for Foods. (1988). *Microorganisms in foods 1: their significance and methods of enumeration*, 2nd edn. University of Toronto Press, Toronto. Currently out of print. New edition expected; details from: http://www.dfst.csiro.au/icmsf/publications.htm.

4. Department of Health. (2000). HSC 2000/002.

5. Haley, R. W. (1995). *J. Hosp. Infect.*, **30**, Suppl., 3.

6. Kressel, A. B. and Kidd, F. (2001). *Infect. Control Hosp. Epidemiol.*, **22**, 414.

7. Verweij, P. E., Bijl, D., Melchers, W. J., De Pauw, B. E., *et al.* (1997). *Infect. Control Hosp. Epidemiol.*, **18**, 128.

8. Mallison, G. F. and Haley, R. W. (1981). In *Nosocomial infections* (ed. R. E. Dixon). Yorke Medical Books, New York.

9. Duckworth, G., Cookson, B., Humphreys, H., and Heathcock, R. (1999). Revised methicillin-resistant *Staphylococcus aureus* infection control guidelines for hospitals. http://www.his.org.uk/work/mrsa21.doc.

10. Millar, M. R., Keyworth, N., Lincoln, C., King, B., and Congdon, P. (1987). *J. Hosp. Infect.*, **10**, 187.

11. Groschel, D. H. (1980). *Ann. N. Y. Acad. Sci.*, **353**, 230.

12. Clark, S., Lach, V., and Lidwell, O. M. (1981). *J. Hosp. Infect.*, **2**, 181.

13. Casewell, M. W., Desai, N., and Lease, E. J. (1986). *J. Hosp. Infect.*, **7**, 250.

14. Whyte, W., Lidwell, O. M., Lowbury, E. J. L., and Blowers, R. (1983). *J. Hosp. Infect.*, **4**, 133.

15. Weinstein, R. A. and Mallinson, G. F. (1978). *Am. J. Clin. Pathol.*, **69**, 130.

16. Tsakris, A., Pantazi, A., Pournaras, S., Maniatis, A., *et al.* (2000). *J. Clin. Microbiol.*, **38**, 3505.

17. Wilson, P. A. and Petts, D. N. (1987). *Lancet*, **i**, 558.

18. Petts, D. N. (1984). *J. Clin. Microbial.*, **19**, 4.

19. De La Rosa, M., Villareal, R., Vega, D., Miranda, C., *et al.* (1983). *J. Clin. Microbiol.*, **18**, 779.

20. Mossel, D. A. A., Eelderink, I., de Vor, H., and Keizer, E. D. (1976). *Lab. Practice*, **25**, 393.

21. Taylor, M. E., Oppenheim, B. A., Chadwick, P. R., Weston, D., *et al.* (1999). *J. Hosp. Infect.*, **43**, 25.

22. Ieven, M., Vercauteren, E., Descheemaeker, P., van Laer, F., and Goossens, H. (1999). *J. Clin. Microbiol.*, **37**, 1436.

23. Borriello, S. P. and Honour, P. (1981). *J. Clin. Pathol.*, **34**, 1124.

24. Curtis, G. D. W., Mitchell, R. G., King, A. F., and Griffin, E. J. (1989). *Lett. Appl. Microbiol.*, **8**, 95.

25. Cooke, E. M., Brayson, J. C., Edmondson, A. S., and Hall, D. (1979). *J. Hygiene (Camb.)*, **82**, 473.

26. Farmer, J. J. 3rd, Silva, F., and Williams, D. R. (1973). *Appl. Microbiol.*, **25**, 151.

27. Flynn, D. M., Weinstein, R. A., Nathan, C., Gaston, M. A., and Kabins, S. A. (1987). *J. Infect. Dis.*, **156**, 363.

28. Hawkey, P. M., McCormick, A., and Simpson, R. A. (1986). *J. Clin. Microbiol.*, **23**, 600.

29. Goto, S. and Enomoto, S. (1970). *Jpn. J. Microbiol.*, **14**, 65.

30. Campbell, M. E., Farmer, S. W., and Speert, D. P. (1988). *J. Clin. Microbiol.*, **26**, 1910.

31. Mead, G. C. and Adams, B. W. (1977). *Br. Poult. Sci.*, **18**, 661.

32. Jawad, A., Hawkey, P. M., Heritage, J., and Snelling, A. M. (1994). *J. Clin. Microbiol.*, **32**, 2353.

33. Kerr, K. G., Denton, M., Todd, N. J., Corps, C. M., *et al.* (1996). *Eur. J. Clin. Microbiol. Infect. Dis.*, **15**, 607.

34. Henry, D. A., Campbell, M. E., Lipuma, J. J., and Speert, D. P. (1997). *J. Clin. Microbiol.*, **35**, 614.

35. Hedges, A. J., Howe, K., and Linton, A. H. (1977). *J. Appl. Bacteriol.*, **43**, 271.

36. Murray, P. R. (1978). *J. Clin. Microbiol.*, **8**, 46.

37. Grant, R. B., Penner, J. L., Hennessy, J. N., and Jackowski, B. J. (1981). *J. Clin. Micrbiol.*, **13**, 561.

38. Prahanth, K. and Badrinath, S. (2000). *J. Med. Microbiol.*, **49**, 773.

39. Ewing, W. H. (1986). *Edwards and Ewing's identification of Enterobacteriaceae*, 4th edn. Elsevier Science, New York.

40. Daw, M. A. and Falkiner, F. R. (1996). *Micron*, **27**, 1.

41. Senior, B. W. (1977). *J. Gen. Microbiol.*, **102**, 235.

42. Achtman, M. (1996). *J. Clin. Microbiol.*, **34**, 1870.

43. Hawkey, P. M. (1999). *J. Hosp. Infect.*, **43**, Suppl., S77.

44. Bennett, P. M., Heritage, J., and Hawkey, P. M. (1986). *J. Antimicrob. Chemother.*, **18**, 421.

Useful websites

1. Association for Professionals in Infection Control and Epidemiology (with link to *American Journal of Infection Control*): http://www.apic.org/

2. Australian Infection Control Association: http://www.aica.org.au/

3. Hospital Infection Society: http://www.his.org.uk (with link to the *Journal of Hospital Infection*)

4. Healthcare Infection Control Practices Advisory Committee (HICPAC): http://www.cdc.gov/ncidod/hip/HICPAC/Hicpac.htm

5. Infection Control Nurses Association: http://www.icna.co.uk/

6. Society for Health Care Epidemiology of America: http://www.shea-online.org/

Chapter 12

Epidemiological methods in the investigation of acute bacterial infections

Stephen R. Palmer

Department of Epidemiology, Statistics and Public Health,
University of Wales, College of Medicine, Health Park, Cardiff,
CF14 4XN

1 Introduction

Epidemiology is the study of the occurrence and causes of disease in populations. In contrast to the clinical situation when an individual patient is the focus of concern, the epidemiological approach relates the disease in the individual to the occurrence or risk of disease in others within the relevant population. This means taking into account not only the microbiological, but all personal, environmental, and social factors which influence the occurrence and presentation of the disease. A well-defined methodology exists (1), which demands specialized skills, but every clinical microbiologist will need to be familiar with certain basic concepts and methods (2) and to take an epidemiological perspective from time to time. Examples include the investigation of sources and modes of transmission in outbreaks, applying public health measures to the control of outbreaks, preventing the spread of sporadic cases of certain infections (such as diphtheria, typhoid, meningococcal meningitis), and devising preventive strategies, for instance for nosocomial legionnaires' disease.

2 Basic concepts in infectious disease epidemiology

2.1 Reservoir of infection

This is the principal habitat of the infectious agent from which it may spread to cause disease. Examples of reservoirs of bacteria are man (example: *Corynebacterium diphtheriae*); animals (*Campylobacter* spp.); soil (*Clostridium tetani*), and water (*Legionella* spp.).

2.2 Source of infection

Infection may be endogenous (cause by the patient's own flora) or exogenous (acquired from another source). The source of an exogenous infection may be different from the reservoir. Thus, in an episode of salmonella food poisoning the reservoir of infection may be commercially reared chickens. However, utensils and surfaces used for preparation of the poultry may cross-contaminate other foods which, when eaten, become the source of infection. When the source of infection is inanimate, such as food or water, it is termed the *vehicle* of infection.

2.3 Mode of transmission

The mechanism by which an infectious agent passes from the reservoir of source of infection to the person is called the mode of transmission. The major categories are:

(a) *Person-to-person* spread from the *primary* case to the *secondary* cases who are *contacts* of primary cases. Within this category possible transmission routes include:
  i.   Faecal–oral spread (e.g. shigellosis).
  ii. Sexual transmission (e.g. syphilis).
  iii. Direct inoculation of blood (e.g. hepatitis B).
  iv. Airborne droplet nuclei (e.g. tuberculosis).
  v.   Droplets (e.g. streptococcal pharyngitis).
  vi. Transplacental and perinatal (e.g. syphilis, gonorrhoea).

(b) *Food-and waterborne* (e.g. salmonella food poisoning, cholera). 'Food poisoning' historically has usually been applied to incidents in which the organism multiplies in the food vehicle before transmission (*Clostridium perfringens*) but all suspected foodborne infections are statutorily notifiable in the UK.

(c) *Insect-borne* transmission via the bite of an infected insect (e.g. Lyme disease caused by *Borrellia burgdorferi* from a tick bite).

(d) *Direct contact* with animals or their products or with the agent in the environment (e.g. anthrax, leptospirosis).

(e) *Airborne* droplet nuclei and aerosols (e.g. legionnaires' disease) or dust (e.g. ornithoisis).

2.4 Occurrence

Cases may be *sporadic* (not known to be related to other cases) or clustered in *outbreaks* (two or more related cases suggesting the possibility of transmission or a common source). Measures of occurrence of infection include the *incidence rate* (rate of appearance of new cases in a defined population, usually expressed as a proportion of the total population, e.g. 10 cases per 100 000 persons per year), *cumulative incidence* or risk, which is the proportion of people who get a disease during a specific period, and *prevalence* (all cases existing at a point or period in time in a defined population). The *attack rate* during an outbreak is a type of cumulative incidence, the proportion of the population at risk who were ill during the period of the outbreak. The *secondary attack rate* is the attack rate in the contacts of primary cases due to person-to-person spread.

An infection which is continuously present in a population is said to be *endemic*, and an increase in incidence above the endemic level is described as an *epidemic* or *pandemic*.

2.5 Incubation period

The time from infection to the onset of symptoms is called the incubation period. For each organism there is a characteristic range within which infecting dose, and portal of entry as well as host factors (such as age) may introduce individual variability.

2.6 Host response

This will depend upon infecting dose, susceptibility (age, sex, other concurrent disease, immunity) as well as existence of other *risk factors* (for example smoking for legionnaires' disease). In any outbreak of infection there will usually be a spectrum of clinical response ranging from no symptoms to fulminant disease and death.

2.6.1 Questionnaire design and administration

In large outbreaks it will not be practicable to interview in-depth all persons affected. Usually a few patients, say five to ten, should be interviewed in-depth to explore all possible exposures. Use these data to draw up a questionnaire (Appendix IV) for subsequent interviews. In some situations it is not possible to interview patients personally, and self-administered questionnaires can be given or posted to patients with a stamped addressed envelope for return. Such questionnaires require especially careful wording to avoid ambiguities. Before administration, try out questionnaires by asking colleagues or office staff to complete them, and then revise the questionnaire. In recent studies, telephone interviews have proved to be satisfactory.

2.7 Analysis and presentation of data

Data from patients must be summarized and compared in order to identify possible common exposures or risk factors. To do this, a line listing is prepared as in Table 1, which is taken from the outbreak investigated using the questionnaire in Appendix IV (3). Each question of interest on the questionnaire should form a

Table 1 Line listing of data from *Salmonella enteritidis* PT6 case-control study

	Age	Sex	Onset date	Raw egg stored in kitchen	Raw egg	Cooked egg	Home made mayonnaise	Chicken
Case	25	M	4/7/99	Y	Y	Y	Y	Y
Control	27	M	NK	Y	N	Y	N	Y

column, and if possible, for each case the data should be recorded as 'Yes', 'No', or 'Not known'. Descriptive data should be summarized by time, place, and person.

2.7.1 Time

The time of crucial importance is the time of onset of disease, since from this and knowledge of the incubation period of the infection the period of exposure to infection can be determined. Do not confuse (as is often done) the date of hospital admission, date of specimen, or date of laboratory test with the date of onset of symptoms. In an outbreak, the dates of onset in cases should be presented graphically, usually in the form of a histogram, though this is often called an *epidemic 'curve'* (Figure 1). The scale of the *x* axis will be determined by the incubation period; hours for *Staphylococcus aureus*, days for salmonellae and most other bacterial infections. The epidemic curve should be drawn immediately data become available, and updated during the course of the outbreak.

The epidemic curve is the most useful and immediate means of assessing the type of outbreak. In point-source outbreaks in which all cases are exposed at a given time (such as a wedding reception), onset of symptoms of all primary cases will cluster within the range of the incubation period (e.g. 6–72 h for salmonella food poisoning). An epidemic curve which extends beyond a single

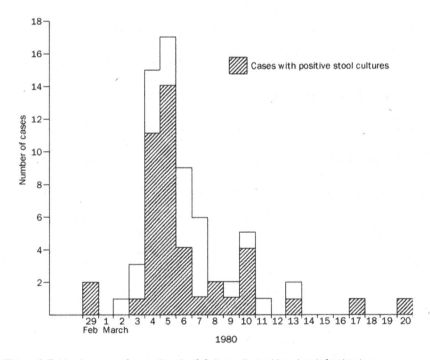

Figure 1 Epidemic curve of an outbreak of *Salmonella typhimurium* infection in a students' hall of residence (5). The major wave of illness from 4–7 March was shown to be due to consumption of cottage pie served March 3 and 4. Subsequent cases which spread out over several incubation periods were thought to be due to person-to-person spread.

incubation period suggests either a continuing or recurring source of infection, or the possibility of secondary transmission (see Figure 1).

2.8 Communicability

The infectious agent may be passed to others over a variable time, the *period of communicability*; in some infections this occurs even from symptomless, temporary, or chronic *carriers* (for example in *Salmonella typhi*).

3 Epidemiological methods

3.1 Descriptive methods

3.1.1 Public health surveillance

Early detection of changes in disease patterns to enable rapid investigation and control is one of the principal aims of population surveillance. The main steps are:

(a) Systematic collection of data.

(b) Analyses of these data to produce statistics.

(c) Interpretation of the statistics to provide information.

(d) Distribution of this information to all those who require it so that action can be taken.

(e) Continuing surveillance to evaluate the action.

A range of data sources may be used (4), but nationally and regionally the core data in the UK continue to be the voluntary reporting of laboratory confirmed cases, collated in England by the Health Protection Agency's Communicable Disease Surveillance Centre, in Wales by the National Public Health Service for Wales and by the Scottish Centre for Infection and Environmental Health in Scotland. Routine outputs are published in the Communicable Disease Review (CDR) and SCIEH Weekly Report (SCIEHs).

3.1.2 Clinical interview

Once an incident has been recognized the investigation and control of both sporadic cases and outbreaks of infection begins with a thorough epidemiological history of the index patients. Routine medical records are seldom sufficient and a careful clinical interview should be undertaken if possible. Data should be recorded accurately, in detail, and retained for future reference.

The data to be collected will be determined by the natural history of the particular infection. In newly recognized infections where the natural history is poorly understood, the questions will have to be wide-ranging and open-ended. Patients should be asked if they have marked calendars, kept diaries, or notes of events and exposures (for example restaurants visited on holiday). When more than one related case is to be interviewed, the main subject headings should be used to draw up a pro-forma to be issued for interviews so that a standard history is obtained from each case. Informal questioning should follow the structured interview to explore possible leads. The following broad categories should be considered when drawing up a data collection form:

Name	*Date of admission*
Address	*Hospital no*
Sex	*Ward and bed*
Age/date of birth	*Attending physician*
Occupation	*Investigations*
Place of work	*Treatment*

Clinical description of disease (nature, onset, severity, duration).

Predisposing factors. Other medical history, smoking, antibiotics, history of immunizations.

Contacts. History of illness in contacts. Identify household and other contacts by name and address for subsequent follow-up if necessary.

Social and recreation. Functions attended, other activities, hobbies, sports, use of recreational pools, etc.

Sexual history. Sexual orientation, names and addresses of partners for contact tracing if appropriate.

Food and drink. Document all food and drink consumed within the period immediately before onset which corresponds to the maximum incubation period for the suspected infection. Before interviewing prepare a checklist of categories of foods, e.g. meats, dairy produce, tins. Record brand names and batch numbers if appropriate.

Exposure to animals. Pets, farm animals, zoos, wildlife.

In outbreaks propagated from person-to-person, the occurrence of cases will be spread over several incubation periods. Mixed outbreaks may also occur. The onset of diseases should be related to other events in the environment which may thereby be implicated as possible sources of infection, for example reduction in hot-water temperatures in a hospital just before a cluster of nosocomial legionnaires' disease (6).

3.1.3 Place

Cases clustering in a particular place of work or neighbourhood, for example, may indicate the existence of a point source of infection or of person-to-person spread. Plotting cases by place of residence or work on a map as a scatter plot, or for example, by hospital ward, may reveal such patterns. In nosocomial outbreaks, movement of patients between wards may hide clusters and therefore it is necessary to identify and plot location at the time of likely exposure.

3.1.4 Person

In communicable diseases, most relevant patient characteristics and exposure factors will be discrete variables (for example, sex) rather than continuous variables (for example, white blood cell count), and will be analysed as proportions of cases or controls who have a particular factor, or as a ratio (for example male : female). Analysis of patient characteristics and histories of exposures (age, sex, medical history, occupation, travel history), may suggest hypotheses about the source and mode of infection. For example, the predominance of patients with gastrointestinal dysfunction in a hospital outbreak of *Salmonella cubana* led to identification of carmine dye used in investigations as the vehicle of infection (7).

4 Analytical methods

Descriptive data may suggest hypotheses about the source of mode of transmission of an infection, but they are not always a sufficient basis for introducing control measures. Furthermore, caution is needed in the analysis and interpretation of data from cases, especially data about place and person. For example, in an outbreak of *Salmonella paratyphi* B bacteriophage type 3a var.4, extending over four years, which exclusively affected holidaymakers visiting Portugal (8), all cases except the last three had eaten at one restaurant in one small village. This restaurant had therefore been considered the most likely source of infection for the first three years, although screening of food handlers failed to identify a carrier. However, when local data was eventually obtained, it was found that the particular restaurant was the only one actually sited on the resort beach and that most if not all visitors would eat at the restaurant. The probable source of infection was found to be raw sewage which was contaminating the beach from a faulty sewer drain. Thus, observations on the cases have to be set against what is expected in the population from which they come: in the example above, all holidaymakers visiting the resort would be expected to eat at the restaurant.

Analytical methods are required to test the hypotheses generated from descriptive data. Broadly, there are two complementary approaches; the microbiological (for example culturing foods remaining from a meal thought to have caused food poisoning) and the epidemiological. Even when microbiological investigations reveal contamination (contaminated food left over from a reception, or legionellae in a hospital cooling tower), this does not in itself identify the source of infection. Epidemiological evidence is still necessary to demonstrate an association between, for example, the contaminated food or the cooling-tower drift and the occurrence of illness. Since, for example, most water stored in large buildings will yield legionellae, but outbreaks are relatively rare, the significance of environmental isolates will need to be determined epidemiologically. Essentially the epidemiological approach is to compare the characteristics of infection persons (cases) with those of a similar group of uninfected persons (controls). Two principal study designs are used, the case-control and the cohort (9). Choice of method in practice is usually determined by what is feasible. Where a cohort can be readily identified, it is usual to undertake a cohort study (e.g. a foodborne outbreak in a wedding party). Where cases occur unpredictably in the wider community a cohort cannot usually be identified readily and a case-control study will be necessary.

4.1 Case-control studies

The use of these should be confined to testing hypotheses which have been generated by careful descriptive epidemiology. If a prior hypothesis has not been clearly and precisely defined case-control studies are seldom productive. Although relatively quick to perform, their design and analysis can be complex, and the practicalities of investigating acute incidents may not allow the ideal design to be followed. Even so, such imperfect studies are often of great help in arriving at answers rapidly during acute episodes. The essential feature of case-control studies is that data on possible sources and risk factors are elicited from both cases and controls retrospectively. Choice of controls is often problematical, but should be determined by the hypothesis being tested. For example, to test the hypothesis that a food item served at a restaurant was the vehicle of infection, controls may be selected from clients of the restaurant who remained well. If the vehicle of infection was turkey, then the proportion of cases eating turkey would be predicted to be higher than the equivalent proportion of controls.

The following aspects of case-control studies need to be carefully considered.

4.1.1 Case definition

With a well-known infection which is readily confirmed microbiologically, case definition is straightforward. However, with newly-recognized diseases this can be difficult. In an investigation of an outbreak of haemorrhagic colitis, a newly-recognized disease eventually attributed to infection with *E. coli* 0157 H7 (10), cases were defined positively by the presence of gross blood in stools, severe abdominal pain, and no fever, and negatively by the absence of other known pathogens in stools. Since it was likely that *E. coli* 0157 H7 produced a spectrum of illness, probably only the severe end of the spectrum was identified by this definition. In a case-control study it is preferable to use such a strict narrow definition of a case.

4.1.2 Possible misclassification of cases and controls

In an outbreak of *Salmonella typhimurium* in a university hostel, a vehicle of infection was not detected by comparing food histories from well and ill persons (6). In this investigation stool samples were obtained from well persons as well as cases, and only when symptomless excretors had been grouped with the ill persons instead of as controls did a statistically significant difference in food histories emerge. To help overcome this problem, controls should be asked about symptoms over the appropriate period and those who may have been unrecognized cases excluded from the study. The feasibility of serotesting, swabbing, or otherwise testing controls to exclude asymptomatic infected persons should be considered in all case-control studies.

4.1.3 Selection of cases and controls

Cases and controls should be representative of the infected and uninfected population from which the cases came. Possible biases in detection of cases, such as considering only those admitted to hospital, may exclude cases who have died of fulminant disease or who have mild illnesses. Risk factors identified on a biased sample may merely reflect those factors which caused the bias, for example admission to hospital. Where possible, cases should be new cases (incident cases) rather than previously interviewed prevalent cases.

Similarly, controls should be representative of the population, and this can be achieved by selecting controls randomly from the well population. However, in practice, taking every nth person on a list (systematic sampling) is often sufficient. A list of persons from which a sample can be chosen is the sampling frame, and sampling frames commonly used include:

(a) Telephone directory.

(b) GP age/sex registers.

(c) Hotel, reception guest lists.

(d) Family members of cases.

(e) Neighbours of cases.

(f) Acquaintances nominated by cases.

(g) Persons investigated by the laboratory but who were negative for the disease in question.

(h) Hospital admissions.

The choice of sampling frame will depend upon the hypothesis being tested.

4.1.4 Data collection

The major drawback of case-control studies is that accurate and complete data may not be available retrospectively. Medical records are notoriously incomplete, and people's recall may be faulty. This latter problem is lessened in acute incidents of short incubation infections since there is usually little delay between the event and the interview. One particular problem is that of rumination bias; because of their illness, cases will have gone over possible exposures in their minds and recall may be biased by their own preconceptions. Also, cases may have been interviewed on many occasions, and this may introduce bias from suggestions made by interviewers as well as prompting a more detailed recall. Therefore, to ensure a systematic approach to questioning cases, and to ensure that controls are given an equal chance of recalling events, cases and controls should be interviewed in the same way, by interview or postal questionnaire, and with the same care. Prompts should be used to encourage recall in controls, for example, relating the time period of interest to significant events. Where possible the exposures should be quantified (for example, portions of a food eaten) so that a dose–response analysis can be done (see later). An increasing strength of association between an exposure and disease strengthens the evidence for a causal link.

4.1.5 Response rate

The loss of cases or controls because of refusal to be interviewed or failure to trace patients can seriously bias survey results. Exposures in those who do not respond may not be similar to those in the responding group. Every attempt should be made to obtain rapidly a good response rate (>85%) using reminder letters, telephone calls, and home visits, since a low response rate may invalidate a study, and a slow response increases the problems of recall bias.

4.1.6 Confounding factors and matching

A confounding factor is one which is not the source of infection, but which is associated both with the cases and independently with the hypothesized source. The association with the occurrence of disease may lead to a misinterpretation of the source of the infection. In the paratyphoid outbreak previously discussed, eating at the beach restaurant was a confounding factor. When confounding factors can be reasonably predicted, they may be excluded by matching controls with cases on those factors. In case-control studies of acute incidents it is common to match controls for sex and age (usually for adults within five years of the case) and often also for neighbourhood of residence. In unmatched studies confounding factors may be dealt with in stratified analysis in which associations between exposure and disease are examined within sub-categories of the confounding variable. This of course depends upon having collected data on the confounding variable.

4.1.7 Number of controls

Often only a small number of cases are identified. To increase the statistical power of the study, the number of controls per case can be increased up to three or four before the efficiency of the study falls. The number of controls is usually determined by practical constraints.

4.1.8 Example: A case-control study (11) of legionnaires' disease associated with a whirlpool

Epidemiological interviews of two patients with legionnaires' disease implicated a single hotel as a possible common source of infection. Retrospective review of illness in guests reports to hotel staff identified 21 further cases of pneumonia over a four month period, 16 of whom had serological evidence of recent infection. Seven other persons met the case definition for Pontiac fever (fever, aches and pains without pneumonia, and a convalescent indirect fluorescent antibody titre of ≥ 64). Interview with these cases suggested the hypothesis that use of the hotel whirlpools or swimming pools might be the source of infection. Control data was needed to test this hypothesis. In order to distinguish between use of whirlpools and other possible hotel-associated risk factors, such as showering and bathing in the hotel rooms, controls would have to be taken from the population of hotel guests, and the use of whirlpools by cases and controls compared. The sampling frame used to select controls was therefore the hotel booking list. In addition, it was considered possible that age, sex, and week of stay could be related both to risk of legionnaires' disease and independently to the use of whirlpools, and *could* therefore be confounding factors. To overcome this possibility, two control groups were selected, one of which was matched for these three possible confounding factors.

The need for matching can be explained as follows. If, for example, age and sex were true confounding factors and cases happened to be older than controls and to have a higher proportion of men, differences between cases and controls in use of the whirlpools could possible be due to (say) older men having a greater susceptibility to 'Legionella and also independently being more likely to use the whirlpools. Without taking into account the possible association of age, sex, and whirlpool use, a false identification of the source might be made. Similarly, if controls were not matched for week of stay, then perhaps if the whirlpools were out of use or a more attractive recreation was available during the time when more controls than cases were at the hotel, a spurious association between cases and whirlpool use would have been produced.

The procedure for selection of matched controls was to define the matching parameters, list all eligible guests from the particular week's records, and then to choose every nth name to give five controls per case. A standard questionnaire was applied to each case and control. Misclassification of controls was a potential problem, since a number of controls reported symptoms which could have been due to *Legionella* infection, and these were excluded from the analysis. Asymptomatic infection could only have been excluded by serotesting all controls, and this was not considered feasible. However, including infected persons as controls would tend to bias results against the hypothesis being tested and would not bias the study to produce falsely positive associations.

The results of the study showed that 17 of 21 cases had used the whirlpools but only 20 of 67 controls had done so (Table 2). This difference was highly statistically significant. There were no significant differences between cases and control in the use of domestic baths and showers. The whirlpools were taken out of use and no further cases occurred.

4.1.9 Sequential case-control studies

Case-control studies can be used sequentially to refine and test hypotheses in a particular outbreak investigation. For example, in an outbreak of *Salmonella*

Table 2 History of exposure to possible sources of *Legionella* infection investigated by a case-control study

Exposure	Cases		Control		Odds ratio
	Exposed	Not exposed	Exposed	Not exposed	
Whirlpool	17	4	20	47	10
Bath	11	9	37	15	0.5
Shower	2	17	14	39	0.3
Drinking tap-water	8	12	37	35	0.6

typhimurium definitive type 124 cases occurred in residents scattered across South East Wales (12). Preliminary questioning suggested a possible source to be sliced ham purchased from delicatessen stores and corner shops rather than from supermarkets. A case-control study of 20 cases and 34 controls showed a significant association (odds ratio for sliced ham was 4.5, 95% CI = 1.1–21.8). It was then hypothesized that these shops had been supplied by ham from a single producer. A second case-control study was performed to obtain more detail about the suppliers of ham to the shops used by cases and controls. Cases were significantly more likely than controls to have purchased ham from a shop supplied by one particular wholesaler (OR = 25.0, 95% CI = 2.3, 1155). Enquiries by environmental health officers discovered that a batch of cooked hams had been cooled in water in a container used to cure raw pork.

4.2 Cohort studies

The essential difference between a case-control study and a cohort study is that the case-control study begins by identifying people with and without the infection and then retrospectively tries to identify factors associated with disease. In cohort studies, groups of people are identified other than by the presence of disease, and then information on disease occurrence is sought. Cohort studies may be prospective, when the disease occurs after the study has begun and the population characteristics have been identified; or retrospective, as is usually the case in investigation of acute incidents. For example, in a food poisoning outbreak at a medical conference, all delegates (the cohort) attending the conference were easily identified and names and addresses obtained from the organizers. Delegates were contacted by postal questionnaires, and data on exposure and illness collected. The total cohort was then divided into two groups according to their exposure to a particular meal. Attack rates in those eating the meal and those not eating the meal were calculated. Once the meal responsible for the food poisoning was identified, attack rates in persons eating particular food items were compared with attack rates in those not eating the items.

As in a case-control study, the hypothesis to be tested by a cohort study will determine the study design. In the outbreak of food poisoning, each food item on the menu was hypothesized to be the vehicle of infection. Each member of the cohort (those attending the meal) was asked about consumption of each food. The attack rate in these persons eating the food (exposed) was then compared with those not eating the food (not exposed). The method can be applied to any hypothesized vehicle of infection and to hypothesized risk factors (factors which are not necessarily the source of infection but contribute to the likelihood of infection). In addition to the factors also relevant to case-control studies (Sections 4.1.1–4.1.5) the following need to be carefully considered.

4.2.1 Defining the population at risk

The descriptive epidemiological enquiry will reveal the population at risk for the infection. Thus, in the previous example, interviews with the first cases of food poisoning revealed that the population at risk comprised of delegates attending a particular conference. In outbreaks where a specific at-risk group cannot be identified, the case-control approach may be more appropriate.

4.2.2 Sampling

If the at-risk population is large, a sample can be investigated and results extrapolated to the total population. In order to do this the sample must be representative. Ideally a random sample should be taken by applying random number tables to the sampling frame. In outbreaks in institutions, a complete list of the population can readily be obtained. An alternative to random number sampling is to select every nth person from the list. Cluster or stratified sampling may sometimes be appropriate.

4.2.3 Case definition

It is usual in cohort studies to seek information on symptoms and to classify persons as cases or not cases according to predetermined definition. Symptoms will need to be precisely defined (e.g. 'by diarrhoea we mean at least three or more loose or water stools in a 24 hour period') so that all respondents understand the questions in the same way. It is seldom practical to confirm a diagnosis microbiologically in such population surveys, and a clinical definition based solely on reported symptoms is usually used.

4.2.4 Example: Cohort studies of an outbreak of *Campylobacter* infection in a residential school (13)

Following a report of an outbreak of *Campylobacter* infection in a residential school, preliminary interviews with a few cases excluded raw milk and foods consumed outside of the school as possible sources of infection. Investigation of the domestic water revealed an unchlorinated borehole supply as a possible source. To test the hypothesis that infection was waterborne, two cohort studies were conducted. All teachers were asked to complete a questionnaire which recorded symptoms and water consumption in the school. The dates of onset of illness in most staff were not sufficiently recent for stool isolation of *Campylobacter* to provide the definition of a case. Instead, a case of illness was defined as the reporting of diarrhoea or abdominal pain for the least 24 hours during the school term. The attack rate in staff drinking water from the suspected source was significantly greater than in the remainder. The pupils were resident in several houses, some of which were supplied with a chlorinated water supply. Cohorts of pupils from the different houses were surveyed by self-administered questionnaire. Attack rates by house corresponded by the distribution of the suspected waster supply (Table 3).

4.3 Statistical analysis of case-control and cohort studies

In both types of study the basic analysis is by a comparison of proportions. For example, in the cohort study (Section 4.2.4) the proportion of staff drinking the unchlorinated water who were ill was 21/39 compared with 2/18 who did not drink the water. The data can be presented in a contingency table (Table 4).

367

Table 3 Attack rates in cohorts of pupils according to water supply to residential houses (14)

Water supply	Total	Ill	Attack rate	Relative risks[a] (95% CI)
Unchlorinated	299	153	51%	3.2
Mixed supply	198	60	30%	1.9
Chlorinated	128	21	16%	–

[a] Compared with chlorinated mains supply.

Table 4 Contingency table of a cohort study (Section 4.2.4) (letters in parenthesis show derivation of values)

	Drank water (exposed)	Did not drink (not exposed)	Total
Ill	21 (a)	2 (c)	23 (a + c)
Well	18 (b)	16 (d)	34 (b + d)
Total	39 (a + b)	18 (c + d)	57 (a + b + c + d)

In cohort studies the ratio of $a/a + b$ is the attack rate of the exposed group. The ratio $(a/a+b)/(c/c+d)$, the ratio of the attack rates in exposed and unexposed groups, is called the *relative risk*. The size of the relative risk is an indication of the causative role of the factor concerned. There is also a dose–response effect, the more unchlorinated the water the greater the relative risk. In case-control studies the ratio $a/a + b$ is not meaningful, since b is an unknown fraction of the total well population who were exposed. However, the cross-product ratio ad/bc, called the *odds* ratio, approximates to the relative risk. It is now normal to present the results of case-control and cohort studies as risk estimates with the 95% confidence intervals, rather than relying on p values alone. If the lower 95% CI is above 1 the nil hypothesis is rejected.

The statistical significance of the comparisons is nevertheless important. The methods used depend on the study design (14). In unmatched case-control studies χ^2 is appropriate. If $(a + b + c + d)$ is <20, or if the expected value of any cell is <5, then it is advisable to use exact probabilities (e.g. Fisher's exact test) rather than χ^2. When controls have been matched to cases, matched analysis should be performed using McNemar's test or the exact binomial probability. Ignoring the matching and using a χ^2 will give a rough estimation of the significance of the differences in proportions. Statistical analysis is usually performed using statistical packages available for microcomputers, but the advice of a statistician should be sought when designing research studies or before using unfamiliar statistical tests.

Two × two analyses may reveal that more than one factor differs significantly between cases and controls. These factors may be causally related to the infection, or they may be confounding factors. Thus, in the cohort study above, drinking water was associated with eating food prepared in the school kitchen. When examined individually, both factors were associated with illness. However, stratification by whether food was eaten produced the following table.

	Food eaten		No food	
	Ill	Total	Ill	Total
Water	20	37	1	2
No water	0	9	2	9

Once the effect of eating food from the school kitchen is controlled, the association of illness with drinking water remains significant. Statistical estimates of the stratified data are usually tested by the Mantel–Haenszel test. More sophisticated analyses using multivariate and log–linear model fitting methods are now being used routinely in analyses of such data. Appropriate analysis of matched case-control studies uses the case-control set as the unit of observation, rather than case versus control groups. McNemar's test, the Mantel–Haenszel test and log–linear model approaches are frequently used.

5 A practical approach to the investigation of an acute incident

The administrative aspects of this approach in hospitals are described in Chapter 11, Section 1.2. This section describes the practical aspects of the investigation (15).

5.1 Identification and confirmation of the problem

5.1.1 Checking information

Inadequate history-taking or clinical examination and investigation, as well as errors in recording and reporting data, can lead to false information being circulated. All epidemiological data should be confirmed by independent enquiry as thoroughly and quickly as possible before action is taken. These data should be accurately recorded and retained for future reference (including possible use as legal evidence).

5.1.2 Checking diagnosis

The possibility of laboratory mistakes, and of equivocal results with some laboratory techniques, requires that laboratory methods should be reviewed and, where appropriate, isolations confirmed by a reference laboratory, which may also be able to help with typing. Isolates and sera should be saved for further typing (Chapter 11, Section 4).

5.1.3 Confirming an outbreak exists

Changes in diagnostic techniques and clinical habits and population structure can cause artefacts in surveillance data, and the media can cause inappropriate public alarm. Prevalence and incidence studies may need to be carried out to confirm a problem exists, and laboratory results reviewed. One useful index of a new problem is the per cent positivity. In an outbreak, not only will the number of cases increase, but the proportion of all tests done which are positive will also increase. An increase in investigations due for example to a new interest or concern of clinicians should only increase the total number of samples submitted. When a problem has been confirmed, interim control measures to be instituted should be considered. At this stage, environmental samples (water, food) which may be required later should be taken.

5.1.4 Communication and designation of responsibilities

It is essential that everyone who needs to know about an acute incident is given early accurate information and knows what tasks they are expected to perform. Professionals and organizations are:

(a) Infection Control Doctor.
(b) Control of Infection Nurse.
(c) Management.
(d) Public Health Physician.
(e) Local Authority Environmental Health Department.
(f) Regional or national epidemiological or microbiological support (e.g. Health Protection agency).
(g) Governmental Health Department.

5.1.5 Patient interviews (see Sections 3.1.2)

In large outbreaks, it will not be practical to interview all cases in-depth. A small number of cases (five to ten) should first be interviewed in-depth to explore possible exposures. It may be helpful to interview a few unaffected persons from the at-risk population as well as any atypical cases or persons with very limited exposures. From these interviews, the population at risk will be defined, and hypotheses of the cause of the outbreak will be generated. An appropriate questionnaire can then be designed (Section 3.2.2).

5.1.6 Defining population at risk

Often this will be obvious: those attending a single function or reception or those living in an institution. Less easy to define are those outbreaks occurring in the general community. Definition of the population is essential in epidemiology, since all investigations and results should be referable to that group and as a preliminary step for case-searching.

5.1.7 Case-searching

Cases presenting at the point of recognition of an outbreak are seldom typical. Vigorous case-finding will be necessary to measure the size of the outbreak, and to increase the power of any proposed case-control study. A preliminary step is to decide on a case definition. This may be approached in two stages. In the first place, a broad case definition is used (pneumonia developing in hospitalized patients); laboratory investigation is then used to reclassify possible cases as confirmed or unconfirmed, for example on the basis of *Legionella* serology). Methods of case-finding, both retrospective and prospective, include:

(a) Review of medical records (GP, hospital, occupational).

(b) Soliciting clinical reports (GPs, hospital doctors, nurses) and statutory notifications.

(c) Review of laboratory data.

(d) Survey of population.

5.1.8 Analysis of case data and formulating a hypothesis

Data should be analysed by time, place, person, and by cross-tabulation, keeping an open mind since new vehicles and new modes of transmission may be identified for old pathogens.

5.1.9 Hypothesis testing

Hypothesis may be tested:

(a) Epidemiologically by case-control or cohort studies.

(b) Microbiologically (testing food samples).

(c) By searching for environmental and other data, e.g. history of water pollution, engineering data, or catering practices.

5.1.10 Monitoring and evaluation of control measures

Microbiological methods such as the use of sewer swabs or water sampling; direct observations, such as kitchen inspection; and epidemiological surveillance should be considered.

References

1. Detels, R., Holland, W. W., McEwan, J., and Omann, G. S. (ed.) (1997). *Oxford textbook of public health*, Vol. 2, *The methods of public health*. Oxford University Press, Oxford.
2. Noah, N. and O'Mahony, M. (ed.) (1998). *Communicable disease epidemiology and control.* John Wiley, Chichester.
3. Hayes, S., Nylen, G., Smith, R., Salmon, R. L., and Palmer, S. R. (1999). *Communicable Dis. Public Health*, **2**, No 1, 66.
4. Palmer, S. R. (1998). In *Communicable disease epidemiology and control* (ed. N. Noah and M. O'Mahony). John Wiley, Chichester.
5. Palmer, S. R., Jephcott, A. E., Rowland, A. J., and Sylvester, D. G. H. (1981). *Lancet*, **i**, 881.
6. Palmer, S. R., Zamiri, I., Ribeiro, C. D., and Gajewska, A. (1986). *Br. Med. J.*, **292**, 1494.
7. Lang, D. J., Kunz, L. J., Martin, A. R., Schroeder, S. A., and Thomson, L. A. (1967). *N. Engl. J. Med.*, **276**, 829.
8. Anonymous. (1982). *Br. Med. J.*, **284**, 1125.

9. Vetter, N. and Matthews, I. (1999). *Epidemiology and public health medicine*. Churchill Livingstone, London.

10. Riley, L. W., Remis, R. S., Helgerson, S. D., McGee, H. B., Wells, J. G., Davis, B. R., *et al.* (1983). *N. Engl. J. Med.*, **308**, 681.

11. Bartlett, C. L. R. Personal Communication.

12. Llewellyn, L. J., Evans, M. R., and Palmer, S. R. (1998). *J. Epidemiol. Community Health*, **i52**, 272.

13. Palmer, S. R., Gully, P. R., White, J. M., Pearson, A. D., Suckling, W. G., Jones, D. M., *et al.* (1983). *Lancet*, **i**, 287.

14. Altman, D. G. (1999). *Practical statistics for medical research*. Chapman & Hall, CRC, London.

15. Gregg, M. B., Dicker, R. C., and Goodman, R. A. (2002). *Field epidemiology* Second Edition. Oxford University Press, New York.

Appendix 1
Staining procedures

1 Gram's stain (Preston and Morrell's modification)

This modification is recommended because it gives reliable results without the need to take great care adjusting the length of decolorization.

1.1 Solutions required

Ammonium oxalate crystal violet

Crystal violet	20 g
Methylated spirit (640P)	200 ml
1% ammonium oxalate in water	800 ml

Iodine solution

Iodine	10 g
Potassium iodide	20 g
Distilled water	1000 ml

Liquor iodi fortis (BP)

Iodine	10 g
Potassium iodide	6 g
Methylated spirit (740P)	90 ml
Distilled water	10 ml

Iodine–acetone

Liquor iodi fortis	35 ml
Acetone	965 ml

Dilute carbol fuchsin

Ziehl–Neelsen's (strong) carbol fuchsin	50 ml
Distilled water	950 ml

1.2 Staining procedure

(a) Flood the slide with ammonium oxalate crystal violet and leave for about 30 sec.

(b) Pour off and wash freely with iodine solution. Cover with fresh iodine solution and leave for about 30 sec.

(c) Pour off the iodine solution and wash freely with iodine–acetone. Cover with fresh iodine–acetone and leave for about 30 sec.

(d) Wash thoroughly with water.

(e) Counterstain with dilute carbol fuchsin for about 30 sec.

(f) Wash with water and blot dry.

The slide must be flooded with each reagent in turn and the previous reagent must be removed thoroughly at each step. Gram-positive organisms stain blue and Gram-negative stain pink.

Other counterstains may be used such as:

Neutral red solution
Neutral red	1 g
1% acetic acid	2 ml
Distilled water	1000 ml

Safranin
| Safranin, saturated alcohol solution (about 2.5 g/100 ml of 95% alcohol) | 10 ml |
| Water | 90 ml |

2 Giemsa stain

2.1 Solutions required

Stock solution
| Giemsa powder | 0.5 g |
| Methyl alcohol, absolute, acetone-free | 33 ml |

Mix thoroughly, allow to sediment, and store at room temperature.

Buffered water, pH 7.2.

Solution A: prepare 0.067 M Na_2HPO_4 by adding 9.5 g of anhydrous salt to 1 litre of distilled water.

Solution B: prepare 0.067 M NaH_2PO_4 by dissolving 9.2 g of anhydrous salt to 1 litre of distilled water.

Mix 72 ml of solution A with 28 ml of solution B and 900 ml of distilled water.

Working solution
| Stock solution | 1 part |
| Buffered water, pH 7.2 | 40 or 50 parts |

2.2 Staining procedure

(a) Air dry the smear, fix with absolute methanol for at least 5 min, and dry again.

(b) Cover the slide with the working Giemsa solution (freshly prepared the same day) for 1 h.

(c) Rinse rapidly in 95% ethyl alcohol to remove excess dye. Dry the slide and examine.

3 Stains for acid-fast bacilli

3.1 Auramine phenol

3.1.1 Solutions required

Staining solution

Auramine 'O'	0.3 g
Phenol	3.0 g
Distilled water	97.0 ml

Decolorizing solution

75% industrial alcohol containing 0.5% NaCl and 0.5% HCl.

Counterstain

Potassium permanganate solution 1 in 1000.

3.1.2 Staining procedure

(a) Stain a smear of sputum (or other appropriate material) with auramine staining solution for 15 min.

(b) Rinse with water and decolorize for 5 min with acid alcohol.

(c) Wash well with water and apply potassium permanganate solution for 30 sec.

(d) Wash well with water and allow to dry.

Examine the dry film with an 8 mm objective lens and high-power eyepiece. Mycobacteria are seen as yellow luminous organisms in a dark field. When such bacilli are seen with the low-power objective check their morphology by observing them under the oil-immersion objective. The method has the advantage that large areas of a film can be scanned in a short time.

3.2 Ziehl–Neelsen

3.2.1 Solutions required

Carbol fuchsin

Basic fuchsin	0.3 g
Ethyl alcohol (95%)	10.0 ml
Phenol, melted crystals	5.0 ml
Distilled water	95.0 ml

Dissolve the basic fuchsin in the alcohol; dissolve the phenol in the water. Mix the two solutions and let it stand for several days before use.

Acid alcohol	
Ethyl alcohol (95%)	97 ml
Hydrochloric acid, concentrated	3 ml
Methylene blue, counterstain	
Methylene blue	0.3 g
Distilled water	100 ml

3.2.2 Staining procedure

(a) Flood the slide with carbol fuchsin and heat slowly until steaming. Use low or intermittent heat to maintain steaming for 3–5 min, and then allow to cool.

(b) Wash briefly with water and decolorize with acid alcohol until no more stain comes off.

(c) Wash with water and counterstain for 30 sec with methylene blue.

(d) Wash with water, blot dry, and examine.

Acid-fast organisms are red; the background and non-acid-fast organisms are blue.

3.2.3 Modification of Ziehl–Neelsen procedure for *Nocardia* spp.

The method is the same as Section 3.2.2 with the exception of the decolorization step. Decolorize with 0.5% sulfuric acid alcohol. Cultures of some *Nocadia* spp. will appear acid-fast when decolorized in this way.

3.3 Kinyoun's acid-fast stain

3.3.1 Solutions required

Kinyoun carbol fuchsin

Basic fuchsin	4 g
Ethyl alcohol (95%)	20 ml
Concentrated phenol	8 ml
Distilled water	100 ml

Acid alcohol

Hydrochloric acid, concentrated	3 ml
Ethyl alcohol (95%)	97 ml

Methylene blue, counterstain

Methylene blue	0.3 g
Distilled water	100 ml

3.3.2 Staining procedure

(a) Flood the slide with Kinyoun carbol fuchsin and let it stain for 2 min.

(b) Wash with water and decolorize with acid alcohol until no more dye is removed.

(c) Wash with water and counterstain with methylene blue for 30 sec.

(d) Wash with water, blot dry, and examine.

Acid-fast organisms stain red; the background and non-acid-fast organisms stain blue.

4 Stains for metachromatic (volutin) granules

4.1 Loeffler's methylene blue

4.1.1 Solutions required

Methylene blue	1 g
Ethyl alcohol (95%)	100 ml

Staining solution

Potassium hydroxide 1% aqueous solution	1 ml
Distilled water	99 ml
Ethanolic methylene blue	30 ml

Mix the reagents in this order. The final reagent must be ripened by oxidation, a process taking several months to complete, but it can be hastened by aeration.

4.1.2 Staining procedure

(a) Heat fix the smear with gentle heat and then flood the slide with the stain.

(b) Leave the stain for 1 min and then wash briefly with water, blot dry, and examine.

Metachromatic granules appear dark blue in a light blue cytoplasm.

4.2 Albert's stain, modified

4.2.1 Solution required

Malachite green	0.2 g
Toluidine blue	0.15 g
Ethyl alcohol (95%)	2 ml
Glacial acetic acid	1 ml
Distilled water	100 ml

Dissolve the dyes in the ethyl alcohol. Mix the acid with the water and add to the dye solution. Allow to stand for 24 h and filter.

4.2.2 Staining procedure

(a) Stain with Albert's stain for 3–5 min.

(b) Wash with water and blot dry.

(c) Stain with Lugol's iodine solution for 1 min.

(d) Wash with water, blot dry, and examine.

The cytoplasm appears light green and the granules blue/black.

4.3 Neisser's stain

4.3.1 Solutions required

Solution A

Methylene blue	0.1 g
Ethyl alcohol (95%)	5 ml
Glacial acetic acid	5 ml
Distilled water	100 ml

Dissolve the dye in the water and add the acid and ethyl alcohol.

Solution B

Crystal violet	0.33 g
Ethyl alcohol (95%)	3.3 ml
Distilled water	100 ml

Dissolve the dye in the ethanol/water mixture. For use mix 20 ml of solution A with 10 ml of solution B.

4.3.2 Staining procedure

(a) Stain with Neisser's stain for 10 sec.

(b) Rinse rapidly with water.

(c) Stain with 0.2% Bismarck brown.

(d) Wash rapidly with water, drain, and blot dry.

The cytoplasm appears light brown and the granules brown/black.

5 Spore stain (Schaeffer and Fulton's method)

5.1 Staining procedure

(a) Flood the slide with 5% aqueous malachite green and steam for 1 min.

(b) Wash under running water.

(c) Counterstain with 0.5% aqueous safranin for 15 sec.

(d) Rinse the slide with water, blot dry, and examine.

Bacterial bodies stain red and spores stain green. This method can be used as a cold stain by allowing the malachite green to act for 10 min.

Appendix 2

Bacteriological media not usually commercially available

1. Transport media

1.1 *Chlamydia* transport medium

The medium described below is that of Richmond (1). Prepare a 0.2 M sucrose buffer as follows:

Sucrose	342.3 g
Dipotassium hydrogen phosphate	10.44 g
Potassium dihydrogen phosphate	5.44 g

Make up to 5 litres and distribute into 500 ml volumes. Autoclave at 10 psi for 15 min and store at 4 °C or less. The transport medium itself is dispensed in 2 ml aliquots in screw-capped bottles; it may be stored frozen at −20 °C. Prepare the medium for dispensing aseptically as follows:

0.2 M sucrose phosphate buffer	500 ml
Streptomycin[a]	50 mg/litre
Vancomycin[a]	100 mg/litre
Amphotericin B[a]	5 mg/litre

[a] Filter sterilized before addition or prepared using sterile water. An alternative medium which contains fetal calf serum is described below (Dr A. E. Jephcott, personal communication).

Earle's saline containing:	
10% sorbitol (w/v)	100 ml
4.4% sodium bicarbonate (w/v)	8 ml
Fetal calf serum	10 ml

The components are mixed together, filter sterilized, dispensed aseptically into 2 ml aliquots, and stored at −20 °C until required.

2 Selective/differential media

2.1 Deoxycholate citrate, crystal violet, cefazolin, rhamnose agar (DCCR)

A selective and differential medium for the isolation of *Enterobacter cloacae*. Most members of the genus *Enterobacter* including *E. cloacae* and *E. aerogenes* are resistant to cefazolin and ferment rhamnose present in the medium. The medium was originally used with a selective enrichment broth, the composition of which was not described (2). Presumptive *E. cloacae* will appear as pink colonies, sometimes mucoid.

Formula	Grams per litre
'Lab-Lemco' powder	5.0
Peptone	5.0
Yeast extract	1.0
Rhamnose	20.0
Sodium citrate	8.5
Sodium thiosulfate	5.4
Ferric citrate	1.0
Sodium deoxycholate	1.0
Neutral red	30 mg
Crystal violet	1 mg
Agar	13.5
pH 7.3 ± 0.2	

Suspend ingredients in 1 litre of sterile distilled water and bring to the boil over a flame using a gauze to prevent rapid heating. The medium should be agitated to prevent charring and *not* autoclaved as the constituents are heat labile. When cooled to 50 °C, 10 mg/litre cefazolin should be added before pouring the plates.

2.2 Deoxyribonuclease, toluidine blue, cefalothin agar (DTBCA)

This is a selective and differential medium for the isolation of *Serratia marcescens* relying on cefalothin or cefazolin for its selective action. Although members of the genera *Klebsiella*, *Enterobacter*, *Citrobacter*, and *Providencia* are not DNase positive, *S. marcescens* and *S. liquefaciens* are, and this characteristic is detected with toluidine blue dye which is pink in the presence of free nucleotides and blue with intact DNA (3). Strains of *Serratia* spp. will be surrounded by a pink halo, the medium being royal blue in colour. Different batches of toluidine blue vary in their dye content so alteration of the amount used in the medium may be necessary (4).

Formula	Grams per litre
DNase agar (Oxoid)	39.0
Toluidine blue O (Sigma Chemical Co. Ltd.)	50 mg[a]
Autoclave at 121 °C for 15 min, pH 7.2	

[a] May be added as 5 ml of an appropriate stock solution. After autoclaving and cooling 1.0 g/litre of cefalothin or cefazolin is added before pouring.

2.3 Leeds *Acinetobacter* medium (LAM)

This medium supersedes Herellea agar which was described in the first edition of this book. LAM recovers more isolates of *Acinetobacter* spp. and is also more selective than Herellea agar (5).

Formula	Grams per litre
Acid casein hydrolysate	15.0
Neutralized soy peptone	5.0
NaCl	5.0
Bacteriological agar No. 1 (Oxoid)	10.0
D-(–) Fructose	5.0
Sucrose	5.0
D-Mannitol	5.0
L-Phenyalanine	1.0
Ferric ammonium chloride	0.4
Phenol red	0.02
Distilled water	1 litre

Adjust to pH 7.0 and autoclave for 15 min at 121 °C and 15 lb/in^2.
Cool to 50–55 °C and add:

Vancomycin hydrochloride	10 mg
Cefsulodin	15 mg
Cefradine	50 mg

Acinetobacter spp. appear as pink colonies against a mauve background. *Stenotrophomonas maltophilia* and *Burkholderia cepacia* (oxidase positive) give colonies of the same colour, but the former produce opaque, flat colonies with a crenated edge, whereas *Acinetobacter* colonies are circular, convex, and smooth.

2.4 MacConkey, inositol, carbenicillin agar (MICA)

Klebsiella spp. are among some of the few genera of the family Enterobacteriaceae that can ferment inositol. Most members of the genus also possess a chromosomally encoded β-lactamase that is capable of hydrolysing carbenicillin. The medium described here was originally developed for isolating *Klebsiella* spp. from faeces, but is equally successful in isolating them from other specimens (6). Colonies of presumptive *Klebsiella* spp. will appear as pink colonies on the medium; carbenicillin-resistant bacteria incapable of fermenting inositol will form translucent colonies. To achieve the highest rate of isolation swabs should be pre-enriched by incubation overnight in Koser's citrate broth, available from most commercial media manufacturers.

Formula	Grams per litre
Sodium taurocholate	5.0
Peptone	20.0
Inositol	10.0
Agar	15.0
Neutral red	50 mg

Autoclave at 121 °C for 15 min, pH 7.5.
When cooled to 50 °C add 10 mg/litre of sodium carbenicillin.

2.5 Nalidixic acid, cetrimide agar

Cetrimide (N-acetyl-N, N, N-trimethyl-ammonium bromide) inhibits the growth of a wide range of Gram-positive and Gram-negative bacteria. *Pseudomonas aeruginosa* and some other species of *Pseudomonas* are resistant. Incorporating magnesium sulfate and dipotassium phosphate (King's Agar Medium A) enhances the production of pyocyanin by *Ps. aeruginosa*. The addition of nalidixic acid inhibits a number of Gram-negative bacteria such as *Serratia* spp. that are resistant to cetrimide, *Ps. aeruginosa* being unaffected by nalidixic acid (7). Care must be exercised in the type of peptone used as only some types (e.g. Bacto peptone) enhance pyocyanin production. Not all strains of *Ps. aeruginosa* will elaborate pigment on this medium, so any oxidase positive colonies appearing should be identified even if not surrounded by the blue/green colour of pyocyanin. Different batches of cetrimide vary in their inhibitory action as commercial preparations are not always pure.

Formula	Grams per litre
Meat peptone	20.0
Dipotassium phosphate K_2HPO_4	0.3
Magnesium sulfate $MgSO_4.7H_2O$	0.3
Cetrimide	0.2
Agar	15.0

Autoclave at 121 °C for 15 min, pH 7.4–7.6.

After sterilization add 15 mg/litre of sterile nalidixic acid (best added as a solution, dissolved with a small amount of dilute NaOH).

2.6 Phenanthroline, C-3911 agar

This is the most selective agar currently available for *Pseudomonas aeruginosa*. Generally the only bacteria growing on it will be *Ps. aeruginosa* (8). As no indicator is included in the medium further identification of presumptive colonies is advisable, although current indications are that resistance to C-390 is a characteristic only found in *Ps. aeruginosa*.

Formula	Grams per litre
Columbia agar	39
C-390[a]	30 mg
o-Phenanthroline	30 mg
Autoclave at 121 °C for 15 min, pH 7.3.	

[a] 9-Chloro-9-[4-(diethylamino)phenyl]-9, 10-dihydro-10-phenylacridine hydrochloride (Norwich Eaton Pharmaceuticals).

2.7 *Proteeae* identification medium

This medium relies on the ability of all species of *Proteeae* (except occasional strains of *Morganella morganii*) to produce a melanin-like pigment from tryptophan, which leads to the development of brown colonies (9). *Proteeae* also degrade tyrosine, although this is not a characteristic uniquely found in *Proteeae*, like the ability to produce the brown pigment. Clindamycin is used to eliminate Gram-positive bacteria and colistin can be used to inhibit almost all species of Gram-negative bacteria (approximately 10% of *Proteeae* will also be inhibited). To prevent swarming extra agar is incorporated in the medium.

Formula	Grams per litre
DL-Tryptophan	5.0
L-Tyrosine	4.0
Agar	8.0
Tryptone soy agar (Oxoid)	40.0
Autoclave at 121 °C for 15 min, pH 7.3.	

When cooled to 50 °C add 5 mg/litre clindamycin sulfate and if desired 100 mg/litre colistin (both as filter sterilized solutions). An alternative method of adding selective antibiotics VCN Selectatabs (Diamed Diagnostics Ltd.) can be used. Final concentrations of antibiotics are 3 mg/litre vancomycin, 7.5 mg/litre colistin, and 12 500 units/litre nystatin; the tyrosine may also be omitted without a great loss of differential properties (10).

2.8 Salt, phenolphthalein, methicillin agar (SPMA)

This medium is an alternative to the more commonly used media for isolating methicillin-resistant *Staphylococcus aureus* listed in Chapter 11, Table 1. Rather than relying on mannitol fermentation, colonies of *S. aureus* are detected by the action of phosphatase on sodium diphenolphthalein diphosphate in the medium, the free phenolphthalein being detected by exposing the plate to ammonia. Selection is provided by 5% NaCl (7.5% is usually used in MSA) and 4 mg/litre methicillin (11). Pre-enrichment in Oxoid No. 2 nutrient broth containing 8% NaCl has been found to be a useful method of increasing isolation rates (12). Multiple swabs from a patient may be examined together in the same container of medium and incubation for longer than 24–48 h may yield extra positive cultures.

Formula	Grams per litre
Sodium chloride	50.0
Columbia agar	39.0

Autoclave at 121 °C for 15 min, pH 7.3.

When cooled to 50 °C add 4 mg/litre methicillin and 100 mg/litre sodium phenolphthalein diphosphate as filtered sterile solutions (phenolphthalein phosphate can be purchased ready prepared from Oxoid Ltd.). Incubate inoculated plates for 18 h and expose to ammonia by placing a few drops of strong ammonia solution (SG 0.880) in the lid of the Petri dish. Presumptive colonies of *Staph. aureus* are pink after exposure for about 1 min and can be subcultured for confirmation of identity. This method is useful for detecting small numbers of MRSA amongst large numbers of coagulase negative staphylococci.

2.9 Toluidine blue deoxynucleic acid agar (TDA)

This medium is used in conjunction with the rapid test for heat stable nuclease (13). The dye toluidine blue is metachromatic which means that it is blue in the presence of intact DNA and pink with free nucleotides.

Formula	Grams per litre
Deoxyribonucleic acid	0.3
Agar	10.0
NaCl	10.0

Add the components to 1 litre of 0.05 M Tris buffer pH 9.0. Add 1 ml of 0.01 M anhydrous $CaCl_2$, and boil until dissolved. Cool to 45 °C and add 3 ml of 0.1 M toluidine blue O dye (Sigma Chemical Co.), then pour the plates. The plates can be used for up to 60 days if stored at 4 °C wrapped in a plastic bag. They should be warmed to 37 °C for 1 h before inoculating; positive and negative controls should be used.

2.10 Vancomycin imipenem agar (VIA)

This is a selective differential medium for the isolation of *Stenotrophomonas maltophilia* (14).

Formula	Grams per litre
MAST ID Mannitol agar	40.6

Adjust to pH 7.0 and autoclave for 15 min at 121 °C and 15 lb/in^2.
Cool to 50–55 °C and add:

Vancomycin	5 mg
Imipenem	32 mg
Amphotericin B deoxycholate	2.5 mg

Stenotrophomonas maltophilia does not produce acid from mannitol and colonies are dark blue/green against a light blue/green background. Vancomycin-resistant enterococci may grow on this medium, but they are easily recognized because they produce smaller, mannitol fermenting (yellow) colonies

References

1. Richmond, S. T. (1987). In *Sexually transmitted diseases, a rational approach to their diagnosis* (ed. E. Jephcott), p. 48. Public Health Laboratory Service, London.
2. Flynn, D. M., Weinstein, R. A., Nathan, C., Gaston, M. A., and Kabins, S. A. (1987). *J. Infect. Dis.*, **156**, 363.
3. Farmer, J. J., Silva, F., and Williams, D. R. (1973). *Appl. Microbiol.*, **25**, 151.
4. Wailer, J. R., Hodel, S. L., and Nuti, R. N. (1985). *J. Clin. Microbiol.*, **21**, 195.
5. Jawad, A., Hawkey, P. M., Heritage, J., and Snelling, A. M. (1994). *J. Clin. Microbiol.*, **32**, 2353.
6. Cooke, E. M., Brayson, J. C., Edmondson, A. S., and Hall, D. (1979). *J. Hygiene (Camb.)*, **82**, 473.
7. Goto, S. and Enomoto, S. (1970). *Jpn. J. Microbiol.*, **14**, 65.
8. Campbell, M. E., Farmer, S. W., and Speert, D. P. (1988). *J. Clin. Microbiol.*, **26**, 1910.
9. Hawkey, P. M., McCormick, A., and Simpson, R. A. (1986). *J. Clin. Microbiol.*, **23**, 600.
10. Haynes, J. and Hawkey, P. M. (1989). *Br. Med. J.*, **299**, 94.
11. Wilson, P. A. and Petts, D. N. (1987). *Lancet*, **i**, 558.
12. Cookson, B. D., Webster, M., and Phillips, I. (1987). *Lancet*, **i**, 696.
13. Barry, A. L., Lachica, R. V. F., and Atchison, F. W. (1973). *Appl. Microbiol.*, **25**, 496.
14. Kerr, K. G., Denton, M., Todd, N., Corps, C. M., Kumari, P., and Hawkey, P. M. (1996). *Eur. J. Clin. Microbiol. Infect. Dis.*, **15**, 607.

Principles of biochemical tests for the identification of bacteria

1. Introduction

The following section describes some of the biochemical tests used to identify medically important bacteria. Most laboratories now use disposable prepared galleries of tests which are read from a colour chart then encoded to give a profile number for use with a computer database. It is still important to understand the underlying principles of the test used to enable any problems encountered to be both recognized and solved.

1.1 Catalase test

Most cytochrome-containing aerobic and facultative anaerobic bacteria possess the enzyme catalase. The major exceptions to this rule are *Streptococcus* spp. which lack the catalase enzyme and the alternative enzyme capable of breaking down hydrogen peroxide, peroxidase, which is usually found in anaerobic bacteria.

In the presence of catalase two molecules of hydrogen peroxide react: one molecule acts as the substrate and is reduced by hydrogen atoms supplied by the other molecule to produce two molecules of water, the donor molecule being oxidized to one molecule of gaseous oxygen. The reaction is detected by trapping the bubbles of oxygen formed in the hydrogen peroxide solution in contact with the bacteria under a coverslip or in a capillary tube.

1.1.1 Precautions

(a) Red blood cells contain catalase, so care must be taken not to take any medium with the bacteria (chocolated blood does not contain catalase).

(b) Do not use platinum loops as they will cause a false positive result.

(c) Hydrogen peroxide solution (30%) is caustic; spills on skin should be quickly washed with 70% ethanol.

(d) Always use fresh hydrogen peroxide and check it with a positive control. Occasional catalase negative strains can be encountered (e.g. *Staphylococcus aureus*) (1).

(e) Routine testing can liberate aerosols so use a method to minimize this such as the capillary tube method.

1.2 Citrate test

This is a test to determine whether a bacterium can utilize citrate as a sole carbon source for growth. It is usually used to help identify Gram-negative bacteria, particularly Enterobacteriaceae. Some bacteria can, in the absence of fermentation of sugars or lactic acid production, use citrate as a sole source of energy. An enzyme, citrate demolase, cleaves citrate to yield oxaloacetate and acetate which can then enter the Krebs cycle. Normally coenzyme A is required to enable citrate to enter the cycle. Pyruvate is then formed which in acid conditions will yield acetate, CO_2 and lactate, or acetoin and CO_2, and in alkaline conditions acetate and formate. Media for the detection of citrate utilization contain ammonium salts which the growing bacteria use as a sole source of nitrogen. These when broken down yield ammonia with alkalinization of the medium. The further utilization of the organic acid produces carbonates and bicarbonates on subsequent decomposition. A typical medium used is Simmon's citrate medium which contains magnesium sulfate (required for activity of citrate demolase), ammonium dihydrogen phosphate, dipotassium phosphate, sodium citrate, sodium chloride, agar, bromothymol blue, and water. The uninoculated medium is green and bacteria unable to utilize citrate as a sole carbon source do not change their colour. A positive result is indicated by a deep Prussian blue colour.

1.2.1 Precautions

(a) A heavy inoculum might give a pale yellow colour in the start; this is *not* a positive result.

(b) When multiple tests are being inoculated glucose or other nutrients may be carried over; therefore flame the loop before inoculating the citrate medium.

(c) If the test is performed in screw-capped tubes the tops should not be tightened down as anaerobic conditions may develop leading to a poor colour change. Some bacteria may require long incubation periods before a colour change develops.

1.3 Decarboxylase and dehydrolase tests

These tests detect enzymes which decarboxylate amino acids yielding alkaline amines. Bacteria possess numerous decarboxylase enzymes with specific substrates. The three enzymes used in identification are ornithine and lysine decarboxylase (ODC and LDC) and arginine dehydrolase (ADH). The process occurs under anaerobic conditions and some of the products such as cadaverine and putrescine are stable when produced under these conditions (2). The alkaline amines produced are detected with pH indicators (in the Moller version of the test bromocresol purple and cresol red). A variety of media exist for the detection of these enzymes (3), Moller's version of the test is the most frequently used.

1.3.1 Precautions

(a) Always inoculate a control tube which lacks any added amino acid; it should remain yellow. A positive colour (purple) invalidates the test.

$$
\begin{array}{c}
NH_2 \\
| \\
CH_2 \\
| \\
(CH_2)_3 \\
| \\
CH_2 \\
| \\
NH_2 \\
| \\
COOH \\
\text{L-Lysine}
\end{array}
\quad\xrightarrow[\text{decarboxylase}]{\text{Lysine}}\quad
\begin{array}{c}
NH_2 \\
| \\
CH_2 \\
| \\
(CH_2)_3 + CO_2 \\
| \\
CH_2 \\
| \\
NH_2 \\
\\
\text{Cadaverine}
\end{array}
$$

$$
\begin{array}{c}
NH_2 \\
| \\
(CH_2)_3 \\
| \\
CH-NH_2 \\
| \\
COOH \\
\text{L-Ornithine}
\end{array}
\quad\xrightarrow[\text{decarboxylase}]{\text{Ornithine}}\quad
\begin{array}{c}
CH_2-NH_2 \\
| \\
(CH_2)_2 \qquad + CO_2 \\
| \\
CH_2-NH_2 \\
\\
\text{Putrescine}
\end{array}
$$

(b) Always layer sterile paraffin oil over the tubes immediately after inoculation and do not attempt to read the tests before they have been incubated for 24 h. Under anaerobic conditions organic acids cannot be oxidized so peptones present in the medium cannot be deaminated; however decarboxylases are active under anaerobic conditions so any pH rise is due to those enzymes' activity.

1.4 Hippurate hydrolysis test

Sodium hippurate can be hydrolysed by some bacteria (e.g. *Streptococcus agalactiae* and *Campylobacter jejuni*) to yield glycine and benzoic acid. Both benzoic acid or glycine can be detected in different versions of the test. The former is usually detected with FeCl$_3$ and glycine with ninhydrin when a deep purple colour is produced (4).

1.4.1 Precautions

When using ninhydrin reagent do not incubate for longer than 30 minutes after adding the reagent as false positive results can occur.

1.5 Hydrogen sulfide test

Sulfur-containing amino acids such as methionine and cysteine can be degraded by some bacteria to liberate hydrogen sulfide. In some cases sodium thiosulfate can also be metabolized to liberate H$_2$S. Hydrogen sulfide is detected by its ability

$$\underset{\text{L-Arginine}}{\begin{array}{c} NH \\ \| \\ CNH_2 \\ | \\ NH \\ | \\ (CH_2)_3 \\ | \\ CH-NH_2 \\ | \\ COOH \end{array}} \xrightarrow[\text{dehydrolase}]{\text{Arginine}} \underset{\text{L-Citrulline}}{\begin{array}{c} NH \\ \| \\ COH \\ | \\ NH \\ | \\ (CH_2)_3 \\ | \\ CH-NH_2 \\ | \\ COOH \end{array}} \xrightarrow[\text{ureidase}]{\text{Citruline}} \underset{\text{L-Ornithine}}{\begin{array}{c} NH_2 \\ | \\ (CH_2)_3 \\ | \\ CH-NH_2 \\ | \\ COOH \\ + \\ 2NH_3 + CO_2 \end{array}} \xrightarrow[\text{decarboxylase}]{\text{Ornithine}} \underset{\text{Putrescine}}{\begin{array}{c} CH_2-NH_2 \\ | \\ (CH_2)_2 \\ | \\ CH_2-NH_2 \\ + \\ CO_2 \end{array}}$$

*This pathway only occurs if ODC is present as well as ADH.

$$\text{Hippuric acid} \rightleftharpoons \text{Benzoic acid + Glycine}$$

to react with metal ions and produce insoluble black sulfides. Ferric ions can be incorporated into media but if lead ions are used (gives increased sensitivity) in the form of lead acetate it is placed on a filter paper strip above the growing bacteria. This is because lead acetate is highly toxic to bacteria.

1.5.1 Precautions

(a) Sucrose in media will suppress the enzyme systems producing H_2S (5), so Triple Sugar Iron agar may give negative results for H_2S production for some species of the H_2S positive salmonellae.

(b) Lead acetate is very toxic to bacteria and paper strips containing it should *not* be allowed to touch the medium.

1.6 Indole test

This test determines the ability of bacterium to cleave the indole ring from tryptophan. Indole positive bacteria possess a series of enzymes collectively known as 'tryptophanase'. These enzymes oxidize tryptophan to intermediates such as indole pyruvic acid which is deaminated to indole, and indole acetic acid which is decarboxylated to skatole (methyl indole). Indole and its related compounds such as skatole and indole acetic acid are detected with an aldehyde in the reagent which causes a condensation of the pyrrole structure present in indole to give rise to an intense red colour quinoidal compound. The most commonly used reagent is *p*-dimethyl aminobenzaldehyde (DMBA). Because this compound will react with a wide range of indole-containing compounds, DMABA is dissolved in amyl alcohol which extracts only indole and skatole. A rapid spot test can be performed using *p*-dimethylaminocinnamaldehyde (DMACA) which is the most sensitive reagent (6).

L-Tryptophan   Indole   Pyruvic acid

1.6.1 Precautions

(a) Certain batches of peptone are low in tryptophan and should be checked for their ability to give a positive test with a positive control bacterium (*E. coli*).

(b) Some bacteria (e.g. *Clostridia* spp.) decompose indole as fast as it is produced and will give a false negative result.

(c) Media for indole testing must not contain any glucose as the acid produced can inhibit tryptophanase (as can media with a low pH); the addition of tryptophan induces the enzyme.

1.7 Methyl red and Voges–Proskauer test

Fermentative bacteria such as Enterobacteriaceae derive their energy from the conversion of sugars such as glucose to pyruvic acid via the Embden–Meyerhof pathway. Pyruvic acid is then utilized usually by either the mixed acid fermentation or the butylenes glycol pathway. A simplified scheme of these pathways is shown below. The methyl red test detects the large amount of mixed acids produced by bacteria using that pathway as methyl red changes colour from orange to red at pH 4.4; above a pH of 6.0 it is yellow. A positive result is indicated by the appearance of a distinct red colour at the surface of the medium after 48 h incubation. A rapid version of the test giving a result after 24 h incubation has been described (7).

The Voges–Proskauer test detects acetoin which is an intermediate produced by bacteria in which butylenes glycol (2,3-butanediol) is the major end-product of glucose fermentation, rather than organic acids. Voges–Proskauer (VP) positive bacteria include *Klebsiella* spp., *Enterobacter* spp., and *Serratia* spp. which also give negative result in the methyl red test. Bacteria which are positive in the methyl red test are not usually positive in the VP test as one pathway only is used (*Proteus mirabilis* and *Hafnia alvei* are exceptions and positive in both tests). Acetoin is detected by KOH oxidizing it to diacetyl which then reacts with the guanidine nucleus present in the meat peptones in the media to produce a pinkish/red colour. The α-naphthol enhances the colour as does gently shaking to expose the media to atmospheric oxygen.

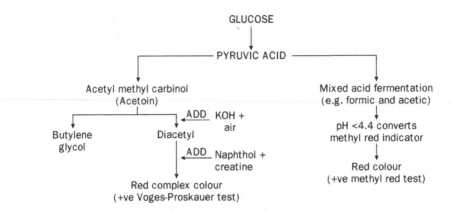

1.7.1 Precautions

(a) Rarely some bacteria known to produce acetoin give a negative VP test; warming the test will give a positive reaction.

(b) Some bacteria can destroy acetoin when it is produced making the test unreliable. It should not be used as the sole test for identification.

1.8 Nitrate reduction test

This test determines the ability of bacterium to reduce nitrate to nitrite, or free nitrogen gas. All members of the Enterobacteriaceae are nitrate positive (except strains of *Enterobacter agglomerans* and *Erwinia* spp.). The test is also used in identifying members of the genera *Neisseria*, *Branhamella*, and *Haemophilus*. In the test bacteria extract oxygen from nitrate form to nitrite and in some cases nitrites are further reduced to N_2, NH_3, or N_2O. The nitrites formed in the process are detected with α-naphthylamine and sulfanilic acid when a red dye (*p*-sulfobenzeneazo-α-naphthylamine) is formed. If on adding the two reagents no colour develops it is possible that either the nitrates have been fully reduced to nitrogen or other products that have escaped or that nitrate has not been reduced and is still present in the medium. The presence of unreduced nitrate is confirmed by adding a small amount of zinc dust which reduces any nitrate present to nitrite with the concomitant development of the red colour. Should the nitrate have been fully reduced no colour will develop on the addition of zinc dust.

1.8.1 Precautions

(a) The red colour produced fades quickly so the results must be interpreted immediately.

(b) The test is very sensitive so always test an uninoculated tube of media to confirm no nitrites are present.

(c) α-Naphthylamine is carcinogenic so the alternative reagent N,N-dimethyl-α-naphthylamine should be substituted whenever possible.

(d) Do not add too much zinc dust as the hydrogen liberated can reduce the nitrite present to NH_3 and give a false negative result.

1.9 ONPG (o-nitrophenyl-β-D-galactopyranoside) test

Bacteria capable of fermenting lactose (an important characteristic in identifying Enterobacteriaceae) possess two enzymes: β-D-galactosidase (intracellular) which cleaves the β-galactosidase-permease which transports the lactose into the cell. Whilst lactose together with a pH indicator can be used to detect the activity of β-D-galactosidase in bacteria with the permease, some bacteria (late lactose fermenters) lack the permease and will not produce the colour change in 24 h as mutants with the enzyme arise on prolonged incubation (8). An alternative substrate ONPG does not require the permease and will detect any bacteria possessing β-D-galactosidase. When ONPG is cleaved in alkaline conditions the yellow product o-nitrophenyl (ONP) is formed.

o-Nitrophenyl-β-D-
galactopyranase
(ONPG, colourless)

o-Nitrophenol (ONP, yellow)

Galactose

1.9.1 Precautions

(a) The ONPG solution must be colourless before use and of the correct pH (7.0–7.5) or the ONP formed will be colourless. Before use the solution must be placed in a 37 °C water-bath to redissolve the phosphate buffer which crystallizes out of solution on storage at 4 °C.

(b) A heavy inoculum must be used or insufficient preformed enzyme will be present.

1.10 Oxidase test

This test determines the presence of the cytochrome oxidase system of enzymes which activate the oxidation of reduced cytochrome by molecular oxygen which then acts as an electron acceptor in the last stage of electron transfer. The enzyme by definition is only found in some bacteria capable of utilizing oxygen as a final hydrogen acceptor to reduce molecular oxygen to H_2O_2 (aerobic, microaerophilic, or facultative anaerobes). All members of the Enterobacteriaceae are negative, whereas some *Pseudomonas* spp., *Neisseria* spp., *Campylobacter* spp., and others are positive. Anaerobic bacteria are invariably negative in the oxidase test. The most frequently used reagent is tetramethyl-*p*-phenylenediamine which produces an intense blue/purple colour (Wurster's blue). An alternative reagent is dimethyl-*p*-phenylenediamine which produces indophenol blue. Both reagents are usually placed on filter paper or a cotton wool swab and the colonies dabbed onto them. A purple colour should appear in 10 seconds.

1.10.1 Precautions

(a) Never use a nichrome wire loop to handle bacteria to be tested for oxidase activity as traces of iron present will catalyse the oxidation of the reagent. Platinum loops can be used but it is better to use paper or cotton wool.

(b) Media containing glucose inhibit oxidase activity. Selective and differential media may also interfere with oxidase activity. Only test colonies from non-selective/differential media, e.g. blood agar, nutrient agar, trypticase soy agar, etc.

(c) The reagents auto-oxidize rapidly so ascorbic acid should be added and the reagent replaced frequently.

1.11 Phenylalanine deaminase test

A small number of bacteria including all the members of the *Proteeae* can deaminate the aromatic amino acid phenylalanine to produce phenyl pyruvic acid. This end-product is detected by adding ferric chloride which chelates with the phenyl pyruvic acid to produce a green colour. The colour fades rapidly so the test must be examined immediately. The API-20E system detects the similar enzyme tryptophan deaminase which has a similar distribution amongst bacteria to phenylalanine deaminase.

Phenylalanine

Phenylpyruvic acid
(detected by the addition of $FeCl_3$ when a green colour develops on exposure to air)

1.12 Urease test

Urease enzymes are widely distributed amongst bacteria and are diverse in their relationships (9). They all catalyse the hydrolysis of urea to form ammonia and carbon dioxide. The ammonia produced causes the medium to become alkaline and this can be detected with a pH indicator. Ureases vary greatly in their rate of hydrolysis of urea and use is made of these differences in buffering the medium used. Stuart's urea broth is highly buffered and so the only urease positive *Proteeae* will produce sufficient ammonia to overcome the buffering system. Christensen's medium is much less buffered than Stuart's medium and urease positive bacteria other than the *Proteeae* will produce a colour change in 24 h (*Proteeae* should produce a positive result in 1–6 h). It is important to remember that only a pH in Christensen's medium to give a false positive result. To eliminate this error if it is thought to have occurred, inoculate a control tube of the medium *without* urea.

$$\begin{array}{c} H_2N \\ \diagdown \\ \qquad C = O \ + \ 2HOH \ \xrightarrow{\text{urease}} \ CO_2 + H_2O + 2NH_3 \\ \diagup \\ H_2N \end{array}$$

References

1. Tu, K. K. and Palutke, W. A. (1976). *J. Clin. Microbiol.*, **3**, 77.
2. Moller, V. (1955). *Acta Pathol. Microbiol. Scand.*, **36**, 158.
3. MacFaddin, J. F. (1980). *Biochemical tests for identification of medical bacteria*, 2nd edn. Williams and Wilkins, Baltimore and London.
4. Hwang, M. and Ederer, G. M. (1975). *J. Clin. Microbiol.*, **1**, 114.
5. Bulmarsh, J. M. and Fulton, J. D. (1964). *J. Bacteriol.*, **88**, 1813.
6. Lowrance, B. L., Reich, P., and Traub, W. H. (1969). *Appl. Microbiol.*, **17**, 923.
7. Barry, A. L., Bernsohn, K. L., Adams, A. P., and Thrupp, L. D. (1970). *Appl. Microbiol.*, **20**, 866.
8. Lowe, G. H. (1962). *J. Med. Lab. Technol.*, **19**, 21.
9. Jones, B. D. and Mobley, H. L. T. (1987). *Infect. Immun.*, **55**, 2198.

Epidemiological questionnaire

A questionnaire used in the investigation of an outbreak of salmonella infection in school children aboard an ocean-going cruise liner.

S.S. UGANDA ENQUIRY

School ....

Name .... Age .... Sex ....

Deck no .... Dormitory name .... Bunk no .... Group no ....

Did you have any of the following symptoms whilst you were on the cruise or within one week of returning from the cruise?

Tick each symptom you suffered and give the date it started. Please be as accurate as possible.

If you suffered more than one bout of illness please give the dates for each one.

Symptoms	Please tick as appropriate			Date of onset of symptoms
Vomiting	Yes	No	Don't know	....
Diarrhoea	Yes	No	Don't know	....
Headache	Yes	No	Don't know	....
Abdominal pain	Yes	No	Don't know	....
Fever/temperature	Yes	No	Don't know	....

If you were unwell on the cruise please put an X or Xs along the line below to show when your illness(es) started.

Put an X along ....

the dotted

line to show ....

when illnesses ....

started   24ᵗʰ   25   26   27   28   1   2   3   4   5   6   7   8   9   10   11

               February   March

Please tick as appropriate

At Naples:

Did you buy any food in the town?	Yes	No	Don't know
Did you drink water or fruit juice in the town?	Yes	No	Don't know
Did you eat locally bought fruit?	Yes	No	Don't know
Did you eat ices/lollipops?	Yes	No	Don't know

Messina:

Did you go ashore?	Yes	No	Don't know
Did you buy food in the town?	Yes	No	Don't know
Did you drink water or fruit juice in the town?	Yes	No	Don't know
Did you eat locally bought fruit?	Yes	No	Don't know
Did you eat ices/lollipops?	Yes	No	Don't know

Alexandria:

Did you go ashore?	Yes	No	Don't know
Did you eat all your packed lunch? (Pork pie, etc.)	Yes	No	Don't know
If not, what did you not eat?			
Did you use your drink token?	Yes	No	Don't know

Haifa:

Did you go ashore?	Yes	No	Don't know
Did you eat all your packed lunch? (chicken)	Yes	No	Don't know
If not, what did you not eat?			
Did you eat anyone else's chicken?	Yes	No	Don't know
Did you eat any local fruit?	Yes	No	Don't know
If yes, what was it?			

Limassol:

Did you go ashore?	Yes	No	Don't know
Did you eat all your packed lunch? (Chicken and bacon pie)	Yes	No	Don't know
If not, what did you not eat?			
Did you eat anyone else's pie?	Yes	No	Don't know
Did you eat any local fruit?	Yes	No	Don't know
If yes, what was it?			

Nauplia:

Did you go ashore?	Yes	No	Don't know
Did you eat all your packed lunch? (Sausage rolls)	Yes	No	Don't know
If not, what did you not eat?			
Did you eat anyone else's sausage rolls?	Yes	No	Don't know
Did you eat any local fruit?	Yes	No	Don't know
If yes, what was it?			

Split:

Did you eat any food in the town?	Yes	No	Don't know

(Please say what you ate, including ice-cream)

....

....

Did you have anything to drink?	Yes	No	Don't know

(Please say what you drank)

....

....

On board ship: **Please tick as appropriate**

Did you drink water from the water fountain?	Yes	No	Don't know

If yes, how many times each day on average

....

Did you drink tap-water?	Yes	No	Don't know
Did you swim in the pool?	Yes	No	Don't know

For breakfast did you have milk on your cereal?

	Every day	Usually	Sometimes	Never
For lunch or dinner did you eat chicken?	Twice	Once	Never	

Did you eat lamb?	Yes	No	Don't know
beef?	Yes	No	Don't know
shepherd's pie?	Yes	No	Don't know
sausages?	Yes	No	Don't know
fish?	Yes	No	Don't know
salads?	Yes	No	Don't know
soup?	Yes	No	Don't know
ice-cream?	Yes	No	Don't know
cakes?	Yes	No	Don't know
fruit?	Yes	No	Don't know
Did you ever have more than one portion per meal?	Yes	No	Don't know
If you did, what were the foods?			
Did you share towels or soap with your friends?	Yes	No	Don't know
Did any of your close friends or dormitory neighbours have diarrhoea?	Yes	No	Don't know

Communicable Disease Surveillance Centre   26th March 1981

61 Colindale Avenue   S.R.P.

Colindale

London NW9 5EQ

Index

Printed in the United States
By Bookmasters